T0092079

HEPATIC ENCEPHALOPATHY, HYPERAMMONEMIA, AND AMMONIA TOXICITY

ADVANCES IN EXPERIMENTAL MEDICINE AND BIOLOGY

Recent Volumes in this Series

HEPATIC ENCEPHALOPATHY, HYPERAMMONEMIA, AND AMMONIA TOXICITY

Edited by

Vicente Felipo
Santiago Grisolia

Instituto de Investigaciones Citologicas de la F. I. B.
Valencia, Spain

SPRINGER SCIENCE+BUSINESS MEDIA, LLC

Library of Congress Cataloging-in-Publication Data

On file

Proceedings of an international symposium on Hepatic Encephalopathy, Hyperammonemia, and Ammonia Toxicity, held January 24–27, 1994, in Valencia, Spain

ISBN 978-0-306-44985-7   ISBN 978-1-4615-1989-8 (eBook)
DOI 10.1007/978-1-4615-1989-8

© 1994 Springer Science+Business Media New York
Originally published by Plenum Press New York in 1994

PREFACE

This volume contains the papers presented at the International Symposium on "Cirrhosis, Hyperammonemia and Hepatic Encephalopathy", held in Valencia, Spain, January 24th–27th, 1994.

Liver cirrhosis and other hepatic dysfunctions such as fulminant hepatic failure and congenital defects of urea cycle enzymes can lead to hepatic encephalopathy, coma and death. Hepatic encephalopathy is one of the main causes of death in western countries.

The ability to detoxify ammonia by its incorporation into urea is diminished by impaired liver function, resulting in increased ammonia levels in blood and brain. Hyperammonemia is considered one of the main factors in the mediation of hepatic encephalopathy and the classical clinical treatments are directed towards reducing blood ammonia levels. However, the molecular bases of the pathogenesis of hepatic encephalopathy and the role of hyperammonemia in this process remain unclear and several hypotheses have been proposed.

To clarify the mechanisms involved in hepatic encephalopathy and hyperammonemia suitable animal models are necessary. The animal models available and the ideal features of an animal model are presented in the initial part of the book.

The following section is devoted to the discussion of the effects of hepatic encephalopathy and hyperammonemia on brain metabolism, trying to clarify the mechanisms involved in these alterations. The use of in vivo magnetic resonance in these studies and the new findings provided by this technology are also included. The interaction between astrocytes and neurons in hepatic encephalopathy and hyperammonemia and the role of cellular hydration in the control of cell metabolism and function are also described.

Altered neurotransmission is an important step in the pathogenesis of hepatic encephalopathy. The effects of hyperammonemia and of hepatic encephalopathy on synaptic transmission and on glutamatergic, GABAergic, serotoninergic and other neurotransmitter systems are reviewed, as well as the possible role of their alterations in the pathogenesis of hepatic encephalopathy and the clinical implications of these findings.

The molecular mechanism of acute ammonia toxicity, of its prevention by L–carnitine and the role of glutamate receptors in this processes is also presented.

The deficiencies in methionine metabolism and S–adenosyl–L–methionine in liver cirrhosis are discussed.

The following part of the book is devoted to the consideration of the diagnosis and therapy of hepatic encephalopathy. The mechanism of action of neomycin and the clinical use of carnitine are discussed. The diagnosis, course and clinical treatment of congenital deficiencies of acetylglutamate synthetase are also reviewed.

The use of gene therapy and the methods of gene delivery for the treatment of congenital deficiencies of ornithine transcarbamylase and of the LDL receptor are also dealt with.

The possibility of using artificial liver support for patients and recent experimental findings using hepatocyte culture bioreactors are discussed. The hepatitis C viral infection after liver transplantation is reviewed.

Finally, the volume concludes with a brief treatment of the central and peripheral effects of exercise–induced hyperammonemia and the possible role of ammonia in the brain in Alzheimer's disease are discussed.

In summary, the book is an updating of the knowledge on some important aspects of the causes, mechanisms and clinical treatments of hepatic encephalopathy, on the effects of hyperammonemia and of the mechanism of ammonia toxicity.

We would like to express our gratitude to all participants for their written contributions and for their enlightened and fruitful discussion, as well as to Forpax S.L. for help in preparing the camera–ready version of the chapters.

We also acknowledge with deep gratitude, the financial support of Sigma–Tau Laboratories, Ministerio de Educación y Ciencia, Ministerio de Sanidad y Consumo y Conselleria de Educación de la Generalitat Valenciana and the Fundación Valenciana de Estudios Avanzados which provided both the facilities for organizing the Symposium and for the sessions.

Vicente Felipo
Santiago Grisolía

CONTENTS

Animal Models of Hepatic Encephalopathy and Hyperammonemia

Kevin D. Mullen, Sigurbjorn Birgisson, Reynaldo C. Gacad, and Hari Conjeevaram

Animal models of chronic liver disease with hyperammonemia are currently available to investigators. Two in particular have been utilized extensively. Carbon tetrachloride induced (CCl₄) cirrhosis in the rat and portacaval shunt in the same species and other animals particularly the dog. In regards to hepatic encephalopathy, however, the CCl₄ cirrhosis rat model seems to display few behavioral changes unless very advanced decompensated cirrhosis is produced. Further work should be done on this model to verify the development of encephalopathy and to improve reproducibility. The portacaval shunt rat on the other hand clearly has a consistent albeit subtle set of behavioral changes. Recent improvements in detecting these changes and more importantly showing reversal or improvement by neomycin or a low protein diet are a major advance. Hopefully, more laboratories will be able to reproduce this reversible change in behavior. Experiences gained from 7 years of using the portacaval shunt rat and other models of liver disease are described.

1. Introduction

The ideal animal model of hepatic encephalopathy (HE) should reproduce at least some of the typical clinical features of this syndrome in humans (Table 1). Since the vast majority of HE seen in every day clinical practice occurs in patients with chronic liver disease it would be ideal for an animal model to be the same. Listed in (Table 2) are a number of fairly satisfactory animal models of HE associated with acute or fulminant hepatic failure. However, even in referral liver transplant centers this is an uncommon setting for HE. Moreover, there are striking differences between HE in fulminant hepatic failure and that seen in patients with chronic liver disease (Table 3). Accordingly, even though animal models of acute liver failure have been very useful in indicating possible mechanisms for the pathogenesis of HE they are far from ideal primarily because it is very difficult to prove that the behavioral changes observed are, in fact, purely due to hepatic encephalopathy.

When considering an ideal animal model of hyperammonemia the basic issue to resolve is what clinical setting of hyperammonemia does the investigator want to reproduce. For instance, requirements for a model to explore the effects of severe hyperammonemia due to urea cycle enzyme deficiencies are very different to the usually more moderate hyperammonemia seen in chronic liver disease. Regardless of the clinical situation of interest, studies of the effects of hyperammonemia in animals are only relevant to humans if the degree and duration of hyperammonemia are at least similar to that seen in patients. This

Division of Gastroenterology MetroHealth Medical Center Case Western Reserve University Cleveland, Ohio USA

Hepatic Encephalopathy, Hyperammonemia, and Ammonia Toxicity
Edited by V. Felipo and S. Grisolia, Plenum Press, New York, 1994

Table 1. Typical clinical features of hepatic encephalopathy

● Occurs predominantly in patients with chronic liver disease
● Often precipitated by defined factors
● Frequently reversible by correction of precipitating factors
● Reversible with neomycin, lactulose or low protein diet
● Associated with abnormal nitrogen and amino acid metabolism
● Wide spectrum of severity

Table 2. Animal models of fulminant hepatic failure

● D–galactosamine induced liver failure in rabbits* and rats*
● Thioacetamide induced liver failure in rats
● Complete hepatic devascularization in many species
● Acetaminophen induced liver failure in dogs* and pigs*
● Total or near total hepatectomy in many species
● Spontaneous hepatitis in Long Evans Cinnamon rats

* = variable reproducibility

Table 3. Features of HE in fulminant hepatic failure

● Often not precipitated by defined factors
● Poor reversibility with any treatment except liver transplant
● Strong association with cerebral edema
● Associated with many complicating metabolic events
● Sometimes associated with episodes of CNS excitation

simple modeling principle is often violated. Many investigators are interested in hyperammonemia because of its potential role in the pathogenesis of HE. The essential prerequisite for studies in this area is that the animal model being utilized display some behavioral changes compatible with HE in humans. Often it is assumed that any or all behavioral changes in an animal model of liver disease are due to HE. However, as in the clinical situation of human HE, the diagnosis of HE is uncertain until other causes of "encephalopathy" are ruled out and a response to empirical HE treatment is observed. In the absence of this approach potentially studies in animal models of liver disease may not be relevant to HE if the animals behavioral changes are not in fact the animal equivalent of human HE. This is true no matter how sophisticated or elegant the investigations performed.

2. Brief Comments on the Limitations of Acute Liver Failure Models

Clearly none of the currently available acute liver failure animal models (Table 2) reproduce the typical clinical features of HE in humans with chronic liver disease (Table 1).

In many studies utilizing these models other causes of "encephalopathy" or "behavioral changes" have not been rigorously excluded. Hypothermia, acidosis, uremia, cerebral edema, massive weight loss (inanition), dehydration and frank starvation due to gross anorexia are all factors that need to be considered as potential contributors to any behavioral changes observed in these models. Recently, more authors have supplied information in manuscripts to ensure that all of these extraneous causes of behavioral changes have been excluded. However, based on our own experience with both the galactosamine and thioacetamide models it is not enough to exclude these factors only once during the early phases of studies (1). An animal model that previously was reliable and reproducible can change utterly in character which can be an enormous problem if it is not realized and the earliest phases of "HE" are being studied. Literally one can end up studying something other than HE unless concurrent controls are always utilized to ensure that the model is behaving and evolving as expected based on prior studies. These types of problems are rarely publishable and yet may account for a lot of the controversy in the literature. Illustrating this point rather well is the recent paper by Peeling et al which suggests that the thioacetamide rat model of liver failure may be unsuitable for studies of HE (2). It has been commented in the past that this model has changed as more laboratories have attempted to us it (1).

3. Animal Models of Chronic Liver Disease

In practical terms despite the longstanding interest in the end to side portacaval shunt dog model very few laboratories are willing or able to handle dog studies. Nonetheless, either surgically created or congenital portosystemic shunts in dogs are frequently associated with behavioral changes compatible with the human equivalent of HE. In particular, veterinary physicians report that congenital portosystemic shunt dogs improve their encephalopathy with low protein diets, or lactulose and neomycin treatment (3). Furthermore, the "encephalopathy" can be precipitated by a high protein diet (4). However, as mentioned above many laboratories cannot handle dogs or do not have access to congenital shunt dogs. Furthermore, there is a great deal of variability in the expression of behavioral changes in dogs subjected to surgically created portosystemic anastomosis (5). Thus dog models will not be discussed further.

4. Portacaval Shunt in the Rat

Extensive studies over the years with the portacaval shunt (PCS) rat model have revealed much of what we know today about ammonia metabolism in liver disease (6). Other than when given an acute ammonia load this model of chronic liver "dysfunction" has been remarkable for the subtle changes in behavior it exhibits. When one of us (KDM) first encountered this model in 1985, he was very dubious about its utility as a model of human HE. Even though the rats observed had been subjected to PCS by a true expert in the field, Dr. Martin Grun, almost no neurobehavioral signs could be detected (7). This led to a huge set of exploratory experiments to try and produce a more florid "encephalopathy" by techniques other than acute ammonia loading. These will be mentioned later. However, in retrospect, the problem we had in measuring any behavioral changes was because our techniques were too insensitive. Excellent work by Bengsston and colleagues (8-10) and other (11,12) unequivocally demonstrated that consistent behavioral changes were present in this model particularly in the area of spontaneous activity in response to a new environment (8-12). Once we reproduced these findings we were surprised to find that no one had ever demonstrated that the behavioral changes in the PCS rat were reversible by measures known to be effective in the treatment of human HE. As mentioned earlier, only by demonstrating this can one start to consider the model to be relevant to human HE. Since then we have

3

Table 4. ANimal models of chronic liver "disease"

ANIMAL MODELS OF CHRONIC LIVER "DISEASE"
● Portacaval shunt in the rat*
● Portacaval shunt in the dog
● Congenital portacaval shunt in the dog
● Carbon tetrachloride induced cirrhosis in the rat*
● Portacaval shunt and bile duct ligation in the rat

* = potentially useful for studies of hyperammonemia and HE.

clearly shown that oral neomycin in the drinking water reverses the reduced spontaneous motor activity of PCS rats in a darkened novel environment (13). These findings have been confirmed by another group of investigators led by Dr. Andres Blei in Chicago using a more sophisticated technique measuring circadian rhythm disturbances in motor activity in PCS rats (14). They have reported that not only does neomycin normalize activity, but so does a low protein diet (15,16). Application of the elegant neurochemical techniques used in the past on brain tissue from PCS rats should now be redone again in PCS rats not only when they have well developed neurobehavioral disturbances, but also when they have been improved by neomycin or a low protein diet. Establishment of correlations between activity and any measured compound will have considerably more weight if the correlations persist through normalization of activity.

A note of caution is in order, however, when using the PCS rat model. The mere construction of a PCS does not ensure that behavioral disturbances will occur. Technical issues such as the size of the PCS stoma (17,18) and the effect of the diet (18) and the length of time after the PCS when the animal is studied can all effect the investigators ability to detect significant behavioral changes (10). Thus in every laboratory it is necessary to prove that behavioral disturbances are present before any inference as to the cause of these changes can be made.

5. Carbon Tetrachloride Induced Cirrhosis in the Rat

This model is reasonably easy to produce with recently described modifications (19). However, a fairly significant number of rats still die during CCl_4 treatment especially if it is decided to treat until ascites is present. Our experience shared by others is that the CCl_4 cirrhosis rat model has few if any detectable behavioral changes unless a very advanced decompensated state is reached (20). Yamamoto et al apparently reached this degree of severity in their studies and reported impressive hyperammonemia and severe behavioral changes about 10 weeks after started CCl_4 treatment (21). Attempts should be made to replicate these findings, but caution needs to be exercised when trying to assess behavior in rats with massive ascites like the authors describe.

The well compensated CCl_4 cirrhosis rat model appears to be useful for investigating the mechanisms of hyperammonemia even though recently the expected reduction in urea cycle enzyme activities were not observed in this model (22). Attempting to produce a more advanced stage of cirrhosis may be of interest, but the complication of ascites and its effects on body weight and interpretation of tracer kinetic studies might limits its usefulness.

6. Portacaval Shunt with Additional Manipulations

Primarily with the idea of producing a more severe encephalopathy the PCS rat (and dogs on some occasions) has been subjected to a variety of manipulations. One potentially useful maneuver was feeding ammonia resins to PCS rats which apparently produced a reversible encephalopathy (23). Ammonia loading by other means (urease injection, ammonia salts IV or IP) clearly causes complete coma, but what this represents in human terms is still unclear to us. Potentially the coma seen is related to ammonia induced cerebral edema, but evidence for this is still sketchy (1). In addition, we are unaware of reports of the reversibility of coma induced by ammonia loading in PCS rats. Normal rats fed ammonia acetate in the diet have hyperammonemia to the same degree as seen in PCS rats and yet are resistent to an acute ammonia load (24) unlike the PCS rat which is the opposite (25). The mechanism of CNS sensitivity to an ammonia load, therefore, is more complex than we realized. Direct neurochemical studies of brain tissue need to be done comparing ammonia acetate/chow fed rats and PCS rats before and after an ammonia load to resolve this interesting phenomenon. Superimposition of acute hepatitis with dimethylnitrosamine on dogs with PCS has been reported to induce severe HE (26). Whether this represents an acute liver failure model is hard to ascertain. Other manipulations used in PCS animals include blood gavage or high protein diets which seem to work in dogs (4) but not rats (7). We, a few years ago, tried partial hepatectomy of PCS rats and inducing cirrhosis with CCl_4 before performing a PCS and neither maneuver caused significant behavioral changes without a massive blood gavage (7). Whether the severe encephalopathy after blood gavage was simply due to hyperammonemia or represented a rodent equivalent of GI bleeding induced HE in humans could not be resolved in this as yet unpublished study.

Finally, a recent manipulation has been to induce acute or subacute cholestasis in the PCS rat by common bile duct ligation (27). This model has not been characterized very well and uncertainty exists as to the nature of the behavioral changes induced by the superimposition of cholestasis. One particularly difficult problem is that this model displays considerable weight loss due presumably to anorexia and malabsorption. Thus in any study of this model in regards to either hyperammonemia or HE the issue of starvation of the animal comes into play. Also if one is unwise enough to try and pair feed to this model the control animal is grossly starved which induces more problems (see next section).

7. Issue of Controls for Experiments with Chronic Liver Disease Models

Particularly in studies of hyperammonemia, growth and amino acid metabolism it is highly desirable to have appropriate control animals to compare to the chronic liver disease model. Any model that displays significant anorexia and weight loss causes great difficulty. Pair feeding of normal control rats who quickly outgrow their anorectic sick chronic liver disease model pair almost by definition starves the normal control. While it might look nice to keep the control animals weight close to the animal model of interest starvation in itself can induce a large array of metabolic changes. Pair feeding animals on a g/100gm body weight basis instead of by giving the pair the absolute weight of the intake of the smaller anorectic animal model of liver disease could improve things. However, the starved pair fed animal will eat most of its chow very fast leaving it to starve for 20–23 hours before the next feeding time. This issue of pair feeding is very difficult to resolve. The easiest solution is to have 2 control groups. One pair fed and the other ad libitum. Statistical analysis is more difficult but the relative effects of starvation versus liver disease can usually be resolved. This, of course, increases the cost of experiments. Other alternatives are to use models of chronic liver disease without anorexia and weight loss (or minimize this in some way) or just use an ad libitum control only and correct data obtained for different body weight, etc.

Scrutinizing many studies it is fairly clear that pair feeding causes more problems than solutions and often totally clouds the interpretation of results.

Traditionally animals are fasted overnight before sacrifice to obtain necropsy tissue and blood. In some studies no statement is made on this issue at all which is unsatisfactory. Even with the variations in eating patterns more consideration should be given to studying animals while still feeding right up to sacrifice since this may maximize differences between liver disease models and controls (eg for blood ammonia, amino acid levels etc.). Regardless of what state the animal is in at sacrifice or blood drawing it is important to have the animals state as similar as possible to when metabolic or behavioral measurements were performed before sacrifice or blood drawing.

8. Measurement of Behavioral Changes

As mentioned earlier what is desired in animal models of chronic liver disease with hyperammonemia is documentation of a behavioral change which can be shown to relevant to HE in humans. Since we can't use psychometric testing or clinical examination in animals other measures have to be used. Detailed testing for various reflexes and responses can be done but these can be very subjectively interpreted (28). Also in a model such as the PCS rat it is very difficult by visual observation or using reflex testing to detect any changes in behavior. Accordingly, the recent use of computerized activity meters (8–10) and devices to measure circadian rhythm of activity (14) in PCS rats are major advances. However, extreme care must be exercised when using data generated from these machines. Some activity meters cannot distinguish stationary twitching movements from purposeful ambulation. Unless animals are directly observed (or a video recording is made) then convulsive activity could be mistaken for an improvement in ambulation after injecting for instance a benzodiazepine receptor antagonist with convulsant properties. Standardization of conditions is obviously critical also. The level of illumination of an open field in which activity is usually measured can dramatically alter results (29). Potentially many other factors identified and some as yet unidentified could modify results with activity meters. To illustrate this point we for a prolonged period of time could not reproduce the reported decrease in spontaneous motor activity in PCS rats described by Bengsston and colleagues (8–10). Only when we realized that he did all his measurements after darkening the open field could we reproduce his results (29). In many papers this point is not mentioned at all. Many investigations may not realize for instance that virtually all of the activity measurements done in acute liver failure models where a variety of benzodiazepine and GABA antagonists were given, were done in bright light (30,31). The rat is a nocturnal animal and usually is far more active in the dark or during the night. The wisdom of using a 10 minutes measurement of activity in bright light in a nocturnal control animal and comparing it to an extremely ill acute liver failure rat can be questioned in these studies. However, in reality the activity meter measurements were used more for demonstrating an objective improvement in ambulation after injection of drugs than to define the presence of "encephalopathy".

Animals like humans have a great deal of variability in activity levels (32). One problem in evaluating behavioral changes in PCS rats is that unless activty levels are measured before the shunt surgery the impact of the PCS on spontaneous motor activity is uncertain. When reasonably large numbers of animals are used and the shunt surgery is optimally performed (by a skilled technician) then the mean value for activity levels (in counts per minutes) are nearly always significantly less in PCS rats compared to unoperated controls or sham rats as long as the activity measurements are done in darkened enclosure. However, in small numbers of animals especially if the shunt stoma is not widely patent (ie a low portosystemic gradient is not present) it may be difficult to show differences between PCS and control animals. There are many factors involved in this problem: [1]) animals subjected to PCS may have been very active pre–operatively and the PCS has reduced the activity by 40–50%. Even with that dramatic reduction there will be little difference to a control rat if the control rat had a low activity level pre–operatively. This problem is lessened by using larger numbers of animals because the impact of a few underactive controls is diluted out by the large numbers of "normally" active controls; [2] It has not been established yet whether rats with high or low activity levels before PCS react differently to creation of a portosystemic shunt. Until this is settled comparing post–PCS activity to pre–PCS is the only reliable way to really establish the impact of the operation on rats. This has been done by Coy et al (14) and Herz et al (12) in the past. Another alternative is to use each animal as its own control which we have done. However, this is only applicable to situations where treatment effects are being evaluated (eg neomycin) (29); [3] A clear attenuation of the behavioral impact of PCS has been noted as animals apparently adapt to the PCS (10,33). Thus care has to be taken not to study animals too long after the shunt procedure or else difficulties will be encountered in observing a reduction in motor activity. One to three weeks is the perfect time to study PCS animals based on a number of published reports (10,33). [4] The shunt technique may be critical also. A wide stoma sutured PCS by an experienced operator (eg Jeanne Gottstein, Martin Grun, Finn Bengsston) appears not only to maximize the effects of portosystemic anastomosis but also tends to be associated with a much slower adaption of the rats (1). Button shunts (23) and shunts in which the anastomosis is secured by cyanoacrylate adhesive have been reported to be more frequently associated with gradual reversal of the effects of portosystemic shunting (17). Whether this is because of reestablishment of collateral blood flow into the liver or other factors has not yet been entirely resolved. Whatever it is important to be aware of the changing status of PCS rats with some of the shunt techniques; [5] Post–operative diet. Rats after PCS are very sensitive to dietary factors. This has been well established in terms of growth and body weight, but could also play a role in activity. If one uses a "starved" pair fed control instead of an ad libitum control it actually accentuates the difference in spontaneous motor activity levels between PCS rat and controls. This is because the starved pair fed control is more active than a normal rat; [6] We have observed a gender difference in terms of motor activity of rats after PCS. Female rats seem to be less affected than male rats (29). However, other studies do not confirm this observation but have not compared male and female rats at the same time (8–10). Female rats in most peoples hands are more active than male rats in animal activity measuring cages (32); [7] Age of rats at time of PCS. Older rats perhaps like their human counterparts appear in our hands to be more effected by PCS than younger rats; [8] Housing conditions. Grouping more than one PCS rat in a cage at a time seems to accentuate shunt effects (34); [9] Coprophagia. Wire bottom cages tend to reduce coprophagia which can inhibit grown in normal rats, but actually seems to improve the status of PCS rats (12).

Listed above are some of the factors known to effect PCS rats. No doubt there are many others may be operative. Some we may be unaware of completely. This serves to illustrate the importance of every laboratory standardizing conditions. Failure to do this leads to discordant results from different laboratories. It has been suggested previously that we should pay more attention to these issues (1,34).

Measurement of evoked potentials (35) or spectral analysis of electroencephalographic patterns (36) represent potentially useful measures of the degree of encephalopathy in animal models with acute liver disease. We are not aware of studies showing convincing changes in these types of measurements in chronic liver disease models. Overall, the sensitivity and specificity of these techniques in diagnosing HE in animal models of liver disease is unknown. How this can be resolved is hard to imagine.

9. Final Comments

The search for more ideal animal models of hyperammonemia and HE in chronic liver disease should continue. Potentially we already have a model, but we just don't realize it (eg.

Table 5. Features of ideal animal model of hepatic encephalopathy

FEATURES OF IDEAL ANIMAL MODEL OF HEPATIC ENCEPHALOPATHY
● Evidence of chronic liver disease / or portosystemic shunt
● Documented behavior changes
● Exclusion of other causes of "encephalopathy"
● Behavioral changes from mild to severe (ie different stages)
● Reversibility of behavioral changes with HE treatment
● Worsening or precipitation of severe behavior changes by precipitating factors
● Hyperammonemia and plasma amino acid profiles similar to human HE
● Alzheimer type II astrocytes present in brain
● Increased brain or CSF glutamine?
● Reproducible model which can be easily standardized
● Low cost
● Not dangerous to laboratory personnel

advanced CCl_4 cirrhosis, PCS rat model with more obvious behavioral changes, ammonia resin in PCS rat etc). Encouragement should be given to investigators to try and develop and validate models fulfilling most if not all the criteria listed in Table 5. Specifically these attempts should be given the chance of being published even if the experiments fail. Otherwise, we will all be repeating experiments perhaps destined to futility without knowing that they were attempted in the past. Even though it might be considered overly provocative we think that no animal model of HE should ever be accepted as a model of HE in chronic liver disease in humans unless it clearly is reversible, precipitated by known factors from human clinic observation, and is reversible by some measure known to improve HE in humans. At present only the PCS rat model has achieved some of these factors. However, it still represents a very mild "encephalopathy" and maybe more relevant to subclinical HE in humans than overt HE. As Gitlin stated in an excellent editorial on subclinical HE (or portal systemic encephalopathy) we still are uncertain as to the relationship between subclinical HE and overt HE (37). Therefore, we should continue to try and develop even better animal models of HE in chronic liver disease.

Acknowledgement: This work was supported in part by grants from the MetroHealth Foundation and National Institutes of Health Grants DK-39527 and MH 433524. None of this work could have been performed without the expert support of Kristine Kaminsky-Russ, Laurie Wills and Arthur McCullough.

References

1. Mullen KD. Optimal animal models for the study of hepatic encephalopathy and nitrogen metabolism. 8th Internat Ammonia Symposium: In Press.
2. Peeling J, Shoemacher L, Gauthier T, Benarroch A, Sutherland GR, Minuk GY. Cerebral metabolic and histological effects of thioacetamide-induced liver failure. Am J Physiol **265**:G572-G578, 1993.
3. Maddison JE. Canine congenital portosystemic encephalopathy. Aust Vet J **65**:245-249, 1988.

4. Bollman JL. The animal with an Eck fistula. Physiological Reviews **41**:607–621.

5. Thompson JS, Schafer DF, Haun J, Schafer GJ. Adequate diet prevents hepatic coma in dogs with Eck Fistulas. Surg Gyn & Obst **162**:126–130, 1986.

6. Cooper AJL, Lai JCK. Cerebral ammonia metabolism in normal and hyperammonemic rats. Neurochemical Pathology **6**:67–95, 1987.

7. Rössle M, Jones DB, Mullen KD, Grun M, Jones EA. Induction of unequivocal encephalopathy in the portacaval shunted rat. Hepatology **6**:1222[A], 1986.

8. Bengtsson F, Nobin A, Falck B, Gage FH, Jeppsson B. Portacaval shunt in the rat: Selective alterations in behavior and brain serotonin. Pharmacol Bioch & Behavior **24**:1611–1616, 1986.

9. Bengtsson F, Nobin A, Falck B, Gage FH, Jeppsson B. Effect of oral branched chain amino acids on behavior and brain serotonin metabolism in portacaval shunted rats. World J Surg **12**:246–254, 1988.

10. Bengtsson F, Bugge M, Brun A, Falck B, Hendriksson JG, Nobin A. The impact of time after portacaval shunt in the rat on behavior, brain serotonin and brain and muscle histology. J of Neurolog Sci **83**:109–122, 1988.

11. Tricklebank MD, Bloxam DL, Kantamaneni BD, Gurzon G. Effect of chronic experimental liver dysfunction and L-tryptophan on behavior in the rat. Pharmacol Biochem Behav **9**:181–189, 1978.

12. Herz R, Sautter V, Robert F, Bircher J. The Eck fistula rat: Definition of an experimental model. Eur J Clin Invest **2**:390–397, 1972.

13. Conjeevaram HS, Nagle A, Katz A, Kaminsky-Russ K, McCullough AJ, Mullen KD. Reversal of Behavioral Changes in Rats Subjected to Portacaval Shunt with Oral Neomycin Therapy. Hepatology: **19**:1245–1250, 1994.

14. Coy DL, Mehta R, Zee P, Salchii F, Turek FW, Blei AT. Portal-systemic shunting and the disruption of circadian locomotion activity in the rat. Gastroenterology **103**:222–228, 1992.

15. Coy D, Zee P, Salchii F, Turek F, Blei AT. Decreased dietary protein ameliorates disrupted circadian rhythm in rats after portacaval anastomosis. Gastroenterology **102**:A776, 1992.

16. Finn B, Sham V, Gottstein J, Blei AT. Neomycin improves a disrupted circadian rhythm in rats after portacaval anastomosis. Hepatogastroenterology 40, 1993.

17. Coy DL, Srivastava A Gottstein J, Butterworth RF, Blei AT. Post-operative course after portacaval anastomosis in rats is determined by the portacaval pressure gradient. Am J Physiol **261**:G1072–G1078, 1991.

18. Jerkins AA, Steele RD. Diet composition and surgical technique influence the post operative recovery of portacaval shunted rats. Hepatology **8**:855–860, 1988.

19. Proctor E, Chatamra K. High-yield micronodular cirrhosis in the rat. Gastroenterology **83**:1183–1190, 1982.

20. Bengtsson F, Bugge M, Vagianos C, Jeppsson B, Nobin A. Brain serotonin metabolism and behavior in rats with carbon tetrachloride-induced liver cirrhosis. Res Experimental Medicine **187**:429–438, 1987.

21. Yamamoto H, Sugihara N. Blood ammonia and hepatic encephalopathy induced by CCl_4 in rats. Toxicol & Appl Pharmacol **91**:461–468, 1987.

22. Snodgrass PJ. Urea cycle enzyme activities are normal and inducible by a high protein diet in CCl_4 cirrhosis of rats. Hepatology **9**:373–379, 1989.

23. Norenberg MD. A light and electron microscopic study of experimental portal-systemic (ammonia) encephalopathy: Progression and reversal of the disorder. Lab Invest **36**:618–627, 1977.

24. Azorin I, Minana MD, Felipo V, Grosolia S. A simple animal model of hyperammonemia. Hepatology **10**:311–314, 1989.

25. Hindtfeldt B, Plum F, Duffy TE. Effect of acute ammonia intoxication or cerebral metabolism in rats with portacaval shunts. J Clin Invest **49**:386–396, 1977.

26. Zeneroli ML, Baraldi M, Ventura E, Vezzelli C, Tofanetti O, Germini M, Casciarri I. Alterations of GABA-A and dopamine D-2 brain receptors in dogs with portal systemic encephalopathy. Life Sci **48**:37–50, 1991.

27. Maddison JE, Dodd PR, Morrison M, Farrell GC. Plasma GABA, GABA like activity and the brain GABA-benzodiazepine receptor complex in rats with chronic hepatic encephalopathy. Hepatology 7:621–628, 1987.

28. Rigotti P, Jonung T, James JH, Edwards LL, Peters JC, Fischer JE. Infusion of branched-chain amino acids and ammonium salts in rats with portacaval shunts. Arch Surg 120:1290–1295, 1985.

29. Conjeevaram HS, Mullen KD, May EJ, McCullough AJ. Gender dependent reduction of spontaneous motor activity and growth in rats subjected to portacaval shunt. Hepatology 19:381–388, 1994.

30. Steindl P, Püspök A, Druml W, Ferenci P. Beneficial effect of pharmacological modulation of the GABA$_A$-Benzodiazepine receptor on hepatic encephalopathy in the rat: Comparison with uremic encephalopathy. Hepatology 14:963–968, 1991.

31. Gammal SH, Basile AS, Geller D, Skolnick P, Jones EA. Reversal of the behavioral and electrophysiological abnormalities of an animal model of hepatic encephalopathy by benzodiazepine receptor ligands. Hepatology 11:371–378, 1990.

32. Robbin TW. A critique of the methods available for the measurement of spontaneous motor activity in: Handbook of Psychopharmacology Vol. 7. Iversen LL, Iversen SD, Snyder SH Eds. Plenum Press, New York, 1977, pp37–82.

33. DeBoer JEG, Oostenbroek J, Van Dongen JJ, Janssen MA, Soeters PB. Sequential metabolic characteristics following portacaval shunts in rats. Eur Surg Res 18:96–100, 1986.

34. Mullen KD, McCullough AJ. Problems with animal models of chronic liver disease: Suggestions for improvement in standardization. Hepatology 9:500–503, 1989.

35. Jones DB, Mullen KD, Roessle M, Maynard T, Jones EA. Hepatic encephalopathy: Application of visual evoked responses to test hypothesis of its pathogenesis in rats. J Hepatol 4:118–126, 1987.

36. Bossman DK, Van Den Buijs CACG, DeHaan JG, Maas MAW, Chamuleau AFM. The effects of benzodiazepine receptor antagonists and partial inverse agonists on acute hepatic encephalopathy in the rat. Gastroenterology 101:771–781, 1991.

37. Gitlin N. Subclinical portal systemic encephalopathy. Am J Gastroenterology 83:8–11, 1988.

Brain Metabolism in Encephalopathy Caused by Hyperammonemia

Richard A. Hawkins and Anke M. Mans

Liver failure, one of the primary causes of death around the world, may occur within days as a result of acute hepatic failure or over many years in chronic conditions such as alcoholic fatty liver or cirrhosis. When the liver fails, or when blood is shunted past the liver, hyperammonemia results and brain function deteriorates: a disorder known as hepatic encephalopathy [1–5]. This syndrome is manifest by signs that range from a rapidly developing sequence of delirium, convulsions and coma in acute hepatic necrosis to a more gradually developing intellectual impairment that may lead to stupor and coma in patients with chronic liver disease. The latter form is more prevalent and may affect millions of people to some degree [6, 7].

The reversibility of the signs in some patients and the absence of damage to neurons suggests that the encephalopathy has a metabolic cause. Brain function is compromised even in the milder stages of portalsystemic encephalopathy [8–10], and becomes more sensitive to drugs and metabolic disturbances that would have no adverse consequences in normal individuals [3–5].

1. Physiology of Ammonia Elimination

Ammonia has long been suspected to be an important factor in the cerebral dysfunction of hepatic failure and in other diseases in which pronounced hyperammonemia occurs [3, 11, 12]. Because of this, reducing the degree of hyperammonemia is one of the primary objectives of therapy [13]. An appreciation of the physiology of ammonia elimination is essential to understanding how high circulating concentrations of ammonia arise during liver dysfunction or due to shunting of blood past the liver.

The normal plasma concentration of ammonia is in the range of 20–50 μM [12]. Normal urea synthesis by the liver, however, requires concentrations in the range of 300–600 μM. Synthesis does not occur at the low concentrations existing in the general circulation because the first enzyme of urea synthesis, carbamyl phosphate synthetase has a low affinity for ammonia [14, 15]. This presents a dilemma because the concentrations necessary for urea synthesis by the liver are toxic for the brain and cannot be permitted to occur in the general circulation without serious consequences [12]. Physiologically this problem is solved by the participation of several tissues in the process of ammonia removal with glutamine as the essential link.

The interaction between the various organs is shown in Figure 1. Amino acids are taken up by peripheral tissues, notably muscle. The amino acids are oxidized by peripheral

Department of Physiology and Biophysics, Finch University of Health Sciences/The Chicago Medical School, 3333 Green Bay Road, North Chicago, IL 60064

Hepatic Encephalopathy, Hyperammonemia, and Ammonia Toxicity
Edited by V. Felipo and S. Grisolia, Plenum Press, New York, 1994

11

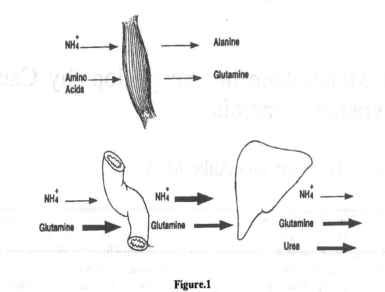

Figure.1

tissues and the nitrogen that results is released as glutamine and alanine. Glutamine is particularly important because it is nitrogen-rich, non-toxic and the predominant amino acid in circulation [16]. Glutamine is, therefore, an ideal vehicle to carry nitrogen to the liver.

The intestinal mucosa, in contrast to most organs of the body, use glutamine in preference to the normal fuels such as free fatty acids and glucose. In the process of oxidizing glutamine the intestinal mucosa produce ammonia [17-19]. Consequently the concentration of ammonia in the hepatic portal blood is raised to 300-600 μM -- concentrations that provide for effective urea synthesis but that would be toxic if they existed in the systemic circulation. Bacterial degradation of urea in the intestinal lumen may also contribute to ammonia [20-24], but this is probably only a small component of total ammonia production [25-28].

The major role of the intestine in ammonia production in the absence of bacterial action was demonstrated in studies of germ-free animals. Nance et al. showed that after portacaval shunting, germ-free dogs developed high plasma ammonia concentrations and a degree of encephalopathy that was comparable to ordinary dogs with portacaval shunts [29]. Furthermore, germ-free dogs showed the same rate of rise in plasma ammonia as normal dogs following the consumption of a blood meal [29]. Shalm and van der Mey found that the circulating levels of ammonia and the onset of hyperammonemic coma following hepatectomy in germ-free and normal rats were indistinguishable [30]. These and other studies [31, 32] demonstrate definitively that hazardous levels of ammonia can be produced without the participation of bacteria.

Thus, the design of multi-organ participation in the disposal of ammonia permits the high concentration of ammonia to be localized only to the hepatic portal vein where it is harmless. The ammonia is delivered directly to the liver which is also organized to metabolize it efficiently [33, 34].

The liver is made of ascini that begin where terminal portal venules and arterioles enter the parenchyma. The ascini extend along the sinusoids and end at the terminal hepatic venule. Perivenous and periportal hepatocytes that make up the ascini are morphologically similar, but they are distinct with respect to their metabolic capabilities [33]. Blood is delivered to the ascini from both the portal vein and the hepatic artery in a ratio of about three- or four-to-one.

The periportal hepatocytes contain all the enzymes necessary for urea synthesis whereas the perivenous cells lack carbamyl phosphate synthetase, and therefore cannot make urea. On the other hand, perivenous cells do contain glutamine synthetase, an enzyme that is completely lacking in the periportal compartment [35, 36]. The first and rate-limiting enzyme of urea synthesis, carbamyl phosphate synthetase, has a relatively high Km in the range of 2,000 μM in rats [37], and even higher in man (3,500 μM) [15] . Because of this the liver requires high ammonia concentrations for urea synthesis [38]. Urea synthesis in periportal cells is made more efficient by a unique system whereby glutamine is hydrolyzed at the site of carbamyl phosphate synthesis to provide even higher ammonia concentrations [14]. This occurs in the periportal hepatocytes, which contain a phosphate-dependent glutaminase, located in the mitochondria (as is carbamyl phosphate synthetase), and stimulated by ammonia. Half-maximal stimulation occurs at ammonia concentrations of about 200-300 μM with maximal stimulation at about 500-600 μM. The functional advantage of this organization is that ammonia, at the concentrations that exist in the portal vein, stimulates liver glutaminase which then operates in positive feedback manner to provide even higher ammonia concentrations at the site of carbamyl phosphate synthesis. One implication of this arrangement is that urea synthesis is at least partially controlled by the intestinal mucosa through its ability to alter the ammonia concentration in hepatic portal blood.

While periportal hepatocytes maintain high intracellular ammonia concentrations, some ammonia may diffuse away. This ammonia is scavenged in the perivenous compartment, which has no capability to make urea, but can incorporate residual ammonia into glutamine by a high-affinity system (Km $\approx$100 μM) [39]. Thus while glutamine is hydrolyzed in the periportal compartment to produce ammonia and glutamate, glutamate and the remaining ammonia are picked up by the periportal cells and resynthesized to glutamine.

The concept that glutamine is degraded and synthesized in two adjacent compartments, arranged in series, has been referred to as the intercellular glutamine cycle [38]. The liver glutamine cycle provides high ammonia concentrations in periportal cells for urea synthesis, and ensures that low concentrations of ammonia are maintained in the peripheral circulation. The overall balance is such that about 90% of the ammonia that enters liver is extracted. About two thirds of the nitrogen in urea originates from portal ammonia and most of the remainder from glutamine.

Hyperammonemia arises whenever hepatocytes become incapable of urea synthesis (e.g. by hepatocellular damage, inborn errors of metabolism, etc.) or when blood is shunted past the liver. In rats with portacaval shunts the liver atrophies to about 50% of its original mass, and the plasma ammonia concentrations rise to levels comparable to those that may be found in the portal vein. It appears that after portacaval shunting the arterial concentration of ammonia must rise until the concentrations are sufficient for the liver to again synthesize urea.

2. Metabolic Signs of Encephalopathy

The mechanism by which liver failure leads to a disturbance in brain function remains obscure, in spite of much information that is now available about the associated metabolic changes. The degree of encephalopathy in humans and rats is reflected by a measurable reduction in the rate of the use of glucose, the principal source of energy, throughout the brain (reviewed in [40]). This diminished rate of energy consumption is most likely explained by a decrement in the activity of brain cells. Because of this relationship a reduction in the rate of brain energy consumption is a convenient measure of diminished cerebral function in experimental animals. There are also various other metabolic changes that may be of etiologic importance. In rats with a portacaval shunt, a model of chronic liver disease which causes liver atrophy, the following changes are found: an increase in plasma and brain ammonia [41], a pronounced change in the plasma amino acid spectrum (decreases in the branched–chain amino acids and threonine and increases in the aromatic amino acids) [42, 43], a large rise in the brain content of aromatic amino acids and glutamine [41, 43], increased permeability of the blood–brain barrier to neutral amino acids [42–45], and increased brain content of serotonin (and its metabolite, 5-HIAA) and norepinephrine [46]. The relationship between these diverse metabolic alterations and encephalopathy remains to be elucidated.

The onset of hepatic encephalopathy occurs soon after portacaval shunting [47]. Brain energy metabolism starts its downward course within six hours and is maximally depressed within one or two days [47, 48]. This reduced rate of energy consumption is maintained for at least several months thereafter [47]. Most of the other abnormalities that are characteristic of the condition are also established by one day, with the exception of the reduction in plasma branched–chain amino acids and threonine, and the increase in brain norepinephrine, which take about two days. The latter changes are, therefore, less likely to be etiologically important.

3. Hyperammonemia Alone Causes Similar Metabolic Abnormalities

While ammonia seems the most prominent candidate for the initiation of the cerebral disturbances associated with hepatic failure, the relationship between hyperammonemia and encephalopathy, however, is puzzling because the blood ammonia levels do not always correlate with the severity of the neurologic signs [4, 11, 12, 49, 50]. Recent experiments showed that hyperammonemia alone could cause several of the metabolic abnormalities associated with portacaval shunting [51, 52]. In these experiments hyperammonemia was induced by intraperitoneal injections of urease rather than through shunting of hepatic portal blood. After two days there was decreased brain glucose consumption, increased transport of tryptophan across the blood–brain barrier, and increased glutamine and aromatic amino acids in brain: the same pattern of metabolic changes as that observed in portacaval shunted rats (Table 1). These experiments showed that ammonia was indeed a major factor in producing these changes.

4. Central Position of Glutamine Synthetase

In the experiments described above on artificially induced hyperammonemia, the decrease in brain energy consumption, and presumably brain function, correlated more closely with increased brain glutamine than with increased plasma ammonia. This was similar to the situation previously described in humans with portalsystemic encephalopathy in which encephalopathy was most closely related with glutamine or one of its metabolites, alpha–ketoglutaramate [53, 54]. The close relationship indicated that glutamine synthesis might be an important connection in the sequence between hyperammonemia and brain dysfunction.

Further experiments showed that glutamine synthesis is indeed an essential step in the adverse response to ammonia. In the absence of net glutamine synthesis hyperammonemia caused no detectable abnormalities [55]. In these experiments glutamine accumulation and hyperammonemia were separated as causes of encephalopathy by raising plasma ammonia levels with a small dose of methionine sulfoximine, an inhibitor of glutamine synthetase. This treatment caused hyperammonemia without an increase in brain glutamine content (Table 1). These hyperammonemic rats, with plasma and brain ammonia levels equivalent to those associated with decreased brain consumption in portacaval shunted rats, behaved normally during the two days of study. There was no depression of cerebral energy consumption, and the concentrations of key intermediary metabolites and high energy phosphates in the brain were normal. Neutral amino acid transport (tryptophan and leucine) and the brain content of

Table 1. Summary of metabolic abnormalities in different hyperammonemic states.

	Portacaval shunt (48h)	Urease treatment (48h)	Methionine sulfoximine (24–48h)
Brain:			
Ammonia	increased	increased	increased
Energy consumption	decreased	decreased	normal
Energy balance	normal	normal	normal
Neutral amino acid transport across blood–brain barrier	increased	increased	normal
Aromatic amino acid content	increased	increased	normal
Glutamine content	increased	increased	normal
Plasma:			
Ammonia	increased	increased	increased
Glutamine	increased	increased	normal
Glucose	normal	normal	normal

Observations on portacaval shunted rats are summarized from [47]. The data on hyperammonemia produced by intraperitoneal injections of urease is from [51] and the data on methionine sulfoximine induced hyperammonemia is from [79].

aromatic amino acids were unchanged. The data suggested that ammonia is benign at concentrations of 1 mM or less if it is not converted to glutamine. Thus, the deleterious effect of chronic hyperammonemia seem to begin with the synthesis of glutamine. The glutamine synthetase reaction, long considered to be a mechanism of ammonia detoxification [3–5, 11, 12, 56, 57], may in fact be the first step causing the metabolic abnormalities.

5. Amelioration of Metabolic Abnormalities

We tested whether the metabolic signs of portalsystemic encephalopathy in rats with portacaval shunts could be prevented or diminished by inhibiting the metabolism of ammonia by glutamine synthetase in the brain, using methionine sulfoximine. We showed that the onset of metabolic signs of encephalopathy caused by portacaval shunting could be prevented to some degree, and that established metabolic abnormalities could be partly reversed, by reducing glutamine synthetase activity in the brain [58]. To do this, a small dose of methionine sulfoximine, sufficient to partially inhibit brain glutamine synthetase, was given to rats either at the time of portacaval shunting or three to four weeks later. The effects on several characteristic cerebral metabolic abnormalities produced by portacaval shunting were measured one to three days after injection of the inhibitor. All untreated portacaval shunted rats had elevated plasma and brain ammonia concentrations, increased brain glutamine and tryptophan content, decreased brain glucose consumption and increased permeability of the blood–brain barrier to tryptophan. In all treated rats brain glutamine content was normalized, indicating inhibition of glutamine synthesis. One day after shunting and methionine sulfoximine administration, glucose consumption, tryptophan transport and brain tryptophan content remained near normal (Table 2). In the three- to four-week shunted rats, studied one to three days after methionine sulfoximine administration, the effect was less pronounced;

Table 2. The effect of reducing glutamine synthetase activity at the time of shunting on the development of the metabolic signs of encephalopathy.

	Portacaval shunt	Portacaval shunt plus methionine sulfoximine
Brain:		
Ammonia	increased	increased
Energy consumption	decreased	normal
Neutral amino acid transport across blood–brain barrier	increased	normal
Aromatic amino acid content	increased	near–normal
Glutamine content	increased	normal
Plasma:		
Ammonia	increased	increased
Glucose	normal	normal

All measurements were taken 24 hours after portacaval shunting. Treated rats were given methionine sulfoximine (15–45 mg/kg) at the time of shunting. See reference [58] for details.

brain glucose consumption and tryptophan content were partially normalized, but tryptophan transport was unaffected (Table 3). The results agree with the earlier conclusion that glutamine synthesis is an essential step in the development of cerebral metabolic abnormalities in hyperammonemic states, and suggest that this step deserves further attention.

6. Possible Mechanisms

Energy reduction. It has been proposed that there may be an energy and metabolite drain, caused by abnormally high rates of glutamine synthesis. It is also conceivable that ammonia interferes with brain energy production by inhibition of the alpha–oxoglutarate dehydrogenase complex or the mitochondrial malate–aspartate shuttle (see [12] for a summary). These hypotheses do not seem to offer an adequate explanation for cerebral dysfunction in chronic hyperammonemia. Such interference with energy production would cause predictable and substantial alterations in the concentrations of several intermediary metabolites, but these changes have not been observed *in vivo* (reviewed in [40]).

Furthermore, while a temporary deficiency in energy production could interfere with cell function, a sustained deficit would result in cell death. The neuropathology of hepatic encephalopathy shows no such evidence. Thus, the finding of reduced cerebral metabolic rates of glucose and oxygen in hepatic encephalopathy must be explained by a reduction in the demand, i.e., the level of work.

The hyperammonemia produced by portacaval shunting does not impose much of a metabolic burden on brain. Even when lethal doses of exogenous ammonia were given, a reduction in phosphocreatine and ATP levels seemed to be a secondary rather than a causal phenomenon [59]. Although the metabolic demand made by increased glutamine synthesis in chronically hyperammonemic rats forms a relatively small percentage of total brain metabolism, it falls entirely on astrocytes which comprise perhaps one third of the total cell volume in brain. While astrocytes do show morphological changes, which may be compensatory to this process, there are no signs of astrocyte cell death, as might be expected in a situation of long–lasting energy failure [60–62]. It is possible that the sustained hyperactivity may disrupt other activities of the astrocytes, such as regulating neurotransmitter uptake and ion homeostasis, and influencing blood–brain barrier transport of essential

Table 3. The effect of reducing glutamine synthetase activity three–four weeks after shunting on established metabolic signs of encephalopathy.

	Portacaval shunt	Portacaval shunt plus methionine sulfoximine
Brain:		
Ammonia	increased	increased
Energy consumption	decreased	near–normal
Neutral amino acid transport across blood–brain barrier	increased	increased
Aromatic amino acid content	increased	partially normalized
Glutamine content	increased	normal
Plasma:		
Ammonia	increased	increased
Glucose	normal	normal

All measurements were taken 3–4 weeks after portacaval shunting. Treated rats were given 30 mg of methionine sulfoximine for a period of 1–3 days before sacrifice. See reference [58] for details.

nutrients. These possibilities remain to be tested.

Inhibition of glutaminase. It has been suggested that ammonia may disturb cerebral function by inhibiting glutaminase [63–65] thereby disrupting the supply of glutamate for glutamatergic neurons [66–68]. Our experiments do not support this hypothesis. Methionine sulfoximine caused hyperammonemia, but the brain content of glutamine and glutamate remained near normal. If there were inhibition of glutaminase by ammonia the glutamate concentration would have been expected to decrease. It is conceivable that the lack of a decrease could be explained if glutaminase was inhibited by ammonia to the same degree that glutamine synthetase was inhibited by methionine sulfoximine. However, in that circumstance production of glutamate from glutamine would have been reduced even more.

Ammonium ion. There are at least two known effects of NH_4^+ on neuronal membranes that could disturb brain function. NH_4^+ can interfere with the generation of inhibitory postsynaptic potentials by inhibiting the Cl^- pump. This occurs at ammonia concentrations similar to those reported here and is maximal at a concentration of 1 mM [69, 70]. At higher concentrations (greater than 2 mM) NH_4^+ can depolarize neurons and interfere with synaptic transmission [69, 70].

In our experiments using methionine sulfoximine the brain concentrations of ammonia were high enough to inhibit the Cl^- pump and, at least in principle, to cause neurons to become more easily excited [71]. However there were no detectable changes in brain glucose consumption or in the concentrations of high–energy intermediates [55]. It is known that neurons adapt to the chronic presence of NH_4^+ and it is possible that the Cl^- pump had recovered by twenty–four hours [72]. Therefore, while it remains conceivable that NH_4^+ directly interferes with nerve cell function in hyperammonemic diseases, the effects may be too subtle to be detected by the techniques used.

Stimulation of blood–brain barrier transport. It is well established that hyperammonemia, whether caused by portacaval shunting or by artificial means, leads to a greater activity of the carrier system that transports neutral amino acids across the blood–brain barrier, as well as to a rise in the brain content of aromatic amino acids [42–44, 51, 73–76]. The permeability of the blood–brain barrier to neutral amino acids and the accumulation of

17

aromatic amino acids are both closely correlated with brain glutamine content [51, 52, 77]. Moreover the elevated rate of transport and the increased accumulation of neutral amino acids caused by hyperammonemia or by portacaval shunting can be reduced by treatment with methionine sulfoximine [76, 78]. Our experiments, in agreement with previous observations, show conclusively that sustained hyperammonemia in the absence of net glutamine synthesis has no effect on either neutral amino acid transport or the accumulation of aromatic amino acids in brain. It may, therefore, be concluded that glutamine synthesis is linked to the stimulation of neutral amino acid transport caused by hyperammonemia as well as to the decrease in cerebral energy metabolism [51, 52]. After portacaval shunting the change in neutral amino acid transport occurs very early, beginning within six hours, and is paralleled by a substantial decrease in cerebral glucose consumption [47]. The relationship between the changes in the permeability of the blood–brain barrier and cerebral dysfunction needs to be clarified.

7. Concluding Comments

It is now evident that hyperammonemia disturbs cerebral function and is an important trigger in the sequence of events leading to hepatic encephalopathy. The absence of a toxic response to hyperammonemia when it is created by inhibiting glutamine synthetase, indicates that ammonia itself is relatively innocuous (at concentrations below 1 mM). It is when ammonia is metabolized that an adverse response is initiated. This does not mean that glutamine itself is toxic, there are many other metabolites and cellular processes to be considered. Nevertheless, the observation that the metabolism of ammonia plays an essential role in causing cerebral dysfunction has important implications for diseases in which hyperammonemia is a characteristic feature like hepatic encephalopathy and some inborn errors of metabolism. Certainly, attention should be focused on the glutamine synthetase reaction and its products in the search for the mechanism of ammonia toxicity.

Acknowledgment: The authors' work was supported by NIH grant NS–16389.

References

1. Adams RD, Foley JM. The neurological disorder associated with liver disease. Res Publ Assoc Nerve Ment Dis 1953;**32:**198–237.
2. Sherlock S, Summerskill WHJ, White LP, Phear EA. Portal–systemic encephalopathy. Neurological complications of liver disease. Lancet 1954;**2:**453–457.
3. Plum F, Hindfelt B. The neurological complications of liver disease. In: Vinken PJ, Bruyn GW, Klawans HL, eds. Metabolic and Deficiency Diseases of the Nervous System. Part I, 27. New York: American Elsevier Publishing Co. Inc., **1976:**349–377.
4. Zieve L. Hepatic encephalopathy: summary of present knowledge with an elaboration on recent developments. In: Popper H, Schaffner F, eds. Progress in Liver Diseases, 6. New York: Grune and Stratton, **1979:**327–341.
5. Hoyumpa Jr. AM, Desmond PV, Avant GR, Roberts RK, Schenker S. Hepatic encephalopathy. Gastroenterology 1979;**76:**184–195.
6. Mendenhall DL. Alcoholic Hepatitis. Clin Gastroenterol 1981;**10:**417–441.
7. Scheig R. That demon rum. Am J Gastroenerol 1991;**86:**150–152.
8. Gilberstadt SJ, Gilberstadt H, Zieve L, Buegel B, Collier Jr. RO, McClain CJ. Psychomotor performance defects in cirrhotic patients without overt encephalopathy. Arch Intern Med 1980;**140:**519–521.
9. Rikkers L, Jenko P, Rudman D, Freides D. Subclinical hepatic encephalopathy: detection, prevalence, and relationship to nitrogen metabolism. Gastroenterology 1978;**75:**462–469.

10. Elsass P, Lund Y, Ranek L. Encephalopathy in patients with cirrhosis of the liver. A neuro-psychological study. Scand J Gastroenterol 1978;**13**:241-247.
11. Butterworth RF, Giguere JF, Michaud J, Lavoie J, Pomier-Layrargues G. Ammonia: key factor in the pathogenesis of hepatic encephalopathy. Neurochem Pathol 1987;**6**:1-12.
12. Cooper AJ, Plum F. Biochemistry and physiology of brain ammonia. Physiol Rev 1987;**67**:440-519.
13. Sherlock S. Chronic portal systemic encephalopathy: update 1987. Gut 1987;**28**:1043-1048.
14. Sies H, Haüssinger D. Hepatic glutamine and ammonia metabolism. Nitrogen redox balance and the intracellular glutamine cycle. In: Haüssinger D, Sies H, eds. Glutamine metabolism in mammalian tissues., New York: Springer-Verlag, **1984**:78-97.
15. Kaiser S, Gerok W, Haüssinger D. Ammonia and glutamine metabolism in human liver slices: new aspects on the pathogenesis of hyperammonaemia in chronic liver disease. Eur J Clin Invest 1988;**18**:535-542.
16. Souba WW, Smith RJ, Wilmore DW. Glutamine metabolism by the intestinal tract. J Parenter Ent Nutr 1985;**9**:608-617.
17. Hanson PJ, Parsons DS. Transport and metabolism of glutamine and glutamate in small intestine. In: Kvamme E, eds. Glutamine and glutamate in mammals, I. Boca: CRC Press, Inc., **1988**:235-253.
18. Souba WW. Glutamine: A key substrate for the splanchnic bed. Annu Rev Nutr 1991;**11**:285-308.
19. Windmueller HG. Metabolism of vascular and luminal glutamine by intestinal mucosa in vivo. In: Gayssubgerm D, Sies H, eds. Glutamine Metabolism in Mammalian Tissues, Berlin: Springer-Verlag, **1984**:61-77.
20. Cholopoff AD. Herkunft und Verteilung des Blutammoniaks nach Untersuchungen an angiostomierten Hunden. Pflüger's Arch ges Physiol 1927;**218**:670-676.
21. Walser M, Bodenloos LJ. Urea metabolism in man. J Clin Invest 1959;**38**:1617-1626.
22. Jones EA, Smallwood RA, Craigie A, Rosenoer VM. The enterohepatic circulation of urea nitrogen. Clin Sci 1969;**37**:825-836.
23. Summerskill WHJ, Wolpert E. Ammonia metabolism in the gut. Am J Clin Nutr 1970;**23**:633-639.
24. Wolpert E, Phillips SF, Summerskill WHJ. Transport of urea and ammonia production in the human colon. Lancet 1971;**2**:1387-1390.
25. Vince A, Down PF, Murison J, Twigg FJ, Wrong OM. Generation of ammonia from non-urea sources in a faecal incubation system. Clin Sci Mol Med 1976;**51**:313-322.
26. Bown RL, Gibson JA, Fenton JCB, Snedden W, Clark ML, Sladen GE. Ammonia and urea transport by the excluded human colon. Clin Sci Mol Med 1975;**48**:279-287.
27. Gibson JA, Park NJ, Sladen GE, Dawson AM. The role of the colon in urea metabolism in man. Clin Sci Mol Med 1976;**50**:51-59.
28. Wrong OM, Vince AJ, Waterlow JC. The origins and bacterial metabolism of faecal ammonia. In: Kasper H, Goebbel H, eds. Falk Symposium 32, Colon and Nutrition, **1981**:133-139.
29. Nance FC, Kline DG. Eck's fistula encephalopathy in germfree dogs. Ann Surg 1971;**174**:856-861.
30. Schalm SW, Van Der Mey T. Hyperammonemic coma after hepatectomy in germ-free rats. Gastroenterology 1979;**77**:231-234.
31. van Leeuwen PAM. Ammonia generation in the gut and the influence of lactulose and neomycin. 1985, University of Maastricht (Thesis)
32. Weber FLJ, Veach GL. The importance of the small intestine in gut ammonium production in the fasting dog. Gastroenterology 1979;**77**:235-240.
33. Jungermann K, Katz N. Metabolic heterogeneity of liver parenchyma. In: Sies H, eds. Metabolic compartmentation, London, New York: Academic Press, **1982**:411-435.
34. Haüssinger D. Nitrogen metabolism in liver: structural and functional organization and physiological relevance. Biochem J 1990;**267**:181-290.
35. Gebhardt R, Mecke D. Heterogeneous distribution of glutamine synthetase among rat liver parenchymal cells *in situ* and in primary culture. Embo J 1983;**2**:567-570.
36. Gaasbeek Janzen JW, Lamers WH, Moorman AFM, De Graaf A, Los JA, Charles R. Immunohistochemical localization of carbamoyl-phosphate synthetase (ammonia) in adult rat liver; evidence for a heterogeneous distribution. J Histochem Cytochem 1984;**32**:557-564.
37. Lusty CJ. Carbamoylphosphate synthetase I of rat-liver mitochondria. Eur J Biochem 1978;**85**:373-383.

38. Häussinger D. Hepatocyte heterogeneity in glutamine and ammonia metabolism and the role of an intercellular glutamine cycle during ureogenesis in perfused rat liver. Eur J Biochem 1983;133:269–275.

39. Deuel TF, Louie M, Lerner A. Glutamine synthetase from rat liver. J Biol Chem 1978;253:6111–6118.

40. Hawkins RA, Mans AM. Brain energy metabolism in hepatic encephalopathy. In: Butterworth RF, Pomier–Layrargues G, eds. Hepatic Encephalopathy, Clifton, NJ: Humana Press Inc., 1989:159–176.

41. Mans AM, Biebuyck JF, Davis DW, Hawkins RA. Portacaval anastomosis: brain and plasma metabolite abnormalities and the effect of nutritional therapy. J Neurochem 1984;43:697–705.

42. Mans AM, Biebuyck JF, Shelly K, Hawkins RA. Regional blood–brain barrier permeability to amino acids after portacaval anastomosis. J Neurochem 1982;38:705–717.

43. James JH, Escourrou J, Fischer JE. Blood–brain neutral amino acid transport activity is increased after portacaval anastomosis. Science 1978;200:1395–1397.

44. Mans AM, Biebuyck JF, Saunders SJ, Kirsch RE, Hawkins RA. Tryptophan transport across the blood–brain barrier during acute hepatic failure. J Neurochem 1979;33:409–418.

45. Sarna GS, Bradbury MW, Cremer JE, Lai JC, Teal HM. Brain metabolism and specific transport at the blood–brain barrier after portocaval anastomosis in the rat. Brain Res 1979;160:69–83.

46. Mans AM, Hawkins RA. Brain monoamines after portacaval anastomosis. Metab Brain Dis 1986;1:45–52.

47. Mans AM, DeJoseph MR, Davis DW, Viña JR, Hawkins RA. Early establishment of cerebral dysfunction after portacaval shunting. Am J Physiol 1990;258:E104–E110.

48. DeJoseph MR, Hawkins RA. Glucose consumption decreases throughout the brain only hours after portacaval shunting. Am J Physiol 1991;260:E613–E619.

49. Sherlock S. Pathogenesis and management of hepatic coma. Am J Med 1958;24:805–813.

50. Lockwood AH. Metabolic encephalopathies: opportunities and challenges. J Cereb Blood Flow Metab 1987;7:523–526.

51. Jessy J, Mans AM, DeJoseph MR, Hawkins RA. Hyperammonemia causes many of the changes found after portacaval shunting. Biochem J 1990;272:311–317.

52. Jessy J, DeJoseph MR, Hawkins RA. Hyperammonemia depresses glucose consumption throughout brain. Biochem J 1991;277:693–696.

53. Vergara F, Plum F, Duffy TE. a–Ketoglutaramate: Increased concentrations in the cerebrospinal fluid of patients in hepatic coma. Science 1974;183:81–83.

54. Hourani BT, Hamlin EM, Reynolds TB. Cerebrospinal fluid glutamine as a measure of hepatic encephalopathy. Arch Intern Med 1971;127:1033–1036.

55. Hawkins RA, Jessy J. Hyperammonemia does not impair brain function in the absence of glutamine synthesis. Biochem J 1991;277:697–703.

56. Krebs HA. Metabolism of amino acids. IV. The synthesis of glutamine in animal tissue. Biochem J 1936;29:1951–1969.

57. Weil–Malherbe H. Significance of glutamic acid for the metabolism of nervous tissue. Physiol Rev 1950;30:549–568.

58. Hawkins RA, Jessy J, Mans AM, De Joseph MR. Effect of reducing brain glutamine synthesis on metabolic signs of hepatic encephalopathy. J Neurochem 1993;60:1000–1006.

59. Schenker S, Brady CE. Pathogenesis of hepatic encephalopathy. In: Conn HO, Bircher J, eds. Hepatic Encephalopathy: Management with Lactulose and Related Carbohydrates, East Lansing, MI: Medi–Ed Press, 1990:15–30.

60. Cavanagh JB, Kyu MH. Type II Alzheimer change experimentally produced in astrocytes in the rat. J Neurol Sci 1971;12:63–75.

61. Norenberg MD. The distribution of glutamine synthetase in the rat central nervous system. J Histochem Cytochem 1979;27:756–762.

62. Zamora AJ, Cavanagh JB, Kyu MH. Ultrastructural responses of the astrocytes to portocaval anastomosis in the rat. J Neurol Sci 1973;18:25–45.

63. Bradford HF, Ward HK. Glutamine as a metabolic substrate for isolated nerve–endings: inhibition by ammonium ions. Biochem Soc Trans 1975;3:1223–1226.

64. Benjamin AM. Control of glutaminase activity in rat brain cortex in vitro: influence of glutamate, phosphate, ammonium, calcium and hydrogen ions. Brain Res 1981;208:363–377.

65. Matheson DF, Van den Berg CJ. Ammonia and brain glutamine: inhibition of glutamine degradation by ammonia. Biochem Soc Trans 1975;**3**:525–528.

66. Bradford HF, Ward HK, Thomas AJ. Glutamine – A major substrate for nerve endings. J Neurochem 1978;**30**:1453–1459.

67. Hamberger A, Hedquist B, Nystrom B. Ammonium ion inhibition of evoked release of endogenous glutamate from hippocampal slices. J Neurochem 1979;**33**:1295–1302.

68. Butterworth RF, Lavoie J, Giguere JF, Layrargues GP, Bergeron M. Cerebral GABA–ergic and glutamatergic function in hepatic encephalopathy. Neurochem Pathol 1987;**6**:131–144.

69. Raabe W. Ammonium decreases excitatory synaptic transmission in cat spinal cord in vivo. J Neurophysiol 1989;**62**:1461–1473.

70. Raabe W. Effects of NH4$^+$ on the function of the CNS. Adv Exp Med Biol 1991;**272**:89–98.

71. Raabe W. Ammonia and postsynaptic inhibition in cat motor cortex. In: Klee MR, Lux HD, Speckmann E–J, eds. Physiology and Pharmacology of Epileptogenic Phenomena, New York: Raven Press, **1982**:73–80.

72. Raabe W. Neurophysiology of ammonia intoxication. In: Butterworth R, Pomier–Layragues G, eds. Hepatic Encephalopathy: Pathophysiology and Treatment, Clifton, NJ: Humana Press, Inc., **1989**:49–77.

73. James JH, Hodgman JM, Funovics JM, Fischer JE. Alterations in brain octopamine and brain tyrosine following portacaval anastomosis in rats. J Neurochem 1976;**27**:223–227.

74. Mans AM, Biebuyck JF, Hawkins RA. Ammonia selectively stimulates neutral amino acid transport across blood–brain barrier. Am J Physiol 1983;**245**:C74–C77.

75. Bachmann C, Colombo JP. Increase of tryptophan and 5–hydroxyindole–acetic acid in the brain of ornithine carbamoyltransferase deficient sparse–fur mice. Pediatr Res 1984;**18**:372–375.

76. Jonung T, Rigotti P, Jeppsson B, James JH, Peters JC, Fischer JE. Methionine sulfoximine prevents the accumulation of large neutral amino acids in brain of hyperammonemic rats. J Surg Res 1984;**36**:349–353.

77. Jeppsson B, James JH, Edwards LL, Fischer JE. Relationship of brain glutamine and brain neutral amino acid concentrations after portacaval anastomosis in rats. Eur J Clin Invest 1985;**15**:179–187.

78. Rigotti P, Jonung T, Peters JC, James JH, Fischer JE. Methionine sulfoximine prevents the accumulation of large neutral amino acids in brain of portacaval–shunted rats. J Neurochem 1985;**44**:929–933.

79. Hawkins RA, Jessy J. Hyperammonemia does not impair brain function in the absence of net glutamine synthesis. Biochem J 1991;**277**:697–703.

In Vivo Brain Magnetic Resonance Imaging (MRI) and Magnetic Resonance Spectroscopy (MRS) in Hepatic Encephalopathy

Chamuleau, R.A.F.M., Vogels, B.A.P.M., Bosman, D.K., Bovée, W.M.M.J.

1. Introduction

Magnetic resonance imaging (MRI) and spectroscopy (MRS) of the living brain have recently been applied during the clinical picture of hepatic encephalopathy (HE) both in patients and experimental animals.

HE is a neuropsychiatric syndrome occurring during severely impaired liver function and/or portosystemic shunting. Hepatic dysfunction may be either chronic (e.g. liver cirrhosis) or acute (e.g. fulminant toxic, allergic or viral hepatitis). In chronic HE a gradual onset is usual, related to a gradual decrease in functioning liver mass or to a gradual progression of portosystemic shunting. Acute on chronic HE can be caused by a specific precipitating event in a cirrhotic patient such as gastrointestinal haemorrhage, infectious disease, overdosage of diuretics or arterial hypotension. Acute HE is most often caused by massive liver cell necrosis, the so called fulminant hepatic failure (FHF) or acute liver atrophy.

The clinical picture of HE consists of a decrease in the level of consciousness accompanied by electroencephalographic and neuromuscular abnormalities. The different stages of HE are given in Table 1 and their development may occur in weeks or months (chronic liver failure) but also in days or even hours (acute on chronic, or FHF). The pathobiochemistry of HE is multifactorial with a variety of circulating neurotoxins that can affect normal brain function.

MRS is a technique which permits chemically specific, non−invasive measurement of several biological important compounds in a volume of interest of living tissue (1−4). Application in vivo without invasiveness is the major advantage. The relative lack of sensitivity in vivo (only tissue concentrations in or near the millimolar range) is its major drawback. The mostly studied nucleus is ^{31}P, which gives information about the intracellular pH and energy metabolism. ^{1}H is more sensitive and more abundant in the body than ^{31}P and therefore might give more information. With suppression of the water signal, which is normally exploited in MRI, a spectrum of a localized region is recorded by ^{1}H−MRS.

Academic Medical Centre. Dept. of Experimental Internal Medicine, G2−130. Meibergdreef 9. 1105 AZ Amsterdam. The Netherlands

Hepatic Encephalopathy, Hyperammonemia, and Ammonia Toxicity
Edited by V. Felipo and S. Grisolia, Plenum Press, New York, 1994

23

Table 1. Clinical grading of hepatic encephalopathy. Adapted from ref. 23.

Stage	Mental state
I	Mild confusion, euphoria of depression, decreased attention, slowing of ability to perform mental tasks, irritability, disorder of sleep pattern.
II	Drowsiness, lethargy, gross deficits in ability to perform mental tasks, obvious personality changes, inappropriate behaviour, intermittent disorientation (usually for time).
III	Somnolent but arousable, unable to perform mental tasks, disorientation with respect to time and/or place, marked confusion, amnesia, occasional fits of rage, speech present but incomprehensible.
IV	Coma

With regard to the pathogenesis of HE MRS has made new contributions mainly in the field of changes in cerebral metabolism and brain cell membrane composition. At higher field strength the resolution can be improved and at 7 T in vivo ^{1}H MRS is able to quantify about 10 different compounds in the cerebral cortex (see Fig 1).

MRI uses the signal of hydrogen nuclei in water molecules to make pictures of anatomical structures, whereas MRS uses much weaker signals from nonwater ^{1}H, ^{31}P, ^{13}C, [23]Na or ^{15}N to obtain spectra which give quantitative information about tissue compounds with relatively crude spatial resolution (1,4). The spatial resolution obtained on whole body systems is of the order of 1 mm for MRI and 1 cm for MRS.

Hepatic failure causes hyperammonemia due to decreased hepatic urea and glutamine synthesis: ammonia diffuses into the brain and has direct neurotoxic effects. In addition ammonia influences cerebral metabolism of glucose (5,6), glutamate, glutamine and gamma–amino butyric acid (GABA) and inhibits the astrocytic re–uptake of glutamate from the extracellular compartment (for review see refs. 7 and 8). Increased cerebral

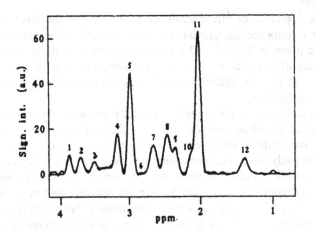

Figure 1. In vivo 7 T ^{1}H–MRS of the cerebral cortex of a conscious rat. 1=creatine, aspartate, 2=glutamine, glutamate, alanine, 3=glycine, inositol; 4=(phospho)–choline; 5=total creatine; 6=aspartate; 7=aspartate, N–acetylaspartate; 8=glutamine, N–acetylaspartate; 9=glutamate; 10=glutamate, glutamine; 11=N–acetylaspartate; 12=lactate.

Table 2. Calculated concentrations* in living normal rat brain.

Compound	Concentration
N–acetyl aspartate	4.8±2
Glutamate	5.0±3
Glutamine	5.6±4
Aspartate	2.2±13
Phosphocreatine + creatine	7.8±2
(Phospho)choline	1.6±2
Lactate	1.4±6

*(mmol/kg w/w) ± two times the Cramer Rao minimum variance bound (%) (ref. 24)

glutamine concentration may influence cell volume (9,10), aromatic amino acid transport, production of glutamate, GABA and alpha–ketoglutaramate (7,8). For this reason much attention has been paid to the majority of these ammonia and glutamine related compounds in the brain. Unfortunately in vivo ^{15}N–MRS is only feasible at very high strength (about 10 T) (11). Therefore studies on the pathobiochemistry of HE in experimental animals and human beings have mainly been done by in vivo brain ^{31}P–MRS and ^{1}H–MRS. At sufficiently high magnetic field (e.g. 7 Tesla) in vivo distinction of cerebral glutamate and glutamine concentrations is possible in experimental animals (see Fig. 1).

2. In Vivo Brain ^{1}H–MRS in Rats

Male Wistar rats 200–300 g (HSD–Zeist), The Netherlands, were used in all experiments. Animal welfare was in accordance with institutional guidelines of the University of Amsterdam. Four groups of rats were studied: normal control rats (n=10), acute liver ischemia (LIS) rats, (n=18), porta caval shunted (PCS) rats (n=10) and PCS rats with ammonium acetate infusion (AI–PCS, n=8)(12).

For acute HE, acute liver ischemia (LIS) was induced by ligation of the celiac trunk one day after porta–caval shunting (PCS). For chronic HE rats with PCS were studied and for subacute HE PCS rats with ammonium acetate infusion (AI–PCS)(12).

All MRS experiments in rats were performed at 300 MHz on a home–built 7 T spectrometer system. Two days before the experiment an ellipsoidal surface coil (axes 13 and 10 mm) was implanted on the skull in order to receive MR signals selectively from the cerebral cortex (13). Water suppression and localization, quantification of spectra and determination of brain cortex concentrations from the peak areas were done as described before, taking the total creatine concentration 7.8 mmol/kg ww in the normal brain as a standard (12). Calculated concentrations of the different compounds in normal brain cortex are given in Table 2 and in Table 3 for HE–rats.

At the end of experiments rats were sacrificed by ether anesthesia and cardiac puncture. Brain analysis of ammonia was performed on neutralized perchloric acid extracts using glutamate dehydrogenase. Table 3 shows brain ammonia concentrations and the measured cerebral cortex concentration of different compounds in rats with different grades of HE: acute, subacute and chronic HE are associated with significantly elevated brain NH_3 concentrations. Different types and different etiologies of HE showed

Table 3. In vivo brain ^{1}H-MRS of different experimental models of HE. Values are means ± SEM. Brain ammonia was measured biochemically at the end of the experiment.

Groups	HE	Brain NH$_3$ (μmol/kg ww)	Glu %	Gln %	Cho %	Lactate %
NORM	none	240±45	100±3	100±12	100±1	100±6
PCS	chronic	500±32	89±3	278±17	88±2	101±12
AI-PCS	subacute	2148±168	83±3	591±84	67±3	174±20
LIS(8h)	acute	1948±171	78±4	550±59	73±0	6317±45

^{1}H-MRS values are expressed as percentage of normal concentration in normal rats. Cho= (phospho)choline compounds.

significant changes in brain glutamate (decrease of about 20%), glutamine (increase of more than 500%), (phospho)choline (decrease of about 30%) and lactate (increase of about 300%).

Increases in brain Gln and lactate and decreases in brain Glu and Phosphocholine have been confirmed by others in PCS rats with hyperammonemia (14,15). Fitzpatrick (15) studied conditions of hyperammonemia in rats by ^{1}H MRS and ^{31}P MRS, while Kanamori (10) used in vivo ^{15}N MRS of hyperammonemic rats studying the activity of cerebral glutamine synthase.

Increased levels of cerebral cortex Gln can be explained either by increased flux through glutamine synthase, the most important ammonia detoxifying enzyme in the brain, or by inhibition of glutaminase by ammonia. The latter possibility seems to be the most likely since glutamine synthase in brain is almost saturated under physiological conditions (8). However, recently Kanamori (11) pointed to the fact that in situ concentrations of other substrates and cofactors of glutamine synthase may limit the activity of this enzyme in brain in vivo.

The increased cerebral cortex lactate concentration, a well known phenomenon during hyperammonemia (14), is positively correlated with brain ammonia concentration and may be explained by the well-known effects of ammonia on phosphofructokinase (stimulation) and on the TCA cycle enzyme isocitrate dehydrogenase (inhibition) (8).

^{1}H-MRS revealed another interesting and to our knowledge new observation: the decrease in cerebral cortex (phospho)choline compounds (Table 3) correlates significantly with the severity of HE. (R = −0.67; P<0.05) (12). The (phospho)choline peak seen in ^{1}H-MRS may originate from several choline containing substances (glycerolcholine, sphingomyelin, phosphatidylcholine, phosphocholine, acetylcholine) and carnitine. Presumably most of these compounds are positioned within the neuronal membrane, suggesting that experimental HE is associated with alterations in the neuronal and astrocytic cell membrane composition.

3. In Vivo ^{31}P-MRS in Rats

Studies on cerebral pH and high energy phosphates of PCS rats with acute hyperammonemia (15,16) and rats with acute liver ischemia (16) have shown no significant changes in intracellular pH or high energy phosphates. Therefore it has been concluded that a change in cerebral cortex high energy phosphates is not an important pathophysiological mechanism during the development of acute and subacute HE.

Table 4. Clinical parameters. Control values are for Number Connection Test (NCT) <35 sec and for plasma ammonia <40 μM.

Patients	Sex	Age yrs	Child (A–C)	NCT (seconds)	Ammonia (μM)	HE grade (0–4)
1	F	23	A	20	98	0
2	F	62	A	40	21	1
3	F	63	A	55	34	1–2
4	F	54	A	50	90	1–2
5	M	51	B	50	23	1–2
6	M	69	B	45	51	1–2
7	M	45	C	100	102	2

4. In Vivo Brain ^{1}H–MRS in Man

In our own clinical studies ^{1}H–MRS spectra of the cerebral cortex of patients were obtained in a 1.5 T Philips Gyroscan (3). A regular 64 MHz ^{1}H head coil was used. By scout imaging a subcortical volume of interest was chosen. Volume selective shimming was performed by optimizing the water signal measured by single shot volume selection.

^{1}H–MR spectra were measured using a 90^0–180^0–180^0 volume selection sequence (17) with a total echotime of 136 ms and presaturation of water. ^{1}H spectra were obtained by Lorentz–Gauss windowing (line broadening about 1.5 Hz), Fourier transformation, linear phase correction and a polynomial baseline correction. Peak areas (see Table 5) were determined by integration of the frequency domain signal. At the day of the ^{1}H–MRS measurement (or within 24 h) clinical grading, (by the level of consciousness, and the number connection test(3), EEG spectral analysis(3) and blood biochemistry (by standard clinical techniques in our hospital) were performed.

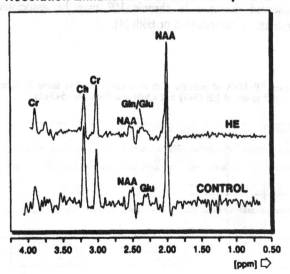

Figure 2. Representative ^{1}H–MR spectra of human cerebral cortex of a normal volunteer and a cirrhotic patient.

Table 5. ^{1}H NMR of cerebral cortex in liver cirrhosis. NAA, N–acetyl aspartate; Cr, (phospho)creatine; PCHO, (phospho)choline. Values are means ± SEM.

| | Controls | Patients Child Classification | | HE | | |
		A	B/C	Grade 0	Grade 1	Grade 2
	(n=5)	(n=4)	(n=3)	(n=1)	(n=5)	(n=1)
(Glu+Gln)/Cr	0.19±0.04	0.90±0.24	0.52±0.07	0.76	0.77±0.21	0.53
NAA/Cr	2.20±0.1	1.80±0.12	1.90±0.02	2.01	1.76±0.08	1.9
PCHO/Cr	1.23±0.09	1.05±0.04	0.96±0.10	1.02	1.08±0.04	0.83

In Table 4 the clinical parameters are shown of the cirrhotic patients studied. Liver cirrhosis varied between Child's classification A and C, whereas HE varied between grade 1 to 2. Two representative proton MR spectra are shown in Fig 2. No clear distinction between glutamate and glutamine was obtained. In Table 5 the relative concentrations of the different compounds are given. There is a significant increase in cerebral cortex glutamine/glutamate concentration during liver cirrhosis and hepatic encephalopathy in comparison to normal controls.

Although under our ^{1}H–MRS measuring conditions at that time it was not possible to make a good distinction between cerebral cortex Glu and Gln, our experimental findings in rats concerning an increase in Gln and a decrease in (phospho)choline were confirmed in mild HE in human beings. We were not able to detect a decrease in cerebral cortex Glu and a consistent increase in cerebral cortex lactate concentration in our patients with mild chronic HE.

Relative to cerebral cortex (phospho)choline compounds there is a tendency to a decrease in cirrhosis and hepatic encephalopathy (Table 5). Since the in vivo (phospho)choline signal is associated with the pool of intermediates involved in membrane turnover, the observed decrease in chronic HE may be associated to variations in myelination, membranous composition or both (4).

Table 6. In vivo brain ^{31}P–MRS of patients with liver cirrhosis. The same 10 patients were grouped in 2 different ways: grade of HE (3+7) and Child classification (5+3+2).

Group	No	pH	P_i/Pcr	ATP (mmol/kg w/w)
Normal	6	7.01±0.01	0.34±0.03	5.98±0.7
HE 0–1	3	7.00±0.01	0.38±0.06	3.67±0.7
HE 1–2	7	7.01±0.01	0.37±0.06	4.47±0.4
CHILD A	5	7.01±0.01	0.43±0.08	4.46±0.6
CHILD B	3	7.00±0.01	0.30±0.06	3.68±0.3
CHILD C	2	7.00±0.00	0.33±0.01	4.49±0.5

In the groups Child B and HE grade 2 there is a significant decrease in N–acetyl aspartate (NAA), suggesting that some neuronal loss may play a role in this subgroup of patients. However, unexpectedly NAA was not significantly decreased in Child C patients, who have more severe liver disease.

Kreis et al were the first to draw attention to a significant decrease (more than 50%) in cerebral myo–inositol (MI) levels in mild chronic HE in man (18,19). According to them to the MI peak contribute: myo–inositol itself (5–7 mmol/L; ≈ 70%), inositol phosphate, phosphatidyl–inositol, IP_3 and IP_4, glycine (±10%). They propose MI as a marker of chronic HE since its concentration is unchanged in patients with well-compensated liver disease. Its deficiency in HE is not well explained. One very interesting aspect is the possible role of MI in major detoxification reactions by its conversion to glucuronic acid, but more studies are needed to shed more light on the role of MI in the pathobiochemistry of HE.

5. In Vivo ^{31}P MRS in Man

Table 6 shows the results of in vivo ^{31}P–MRS of the brain cortex of 10 patients with liver cirrhosis of different severity and mild degree of HE. Cerebral cortex values are compared to those of 6 control volunteers of comparable mean age.

Although there was a tendency to a somewhat lower cortical ATP concentration (controls 5.98±0.7 versus 3.67±0.7 in HE patients) this difference was not significant (Student's T–test).

In addition classifying the same 10 patients according to Child's classification no significant differences in pH, P_i/Phosphocreatine ratio and ATP were observed; these observations are in agreement with the experimental data in rats (15,16).

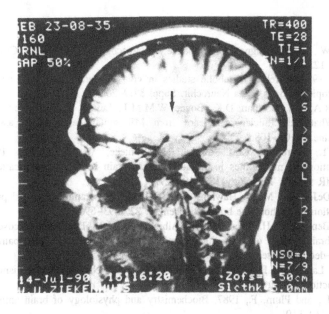

Figure 3. MRI of a patient with liver cirrhosis and HE grade 1. Notice the high intensity of the globus pallidus.

6. MRI in Man

At the start of our MRS measurements in man a region of interest in the cerebral cortex was chosen by MRI. Careful examination of these pictures showed an hyperintensity in the globus pallidus of all patients with significant degree of HE (Fig 3). Hyperintense globus pallidus on T_1-weighted MRI is present in most patients with advanced liver disease. The nature of the globus pallidus lesion is unknown: possibilities are accumulation of lipid deposits or toxic substances reaching the brain by porto-systemic shunting and changing the amount of paramagnetic compounds of this cerebral region. Brunberg (20) and Pujol (21) suggest a direct relation between impaired liver-function and increased intensity of the globus pallidus, whereas others (22) suggest a relation with the severity of HE. Several groups report on the reversibility of this phenomenon after liver transplantation (20,21).

7. Conclusion

In vivo brain ^{1}H MRS and ^{31}P MRS in the study of the pathobiochemistry of HE, have in an elegant way partly confirmed already known changes in cerebral cortex compounds studied by classic biochemical techniques: increase in ammonia, Gln and lactate, and a decrease in Glu. New findings have been the absence of important changes in cerebral high energy phosphate compounds and a decrease in (phospho)choline, myoinositol and probably N-acetylaspartate, suggesting that more structural changes, especially in brain cellular membranes and blood-brain barrier, may play a role in the pathogenesis of HE than has been assumed before in vivo MRS and MRI were introduced in the field of HE.

References

1. Prichard, J.W., 1992, Magnetic resonance spectroscopy of the brain, Clin. Chim. Acta **206**:115-123.
2. Behar, K.L., 1993, Cerebral metabolic studies in vivo by combined ^{1}H/^{31}P and ^{1}H/^{13}C NMR spectroscopic methods, Acta Neurochir. Suppl **57**:9-20.
3. Chamuleau, R.A.F.M., Bosman, D.K., Bovée, W.M.M.J., Luyten, P.R., and den Hollander, J.A., 1991, What the clinician can learn from MR glutamine/glutamate assays, NMR in biomedicine. **4**:103-108.
4. Michaelis, T., Merboldt, K.M., Bruhn, H., Hänicke, W., Frahm, J., 1993, Absolute concentrations of metabolites in the adult human brain in vivo: quantification of localized proton MR spectra, Radiology **187**:219-227.
5. Jessy, J., DeJoseph, M.R., Hawkins, R.A., 1991, Hyperammonemia depresses glucose consumption throughout the brain, Biochem. J. **277**:693-696.
6. Hilgier, W., Benveniste, H., Diemer, N.H., Albrecht, J., 1991, Decreased glucose uitilization in discrete brain regions of rat in thioacetamide-induced hepatic encephalopathy as measured with 3H-deoxyglucose, Acta Neurol. Scand. **83**:353-355.
7. Meijer, A.J., Lamers, W.H., Chamuleau, R.A.F.M., 1990, Nitrogen metabolism and ornithine cycle function, Physiol. Rev. **70**:701-748.
8. Cooper, A.J.L., and Plum, F., 1987, Biochemistry and physiology of brain ammonia, Physiol. Rev., **67**:440-519.

9. Takahashi, H., Koehler, R.C., Brusilow, S.W., Traystman, R.J., 1991, Inhibition of brain glutamine accumulation prevents edema in hyperammonemic rats, Am. J. Physiol. **261:** H825–H829.

10. Hawkins, R.A., Jessy, J., Mans, A.M., DeJoseph, M.R., 1993, Effect of reducing brain glutamine synthesis on metabolic symptoms of hepatic encephalopathy, J. of Neurochemistry, **60:**1000–1006.

11. Kanamori, K., Parivar, F., and Ross, B.D., 1993, A ^{15}N NMR study of in vivo cerebral glutamine synthesis in hyperammonemic rats, NMR in Biomedicine **6:**21–26.

12. Bovée, W.M.M.J., van Dijk, J., Slotboom, H., Bosman, D.K., and Chamuleau, R.A.F.M., 1993, In vivo proton NMR of the brain, in: Surviving Hypoxia Ed. P.W. Hochachka, P.L. Lutz et al, CRC Press, London, Tokyo, p.65–73.

13. Bosman, D.K., Deutz, N.E.P., de Graaf, A.A., v.d. Hulst, R.W.N., van Eijk, H.M.H., Bovée, W.M.M.J., Maas, M.A.W., Jörning, G.G.A., and Chamuleau, R.A.F.M., 1990, Changes in brain metabolism during hyperammonemia and acute liver failure: results of a comparative ^{1}H–NMR spectroscopy and biochemical investigation, Hepatology **12,2:**281–290.

14. Hindfelt, B., Plum F., and Duffy, T.E., 1977, Effect of acute ammonia intoxication on cerebral metabolism in rats with portacaval shunts, J. Clin. Invest. **59:**386–396.

15. Fitzpatrick, S.M., Behar, K.L., and Shulman, R.G., 1989, In vivo NMR spectroscopic studies of cerebral metabolism in rats after portal–caval shunting, in: Hepatic Encephalopathy Ed:R.F.Butterworth and G. Pomier Layrargues, Human Press Clifton, New Jersey:177–187.

16. Deutz, N.E.P., Chamuleau, R.A.F.M., de Graaf, A.A., Bovée, W.M.M.J., and de Beer, R., 1988, In vivo ^{31}P NMR spectroscopy of the rat cerebral cortex during acute hepatic encephalopathy, NMR in Biomedicine **1,101:**1–106.

17. Bottomley, P.A., 1984, Selective volume method for performing localized NMR spectroscopy, U.S. Patent 4480228.

18. Kreis, R., Ross, B.D., Farrow, N.A., Ackerman, Zvi, 1992, Metabolic disorders of the brain in chronic hepatic encephalopathy detected with H-1 MR spectroscopy, Radiology, **182:**19–27.

19. Kreis, R., Farrow, N.A., and Ross, B.D., 1990, Diagnosis of hepatic encephalopathy by proton magnetic resonance spectroscopy, Lancet. **336:**635–636.

20. Brunberg, J.A., Kanal, E., Hirsch, W., and van Thiel, D.H., 1991, Chronic acquired hepatic failure: MR imaging of the brain at 1.5 T, AJR **157:**1111–1116.

21. Pujol, A., Pujol, J., Graus, F., et al., 1993, Hyperintense globus pallidus on T_1–weighted MRI in cirrhotic patients is associated with severity of liver failure, Neurology, **43:**65–69.

22. Zeneroli, M.L., Cioni, G., Crisi, G., Vezelli, C., and Ventura, E., 1991, Globus pallidus alterations and brain atrophy in liver cirrhosis patients with encephalopathy: a MR imaging study, Magn. Reson. Imaging **9:**295–302.

23. Ferenci, P., 1991, Hepatic Encephalopathy, in: Oxford textbook of Clinical Hepatology, vol 1, Ed: N. McIntyre, J.P. Benhamou, J. Bircher, M. Rizzetto, J. Rodes, Oxford University Press, Oxford, New York, Tokio, p.473–483.

24. Van den Bos, A., 1982, Parameter estimation, in: Handbook of Measurement Science, Seidenham, P.H., Ed., Vol.1, John Wiley & Sons, New York, p.331.

Role of the Cellular Hydration State for Cellular Function: Physiological and Pathophysiological Aspects

Dieter Häussinger and Wolfgang Gerok

1. Introduction

In recent years it became clear that the regulation of cell function involves another important controlling parameter, i.e. the cellular hydration state. Cellular hydration can change within minutes under the influence of hormones, nutrient supply and oxidative stress and such a short-term modulation of cell volume within a narrow range acts per se as a potent signal which modifies cellular metabolism and gene expression. The interaction between cellular hydration and cell function was most extensively studied in liver cells, but evidence is increasing that modulation of cell function in response to alterations of cellular hydration is a general mechanism. Disturbances of cellular hydration as a pathogenetic factor for the development of hyperammonemia and hepatic encephalopathy have not yet been considered, but very recent evidence suggests interesting aspects for the understanding of hyperammonemic states. Thus, the article will briefly review the current state of knowledge regarding the interaction between hepatocellular volume and liver function and then discuss some pathophysiological conditions in which disturbances of cellular volume could be of pathogenetic relevance.

2. Physiological Modulators of Cellular Hydration

One of the most important challenges for cell volume homeostasis is the cumulative uptake of osmotically active substances, such as amino acids, which is largely accomplished by specific Na^+-dependent transport systems in the plasma membrane (for review see [1]). These transport systems can build up intra/extracellular amino acid concentration gradients up to 20 by utilizing the energy of the transmembrane electrochemical Na^+ gradient. The accumulation of amino acids inside the cells leads to rapid cell swelling. This is illustrated in fig. 1 at the example of glutamine uptake into hepatocytes via the Na^+ coupled amino acid transport system N. Infusion of glutamine into isolated perfused rat liver creates within about 12 min an intra/extracellular glutamine concentration gradient of about 12. As a result of the accumulation of glutamine together with Na^+ (which is in turn exchanged against K^+ at Na^+/K^+ ATPase and explains the net K^+ uptake during the first 2 min of glutamine addition in fig. 1), hepatocytes in situ swell by about 10% within the first 2 min of glutamine addition. Most importantly, this increase of hepatocellular hydration is maintained as long as the amino

Medizinische Universitätsklinik. Hugstetterstrasse 55, D–79106 Freiburg Germany. Tel: 0761 2703634. Fax: 0761 2703205

Hepatic Encephalopathy, Hyperammonemia, and Ammonia Toxicity
Edited by V. Felipo and S. Grisolia, Plenum Press, New York, 1994

33

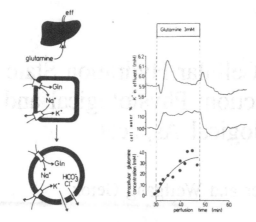

Figure 1. Effect of glutamine (3 mM) addition to influent perfusate of isolated, single– pass perfused rat liver on intracellular glutamine accumulation, cell volume and volume– regulatory K⁺ fluxes. Addition of glutamine to portal perfusate leads to rapid cell swelling due to cumulative, Na⁺–dependent uptake of glutamine into liver cells. The initial net K⁺ uptake is explained by exchange of cotransported Na⁺ against K⁺ by Na⁺/K⁺ ATPase. Glutamine– induced cell swelling during the first 2 min of glutamine infusion activates volume regulatory K⁺ (plus Cl⁻ and HCO₃⁻) efflux. This volume–regulatory response prevents further cell swelling despite continuing glutamine accumulation inside the cell until a steady state intracellular glutamine concentration of about 35 mM is reached. However, the liver cell remains in a swollen state as long as glutamine is infused. This degree of cell swelling modifies cellular function. From [46].

acid is present, despite subsequent activation of a volume regulatory net K⁺ efflux. The latter does not restore liver cell volume; it only prevents cell swelling to become excessive as it would otherwise be predicted from the continuing accumulation of glutamine inside the cell. The degree of amino acid–induced cell swelling seems largely to be related to the steady state intra/extracellular amino acid concentration gradient. This gradient and accordingly the degree of amino acid–induced cell swelling is modified by hormones and the nutritional state by (a) regulating the expression of concentrating transport systems in the plasma membrane, (b) modifying the electrochemical Na⁺ gradient as a driving force for Na⁺ coupled transport and (c) by altering intracellular amino acid metabolism.

Also hormones are potent modulators of liver cell volume [2]. Whereas cumulative substrate transport into hepatocytes lead primarily to cell swelling with secondary activation of volume–regulatory ion transporters, hormones primarily affect the activity of volume–regulatory transport systems with cell volume changes being the consequence. In liver, insulin stimulates Na⁺/H⁺ exchange, Na–K–2Cl–cotransport and the Na⁺/K⁺ ATPase; i.e. transport systems which are turned on for regulatory volume increase in a variety of tissues. This results in an insulin–induced accumulation of K⁺, Na⁺ and Cl⁻ inside the cells and consequently cell swelling. Glucagon activates Na⁺/K⁺ ATPase, but simultaneously decreases cellular K⁺ in isolated perfused rat liver, due to a simultaneous opening of Ba⁺⁺– and quinidine–sensitive K⁺ channels. Thus, glucagon may lead to a depletion of cellular Na⁺, K⁺ and Cl⁻, resulting in cell shrinkage. Indeed, in both, perfused livers and isolated hepatocytes, insulin increases and glucagon decreases cellular volume within minutes by about 12%, each. Modulation of cell volume by insulin and glucagon is not a pharmacological phenomenon because halfmaximal hormone–effects on cell volume are observed at their physiological portal concentration. Also other hormones can induce hepatocellular shrinkage (e.g. adenosine, extracellular ATP, vasopressin, serotonin) or swelling (e.g. bradykinin, α–adrenergic compounds).

Oxidative stress exerted by hydrogen peroxides induces hepatocellular shrinkage due to an opening of K⁺ channels [3]. Evidence has been presented that the balance between intracellular metabolic H₂O₂ generation and its removal by detoxication systems such as catalase and glutathione peroxidase is one determinant for hepatocellular K^+ balance and accordingly cell volume [4].

3. Regulation of Cellular Function by the Cellular Hydration State

Recent evidence suggests that the dynamic alterations of cellular hydration which occur physiologically under the influence of hormones and substrates exert per se within minutes profound effects on cellular function (table 1). This was shown in experiments mimicking hormone– and substrate–induced cell volume changes by anisotonic exposure of the cells. Thus, alterations of cell volume represent another principle of metabolic control [2,5] and substrates and hormones such as insulin and glucagon exert their influence on metabolism in part by changing cellular hydration. Cell swelling stimulates protein, and glycogen synthesis and simultaneously inhibits proteolysis and glycogenolysis (table 1); opposite metabolic patterns are triggered by cell shrinkage. The metabolic changes listed in table 1 suggest that cell swelling acts like a proliferative anabolic signal, whereas cell shrinkage is catabolic. Indeed, this anabolic signal is also set when the cells swell under the influence of amino acids or insulin. Thus, alterations of cellular hydration in response to physiological stimuli are an important and until recently unrecognized signal which helps to adapt cellular metabolism to alterations of the environment (substrate, tonicity) and hormones. Consequently, the role of Na^+–dependent amino acid transport systems in the plasma membrane can no longer merely be identified with amino acid translocation; these transporters rather act as a transmembrane signalling system triggering cellular function by altering cellular hydration in response to substrate delivery [2,5]. Such a signalling role may shed a new light on the long known heterogeneity of transport systems among different cell types and their different expression during development (for reviews see [1]), rendering specific amino acids as a more or less potent signal. Likewise, transmembrane ion movements under the influence of hormones are an integral part of hormonal signal transduction mechanisms with alterations of cellular hydration acting as another "second messenger" of hormone action [2]. However, the exact place of hormone–induced cell volume changes in the hierarchy of postreceptor events of intracellular signalling and its interplay with other known hormone–activated messenger systems remains to be established.

Table 1. Liver cell swelling as an anabolic signal.

CELL SWELLING

Increases	Decreases
protein synthesis	proteolysis
glycogen synthesis	glycogenolysis
lactate uptake	glycolysis
amino acid uptake	
glutamine breakdown	glutamine synthesis
glycine oxidation	
ketoisocaproate oxidation	
acetyl–CoA carboxylase	
urea synthesis from amino acids	urea synthesis from NH_4^+
glutathione (GSH) efflux	biliary GSSG release
taurocholate excretion	
into bile	
actin polymerization	
pH in vesicular compartments	cytosolic pH
mRNA levels of c–jun, ornithine	mRNA levels for PEPCK
decarboxylase, β–actin, tubulin	
	viral replication
	synthesis of viral protein

The role of cellular hydration as a signal for cellular function may be seen in analogy to metabolic regulation by $[Ca^{++}]_i$ or pH_i. As for cell volume regulation, cells possess potent mechanisms to keep the intracellular calcium and proton concentration within a narrow range, otherwise the cell will die. However, these homeostatic mechanisms can also be used to produce small, i.e. "physiological" changes of cellular hydration, $[Ca^{++}]_i$ or pH_i, which then act to regulate cell function. Only a few examples on the importance of hydration changes for cellular function will be addressed below.

3.1. Cellular Hydration and Protein Turnover

Hepatic proteolysis is under the control of amino acids and hormones, such as insulin and glucagon, but the underlying mechanism remained obscure [6,7]. It recently became clear that hypoosmotic cell swelling inhibits proteolysis in liver, whereas conversely, hyperosmotic cell shrinkage stimulates protein breakdown under conditions when the proteolytic pathway is not already fully activated [8,9]. Indeed, cellular hydration was identified as a major site of proteolysis control [8]. The known antiproteolytic effect of insulin and several (but not all) amino acids, such as glutamine, alanine and glycine can be ascribed to the accompanying cell swelling, whereas stimulation of proteolysis by glucagon is apparently mediated by cell shrinkage [8,9]. This was evidenced by the fact that the effects of glutamine, IGF-1, glycine, insulin and glucagon on proteolysis are quantitatively mimicked when the cell volume changes in response to these effectors are induced to the same degree by anisotonic exposure. Further, when insulin-induced cell swelling is prevented in presence of inhibitors of the Na^+/H^+ antiporter and the $Na^+-K^+-2Cl^-$ cotransporter, the antiproteolytic activity of the hormone disappears. There is a close relationship between the proteolytic rate and hepatocellular hydration, regardless of whether the latter is modified by hormones, glutamine, glycine, bile acids, the K^+ channel blocker Ba^{++} or anisotonic exposure (fig. 2). The nutritional state exerts its control on proteolysis by altering the swelling potencies of hormones and amino acids. For example, in the fed state the antiproteolytic effect of glycine is only about one third compared to that found after 24h starvation due to an about 3-fold higher swelling potency of glycine during starvation. This is the consequence of an up-regulation of the glycine-transporting amino acid transport system A in starvation. Likewise, both the swelling potency and the antiproteolytic effect of insulin are in parallel diminished following starvation to about one third.

The mechanism how cellular hydration exerts control on proteolysis is not settled, however, the proteolysis control by the hepatocellular hydration state depends on an intact microtubulus system [10] and may involve alterations of lysosomal acidification [11].

Liver cell swelling not only inhibits proteolysis, but simultaneously stimulates protein synthesis, whereas cell shrinkage triggers the inhibition of protein synthesis and stimulation of proteolysis [12].

3.2. Cellular Hydration and the Cytoskeleton

Cell swelling, either induced by hypoosmotic exposure, insulin or glutamine leads within one minute to an increased polymerization state of β-actin [13] and increases the stability of microtubules [10]. Microtubules apparently play an important role in transducing some metabolic alterations in response to changes of cellular hydration. For example, disruption of microtubules by colchicine abolishes the cell swelling-induced inhibition of proteolysis [10] and the stimulation of transcellular bile acid transport in liver [141]. However, other pathways which are activated in response to cell swelling, such as stimulation of glycine oxidation or of the pentose phosphate shunt are not affected following microtubule disruption. Cell swelling also increases the mRNA levels for β-actin and tubulin [10,13].

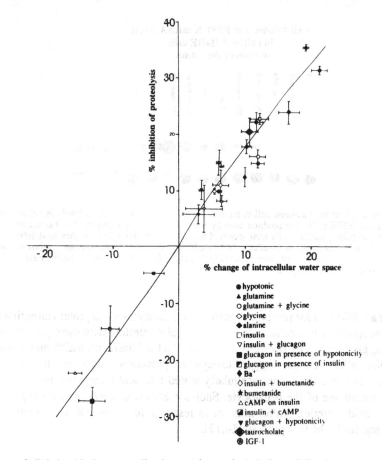

● hypotonic
▲ glutamine
○ glutamine + glycine
◇ glycine
◆ alanine
□ insulin
▽ insulin + glucagon
■ glucagon in presence of hypotonicity
▨ glucagon in presence of insulin
◆ Ba⁺
◇ insulin + bumetanide
★ bumetanide
△ cAMP on insulin
▨ insulin + cAMP
▼ glucagon + hypotonicity
◆ taurocholate
⊛ IGF-1

Figure 2. Relationship between cell volume and proteolysis in liver. Cell volume in perfused liver was determined as intracellular water space and proteolysis was assessed as [³H]leucine release in effluent perfusate from perfused livers from rats, which were prelabelled in vivo by intraperitoneal injection of [³H]leucine 16h prior to the perfusion experiment. Cell shrinkage stimulates proteolysis, whereas cell swelling inhibits. It should be noted that proteolysis is already maximally activated in the absence of hormones and amino acids and cannot be further stimulated by hyperosmotic or glucagon–induced cell shrinkage. The proteolysis–stimulating effect of these cell-shrinking maneuvres, however, becomes apparent when proteolysis is preinhibited by either amino acids or insulin. Cell volume changes were induced by insulin, cAMP, glucagon, amino acids, Ba⁺⁺ or anisoosmotic exposure. Modified from [8].

3.3. Cell Volume and the Acidification of Intracellular Compartments

Recent studies on acridine orange fluorescence in hepatocytes showed that an increase of cellular hydration is accompanied by a rapid alkalinization of acidic cellular compartments, suggestive for lysosomal alkalinization [11,15]. Since autophagic proteolysis, which makes up about 70% of total hepatocellular proteolysis, is critically dependent on a low intralysosomal pH (i.e. around 5), the possibility must be envisaged that cell swelling somehow interferes with the activity of vacuolar type H^+–ATPases, thereby triggering an inhibition of proteolysis. Swelling–induced pH shifts were also observed with respect to the fluorescence of endocytosed FITC–dextran [15]. This high molecular weight (70 kD) fluorescent probe is taken up by fluid phase endocytosis and accumulates not only in endocytotic vesicles, but –following fusion with other vesicular compartmnts– also in autophagosomes and Golgi–derived vesicles. Cell swelling increases the pH in this FITC–dextran accessible endocytotic compartment, but simultaneously lowers the cytosolic pH; opposite pH changes occur in response to cell shrinkage [15]. Given the important role

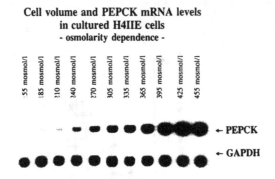

Figure 3. Effect of anisotonic cell volume modulation on PEPCK mRNA levels in cultured rat hepatoma H4IIE cells. The medium tonicity was changed by adjusting the NaCl concentration in the incubation media. Cells were exposed to anisotonicity for 6 h; thereafter total RNA was isolated and subjected to Northern blot analysis for phosphoenolpyruvate carboxykinase (PEPCK) and glyceraldehyde phosphate dehydrogenase (GAPDH). 15 µg total RNA were loaded in each lane. From ref. [20].

of vacuolar acidification for receptor–ligand sorting, exocytosis and protein targeting [16], one is tempted to speculate that cellular hydration may also interfere with these processes. Indeed, cell swelling gives rise to an IP_3 signal followed by a Ca^{++} transient, which may together with the vacuolar alkalinization trigger exocytotic processes, such as the hypothesized swelling–induced insertion of intracellularly stored bile acid transporter molecules into the canalicular membrane of the hepatocyte. Such a mechanism would explain the doubling of V_{max} of bile acid secretion within minutes in response to a 10–15% cell swelling and the colchicine sensitivity of this process [14,17].

3.4. Cellular Hydration and Gene Expression

Cellular hydration modifies cellular metabolism also on a long–term time scale by modifying gene expression. Examples are the rapid increases of mRNA levels for β–actin, tubulin, ornithine decarboxylase and c–jun in response to liver cell swelling [10,13,18,19]. Cellular hydration also affects the expression of phosphoenolpyruvate carboxykinase (PEPCK) (fig. 3); PEPCK mRNA levels markedly increase in response to cell shrinkage but decrease in response to cell swelling in both, the intact perfused rat liver and in cultured rat hepatoma H4IIE cells [20]. Regulation of PEPCK mRNA by cellular hydration occurs at the level of transcription and does not involve protein kinase C activation or changes in cAMP levels. The regulatory elements and factors, however, remain to be established. In fibroblasts, amino acid deprivation leads to a cycloheximide–sensitive adaptive increase in the activity of the amino acid transport system A. This adaptive increase is potentiated by hyperosmotic cell shrinkage and counteracted by hypoosmolar cell swelling [21], indicating that cell volume modifies the expression of amino acid transport systems. The mechanisms how cell volume changes affect gene expression are largely unclear, but changes in the ionic composition, the cytoskeleton and of protein phosphorylation are likely candidates.

Alterations in gene expression, however, may also in turn affect cellular volume. This was shown by an increase in the resting state cell volume by about 30% following expression of ras–oncogene in NIH fibroblasts [22]. The growth factor–independent proliferation of the ras oncogene expressing cells is sensitive to amiloride and furosemide, i.e. to blockers of Na^+/H^+ antiport and Na–K–2Cl cotransport, suggesting a role of cell swelling induced by activation of these transporters for cell proliferation. Also in lymphocytes, mitogenic signals activate these transporters and may shift the set–point of cell volume regulation to higher resting values [23]; this cell volume increase may be an important prerequisite for cellular proliferation.

3.5. Signals Linking the Cellular Hydration State to Cellular Function

This issue is far from being settled. However, several potential mechanisms linking alterations of cellular hydration to respective functional changes have been described. Clearly, no single mechanism can be expected to account for all the diverse metabolic effects occuring in response to hydration changes of the cell. Alterations of cellular hydration will influence membrane stretch, membrane–bound signalling systems and the cytoskeleton, protein phosphorylation, will alter the ionic interior of the cell as well as the extent of macromolecular crowding in the cytosol (for reviews see [2,5,25–29]. Depending on the metabolic pathway under study the relative importance of these above mentioned potential mechanisms may vary. A model has been presented postulating that the extent of macromolecular crowding, i.e. the cytosolic protein concentration will determine the tendency of intracellular macromolecules to associate with the plasma membrane and to determine their enzymatic activity [29]. It is well conceivable that alterations of cellular hydration may also interfere with the activity of protein kinases and phosphatases, which are not only involved in the regulation of volume–regulatory responses, but also in the regulation of metabolism.

4. Pathophysiological Aspects

4.1. Protein–catabolic States

The finding that cellular hydration affects both protein degradation and synthesis in opposite directions sheds a new light on the understanding of protein–catabolic states in disease. Indeed, a close relationship between the cellular hydration state in skeletal muscle and the negativity of nitrogen balance was shown in the severely ill patient, irrespective of the underlying disease (fig. 4). From this, it was hypothesized that cell shrinkage in skeletal

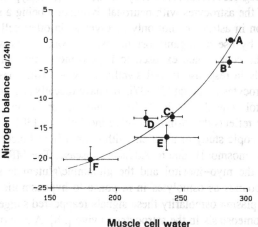

Figure 4. Whole body nitrogen balance and cellular hydration of skeletal muscle. Data were obtained in humans. A: healthy subjects (n=17); B=liver tumors (n=5), C and D= polytrauma day 2 (C) and day 9 (D) after trauma (n=11); E=acute necrotizing pancreatitis (n=6); F= burn patients (n=4). From [31].

muscle and liver may be the common end-path triggering protein catabolism in a variety of diseases [30]. Although this implies that the extent of cellular hydration determines the extent of nitrogen wasting irrespective of the underlying disease, the pathogenetic mechanisms leading to cell shrinkage may well be multifactorial and heterogeneous and could involve disease–specific components. It is conceivable that the physician interferes already empirically with the cellular hydration state, when he tries to overcome protein–catabolic states by infusion of amino acids.

4.2. Cholestatic Diseases

Ursodesoxycholic acid is used to treat cholestatic diseases, such as primary biliary cirrhosis, but the mechanism of its action is poorly understood. Indeed, tauroursodesoxycholic acid was shown to induce liver cell swelling and the latter apparently stimulates the excretion of endogenous bile acids due to a swelling–induced increase of V_{max} of bile acid excretion [14].

4.3. Hepatic Encephalopathy

The pathogenesis of portosystemic HE (PSE) is still unclear, although a variety of mechanisms have been implicated such as the action of ammonia and other neurotoxins, disturbances of the blood–brain barrier and alterations of various neurotransmitter systems and their receptors (for review see [31,32]). In PSE, no morphological abnormalities of the neurons are detectable, but astrocytes exhibit signs of Alzheimer type II degeneration. These Alzheimer type II changes can be induced even in cultured astrocytes in vitro by addition of ammonia, thereby underlining the pathogenetic role of this neurotoxin [33]. Astrocytes are the only cellular compartment in the brain capable of glutamine synthesis [34], which is the major pathway for cerebral ammonia detoxication. Whereas brain edema in HE of acute liver failure is common (80%) and eventually determines the patients final outcome, low grade (I–III) PSE in chronic liver disease is generally not considered to involve brain swelling. However, recent data on ¹H–MR spectroscopy suggest that glial swelling is an early event in PSE with potential pathophysiological relevance, thereby strenghtening the hypothesis that PSE may be a primary disorder of the astrocytes with neuronal dyfunction being a secondary event [33]. Cell volume regulation in astrocytes not only involves as in other cell types ion fluxes, but is also accomplished by use of organic osmolytes, i.e. compounds which are specifically accumulated inside the cells, when exposed to hyperosmotic environments or specifically released from the cells in response to cell swelling. Myo–inositol has been identified as a major osmolyte in astrocytes in the rat [35–37]. We have recently succeeded in demonstrating that the myo–inositol signal obtained from human brain in vivo by means of ¹H–MR–spectroscopy reflects this osmo–sensitive inositol pool [38]. Evidence for this came from an MR–spectroscopic study of a patient with normal liver function, but severe plasma hypoosmolarity (222 mosmol/l) due to Addison's disease. The MR–spectrum showed the complete absence of the myo–inositol and the glutamine/glutamate signal, indicating the release of these compounds as osmolytes in response to hypoosmotic glial swelling. Upon restoration of normal plasma osmolarity these signals reappeared suggesting the recovery of normal cell volume homeostasis in the astrocytes in vivo [38]. A role of brain myo–inositol, which is detected by MR–spectroscopy is also augmented by recent animal experiments, which showed a decrease of the myo–inositol content in the brains removed from rats, which were made experimentally acutely hyponatremic [39]. The role of myo–inositol as an osmolyte in the human brain is further augmented by the demonstration that hypernatremia, which is expected to lead to cell shrinkage and to favour osmolyte accumulation in the astrocytes, is indeed associated with an increased myo–inositol signal as detected by ^{1}H–NMR–spectroscopy [40]. PSE patients, even at a preclinical latent stage, exhibit a marked decrease of the myo–inositol and an increase of the glutamine signal in the brain [38,41,42]; similar alterations could also be induced in the rat following portocaval shunting [43]. These findings are interpreted to reflect glial swelling due to a hyperammonemia–induced glutamine accumulation in the astrocytes already at early stages of PSE. Since no significant neuropsychiatric abnormalities were observed in our patient with severe hypoosmolarity in contrast to the patients with PSE, it appears that a "deficiency" of cerebral myo–inositol per se does not predict major encephalopathy symptoms. The myo–inositol loss, however, indicates glial swelling, which may affect astroglial gene expression and lead to sustained disturbances of astrocyte function, with not yet known consequences for glial–neuronal communication. In line with this, cultured astrocytes swell under the influence of ammonia [45] as do hepatocytes [unpublished observation] and ammonia toxicity was shown to be reduced by inhibitors of astroglial glutamine synthetase [45], which also prevents cell swelling. It should be emphasized that cell volume fluctuations as a trigger of cell function are a physiological mechanism for metabolic regulation and the corresponding intracellular signalling events are already activated when cell volume changes by $\pm 5\%$ or less. Thus, in the astrocyte, swelling as indicated by inositol release may have important functional consequences even in the absence of detectable increases of intracranial pressure. Indeed, swelling–effects on astrocytes could well explain several established phenomena in PSE, such as disturbances of cerebral glucose metabolism, alterations of blood–brain permeability and of glial cytoskeletal proteins. Because astrocyte swelling may not only be triggered by ammonia, but also by hormones and mediators of inflammation, such as oxidative stress, it is not surprising that many investigators failed to show a correlation between plasma ammonia levels and the severity of PSE. According to own anectodal observations, successful treatment of hepatic encephalopathy is associated with a recovery of myo–inositol signal in the [1]H–MR–spectrum. Taken together, the available evidence suggests glial swelling to be an early event in PSE. Whether this is of pathogenetic relevance for PSE or just an epiphenomenon remains to be established. However, the latter appears to be rather unlikely in view of the remarkable functional consequences occurring upon minor alterations of cellular hydration in other cell types.

4.4. Cell Volume and Viral Replication

Cellular hydration is not only an important site of control for the expression of cell-specific genes, but also strongly influences viral replication [47]. This was shown in primary cultured hepatocytes from ducks, which were infected in vivo with the duck hepatitis B virus (DHBV) 10 days prior to hepatocyte isolation. Following hyperosmotic cell shrinkage, synthesis of viral DNA, RNA and viral proteins was enhanced by about 5–fold, whereas hypoosmotic cell swelling inhibited viral replication and the synthesis of viral protein by about 50%. Interestingly, cell shrinkage increased viral protein synthesis, whereas the synthesis of host cell proteins was decreased. The reason for the host cell– volume dependent replicative activity of the viruses is not yet clear, but may reside in a cell volume–dependent formation or activation of transcription factors which can bind to the regulatory elements in viral DNA.

Acknowledgements: Our own work reported herein was supported by Deutsche Forschungsgemeinschaft through Sonderforschungsbereich 154, the Gottfried Wilhelm Leibniz–Programm, the Schilling Stiftung and the Fonds der Chemischen Industrie.

References

1. Kilberg M. & Häussinger, D., eds. (1992) Mammalian amino acid transport: mechanisms and control. Plenum Press New York.
2. Häussinger D. & Lang, F. (1992) Cell volume and hormone action. Trends Pharmacol. Sci. 13:371–373.
3. Hallbrucker, C., Ritter, M., Lang, F., Gerok W. & Häussinger, D. (1993) Hydroperoxide metabolism in rat liver. K$^+$ channel opening, cell volume changes and eicosanoid formation. Eur. J. Biochem. 211:449–458.
4. Saha, N., Schreiber, R., vom Dahl, S., Lang, F., Gerok, W. & Häussinger, D. (1993) Endogenous hydroperoxide formation, cell volume and cellular K$^+$ balance in perfused rat liver. Biochem J. 296:701–707.
5. Häussinger, D. & Lang, F. (1991) Cell volume in the regulation of hepatic function: a new mechanism for metabolic control. Biochim. Biophys. Acta 1071:331–350.
6. Mortimore, G.E. & Pösö, A.R. (1987) Intracellular protein catabolism and its control during nutrient deprivation and supply. Ann. Rev. Nutr. 7:539–564.
7. Seglen, P.O. & Gordon, P.B. (1984) Amino acid control of autophagic sequestration and protein degradation in isolated rat hepatocytes. J. Cell. Biol. 99:435–444.
8. Häussinger, D., Hallbrucker, C., vom Dahl, S., Decker, S., Schweizer, U., Lang, F. Gerok, W. (1991) Cell volume is a major determinant of proteolysis control in liver. FEBS Lett. 283:70–72.
9. Vom Dahl, S., Hallbrucker, C., Lang, F., Gerok, W. & Häussinger, D. (1991a) Regulation of liver cell volume and proteolysis by glucagon and insulin. Biochem. J. 278:771–777.
10. Häussinger, D., Stoll, B., vom Dahl, S., Theodoropoulos, P.A., Markogiannakis, E., Gravanis, A., Lang, F. & Stournaras, C. (1994) Microtubule stabilization and induction of tubulin mRNA by cell swelling in isolated rat hepatocytes. Biochem. Cell. Biol. 72:12–19.
11. Völkl, H., Friedrich, F., Häussinger, D. & Lang, F. (1993) Effect of cell volume on acridine orange fluorescence in hepatocytes. Biochem. J. 295:11–14.
12. Stoll, B., Gerok, W., Lang, F. & Häussinger, D. (1992) Liver cell volume and protein synthesis. Biochem. J. 287:217–222.
13. Theodoropoulos, T., Stournaras, C., Stoll B., Markogiannakis, E., Lang, F., Gravani, A. & Häussinger, D. (1992) Hepatocyte swelling leads to rapid decrease of G–/total actin ratio and increases actin mRNA levels. FEBS Lett. 311:241–245.
14. Häussinger, D., Saha, N., Hallbrucker, C., Lang, F. & Gerok, W. (1993) Involvement of microtubules in the swelling–induced stimulation of transcellular taurocholate transport in perfused rat liver. Biochem. J. 291:355–360.
15. Schreiber, R., Stoll, B., Lang, F. & Häussinger, D. (1994) Effects of anisotonicity on intracellular pH in isolated rat hepatocytes as assessed by BCECF and FITC–dextran fluorescence. Biochem. J. in press.
16. Tager, J.M., Aerts, J.M.F.G., Oude–Elferink, R.J.A., Groen, A.K., Holle mans, M. & Schram, A.W. (1988) pH regulation of intracellular membrane flow. In: pH Homeostasis (Häussinger, D., Ed.) pp.123–162, Academic Press London.
17. Häussinger, D., Hallbrucker, C., Saha, N., Lang, F. & Gerok, W. (1992) Cell volume and bile acid excretion. Biochem. J. 288:681–689.
18. Finkenzeller, G., Newsome, W.P., Lang, F. & Häussinger, D. (1994) Increase of c–jun mRNA upon hypoosmotic cell swelling of rat hepatoma cells. FEBS Lett. 340:163–166.
19. Tohyama, Y., Kameji, T. & Hayashi, S. (1991) Mechanisms of dramatic fluctuations of ornithine decarboxylase activity upon tonicity changes in primary cultured rat hepatocytes. Eur. J. Biochem. 202:1327–1331.
20. Newsome, W.P., Warskulat, U., Noe, B., Wettstein, M., Stoll, B., Gerok,W. & Häussinger, D. (1994) Modulation of phosphoenolpyruvate carboxykinase mRNA levels by the hepatocellular hydration state. Biochem. J. in press.
21. Gazzola, G.C., Dall'Asta, V., Nucci, F.A., Rossi, P.A., Bussolati, O., Hoffmann, E.K. & Guidotti, G.G. (1991) Role of amino acid transport system A in the control of cell volume in cultured human fibroblasts. Cell. Physiol. Biochem. 1:131–142.

22. Lang, F., Ritter, M., Wöll, E., Weiss, H., Häussinger, D., Maly, K. & Grunicke, H. (1992) Altered cell volume regulation in ras oncogene expressing NIH fibroblasts. Pflügers Arch. Physiol. **420**:424–427.

23. Bianchini, L. & Grinstein, S. (1993) Regulation of volume–modulating ion transport systems by growth promoters. In: Interaction of cell volume and cell function (Lang, F. & Häussinger, D., eds.) pp.249–277, Springer Verlag Heidelberg.

24. Grinstein S., Furuya, W. & Bianchini, L. (1992) Protein kinases, phosphatases, and the control of cell volume. News Physiol. Sci. **7**:232–237.

25. Halestrap, A.P. (1993) The regulation of organelle function through changes of their volume. In: Interactions of cell volume and cell function (Lang, F. & Häussinger, D., eds.) pp.279–307, Springer Verlag Heidelberg.

26. Hoffmann, E.K., Simonsen, L.O. & Lambert, I.H. (1993) Cell volume regulation: intracellular transmission. In: Interactions of cell volume and cell function (Lang, F. & Häussinger,, eds) pp.187–248, Springer Verlag Heidelberg.

27. Lang, F. & Häussinger, D., eds. (1993) Interaction of cell volume and cell function. Springer Verlag Heidelberg.

28. McCarty, N.A. & O°Neil, R.G. (1992) Calcium signalling in cell volume regulation. Physiol. Rev. **72**:1037–1061.

29. Minton, A.P., Colclasure, G.C. & Parker, J.C. (1992) Model for the role of macromolecular crowding in regulation of cellular volume. Proc. Nat. Acad. Sci. **89**:10504–10506.

30. Häussinger, D., Roth, E., Lang, F. & Gerok, W. (1993) Cellular hydration state: an important determinant of protein catabolism in health and disease. Lancet **341**:1330–1332.

31. Ferenci, P., Püspök, A., Steindl, P. (1992) Current concepts in the pathogenesis of hepatic encephalopathy. Eur. J. Clin. Invest. **22**:573–581.

32. Lockwood, A.H. (1992) Hepatic encephalopathy. Butterworth–Heinemann Boston.

33. Norenberg, M.D., Neary, J.T., Bender, A.S. & Dombro, R.S. (1992) Hepatic encephalopathy: a disorder in glial–neuronal communication. Progress Brain Res. **94**:261–269.

34. Martinez–Hernandez, A., Bell, K.P. & Norenberg, M.D. (1977) Glutamine synthetase: glial localization in brain. Science **195**:1356–1358.

35. Kimelberg, H.K., O`Connor, E.R. & Kettenmann, H. (1993) Effects of swelling on glial cell function. In: Interactions cell volume and cell function (Lang, F., Häussinger, D., eds,) pp.158–186, Springer Verlag Heidelberg.

36. Lien, Y.H.H., Shapiro, J.L. & Chan, L. (1990) Effects of hypernatremia on organic brain osmoles. J. Clin. Invest. **85**:1427–1435.

37. Murphy S. ed. (1993) Astrocytes–Pharmacology and function. Academic Press San Diego.

38. Häussinger, D., Laubenberger, J., vom Dahl, S., Ernst, T., Bayer, S., Langer, M., Gerok, W. & Hennig, J. (1994). Proton Magnetic Resonance Spectroscopic Studies on Human Brain Myo-inositol in Hypoosmolarity and Hepatic Encephalopathy. Gastroenterology, in press.

39. Sterns, R.H., Baer, J., Ebersol, S., Thomas, D., Lohr, J.W., Kamm, D.E. (1993) Organic osmolytes in acute hyponatremia. Am. J. Physiol. **264**:F833–F836.

40. Lee, J.H., Ross, B.D. (1993) Quantitation of idiogenic osmoles in human brain. Abstr. Commun. 12th Ann. Meet. Soc. MR Med. 1993; 1553.

41. Kreis, R., Farrow, N.A. & Ross, B.D. (1990) Diagnosis of hepatic ence phalopathy by proton magnetic resonance spectroscopy. Lancet **336**:635–636.

42. Kreis, R., Ross, B.D., Farrow, N.A. & Ackerman, Z. (1992) Metabolic disorders of the brain in chronic hepatic encephalopathy detected with H–1 MR spectroscopy. Radiology **182**:19–27.

43. Moats, R.A., Lien, Y.H.H., Filippi, D. & Ross, B.D. (1993) Decrease in cerebral inositols in rats and humans. Biochem. J. **295**:15–18.

44. Norenberg, M.D., Baker, L., Norenberg, L.O.B., Blicharska, J., Bruce–Gregorius, J.H. & Neary, J.T. (1991) Ammonia–induced astrocyte swelling in primary culture. Neurochem. Res. **16**:833–836.

45. Hawkins, R.A., Jessy, J., Mans, A.M. & De Joseph, M.R. (1993) Effect of reducing brain glutamine synthesis on metabolic symptoms of hepatic encephalopathy. J. Neurochem. **60**:1000–1006.

46. Häussinger, D., Lang, F. Bauers, K. & Gerok, W. (1990) Interactions between glutamine metabolism and cell volume regulation in perfused rat liver. Eur. J. Biochem. **188**:689–695.

47. Offensperger, W.B., Offensperger, S., Stoll, B. Gerok, W. & Häussinger, D. (1994) Effect of anisotonic exposure on duck hepatitis B virus replication. Hepatology, in press.

Astrocyte–Neuron Interactions in Hyperammonemia and Hepatic Encephalopathy

Jan Albrecht and Lidia Faff

1. Introduction

It has been known for a long time that hepatic encephalopathy (HE) and other cerebral disorders related to hyperammonemia (HA) are manifested by pronounced neuropathological changes that primarily affect astrocytes, leaving the other cell types of the CNS relatively intact. In 1912, von Hösslin and Alzheimer (1) were the first to note the occurrence in the brain of a patient with pseudosclerosis, of large, pale astrocytes with enlarged, lobulated nuclei. These cells, later consistently defined as Alzheimer type II cells, were convincingly associated with HE by Adams and Foley (2). Since then the literature has become flooded with reports of HE– induced astroglial changes, which beside the appearance of degenerated forms of these cells include diffuse proliferation of protoplasmic astrocytes: for excellent reviews on this subject the reader is referred to the articles of Diemer (3) and Norenberg (4). However, until recently, these glial changes have been considered as unrelated to the neurological symptoms of HE. This was not unexpected, as at that time astrocytes were considered to perform only static, supportive functions.

In the early sixties, the Wealsch group demonstrated that brain lacks a number of enzymes involved in the urea cycle and therefore the glutamine synthetase (GS)–mediated amidation of glutamate (GLU) to glutamine (GLN) remains the only significant route of ammonia metabolism (5,6), and recent studies performed with the use of more sophisticated metabolic tracing techniques fully confirmed this conclusion (cf. ref. [7]). In the late seventies, Norenberg and colleagues provided immunocytochemical evidence that GS is an astroglia–specific enzyme (8,9), showing that astrocytes are the cells in which the neutralization of endogenous and blood–derived ammonia takes place. In another breakthrough study of the late seventies, Cotman group demonstrated that GLN can serve as a precursor for the releasable, neurotransmitter pool of GLU (10). More recently, studies performed on astrocytic cultures confirmed that astrocytes are the GLN–exporting cells (11–13), and studies on "sandwich" cocultures of astrocytes and neurons using [^{13}C] NMR spectroscopy directly demonstrated that astroglia–derived GLN is metabolized in nerve cells to GLU and GABA (14, and references therein). These important discoveries made it clear that GS–mediated GLN synthesis, the process that couples the metabolism of ammonia in astrocytes to the synthesis of amino acid neurotransmitters in the nerve cells, is at once a major area of functional interaction between astrocytes and neurons and the main target of ammonia entering the brain in hyperammonemic conditions. It is therefore not surprising that

Department of Neuropathology, Medical Research Centre, Polish Academy of Sciences, 00–704 Warsaw Dworkowa 3, Poland

Hepatic Encephalopathy, Hyperammonemia, and Ammonia Toxicity
Edited by V. Felipo and S. Grisolia, Plenum Press, New York, 1994

45

the fate of cerebral GS and of the various aspects of GLN metabolism have attracted the attention of a vast majority of research groups investigating the pathomechanism of HE. The often discrepant data regarding GS activity and the controversies around the role of enhanced GLN content accompanying HE (beneficial or detrimental, cf. ref. [15]) are subject of first hand reviews presented during this symposium by Drs. Hawkins and Butterworth, and will not be dealt with in this chapter. Instead, the first section of this review deals with a closely related subject: We discuss the responses to hyperammonemic conditions, of other metabolic reactions participating in the synthesis and metabolism of GLU, also involving an interplay between the different cell compartments of the CNS, including astrocytes and neurons. We then turn the readers' attention to what is known or suspected about the effects of HE and/or HA on the two direct neuromodulatory functions of astrocytes: clearance of ions and neurotransmitters released from the neurons. We will also shortly dwell on the possible implications of ammonia–induced release of a putative gliotransmitter taurine. It is important to note here that, we did not pretend to discuss, or even to list all the metabolic changes ever found to occur in astrocytes affected by ammonia or HE: exhaustive reviews on this so broadly understood subject have recently been published (16,17). The scope of this chapter will be confined to changes that directly pertain to the crosstalk between astrocytes and neurons, and in consequence, are likely to contribute to changes of neural transmission.

2. Compartmentation of the Effects of HE and HA on the Enzymes Coupling Energy Metabolism to the Synthesis of Neurotransmitter GLU. Studies with Synaptic and Nonsynaptic Mitochondria

2.1 Astrocytic Tricarboxylic Acid Cycle (TCA) Constituents as Putative Precursors of Neurotransmitter GLU

There is considerable evidence to suggest that GLN is not the only astroglia–derived precursor of neurotransmitter GLU; this role has also been ascribed to a number of TCA intermediates. It has been demonstrated that glutamatergic nerve cell terminals vividly take up and metabolize to GLU, 2–oxoglutarate (2–OG) (18–20) and malate (18). As to the astrocytic side of the synaptic cleft, cultured astrocytes have been shown to actively release citrate (21). According to most recent accounts, the intimate relationship between the TCA cycle constituents and GLU synthesis also involves the utilization of GLN: Schousboe group proposed that GLU produced in synaptic mitochondria from GLN in the glutaminase–mediated reaction is not directly introduced into the neurotransmitter pool but has to go through two transaminations in the malate–aspartate shuttle (22,23).

Fig. 1 summarizes the present views regarding the relationship between synaptic GLU and its precursors and metabolites. As can be seen, the process of GLU synthesis involves a cooperative action of a number of mitochondrial enzymes located, respectively, in astrocytes and nerve terminals.

2.2 Rationale for Selecting the Subject and Experimental Approaches

Disturbances of energy metabolism and glutamatergic neurotransmission are considered to be significant contributors to the pathomechanism of HE. Therefore, it was most tempting to assume that the disturbances involve the activities of the mitochondrial enzymes that couple the two processes on the astrocytic and synaptic side of the synaptic cleft. We chose to test this assumption by measuring some of the enzyme activities shown in Fig. 1,

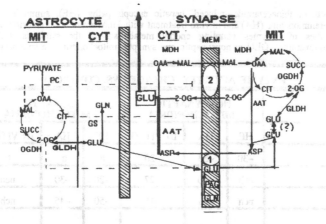

Figure 1. Astrocytic and synaptic enzymes involved in the metabolism of synaptic GLU and its precursors.
CYT – cytoplasm, MEM – inner mitochondrial membrane, MIT – mitochondrial matrix, AAT – aspartate aminotransferase, GlDH – glutamate dehydrogenase, GS – glutamate synthetase, MDH – malate dehydrogenase, OGDH – 2-oxoglutarate dehydrogenase, PAG – glutaminase, ASP – aspartate, CIT – citrate, GLU – glutamate, GLN – glutamine, MAL – malate, OAA – oxaloacetate, 2-OG – 2-oxoglutarate, Suc–CoA – succinyl–Coa
1 – ASP/GLU carrier
2 – Dicarboxylate carrier

separately in mitochondria derived from the nerve endings (synaptic mitochondria) and in nonsynaptic mitochondria, which have been reported to be considerably enriched in astrocytic mitochondria (24,25).

As frequently mentioned during this Symposium, there are controversies in the literature as to the relative contribution of ammonia vs. other toxins to the pathomechanism of HE (for an excellent review on this subject see also ref. [26]). To account for this, we have compared the effects produced in two in vivo models: 1) "genuine" HE produced by three i.p. injections of a hepatotoxin – thioacetamide (27–29) and 2) simple hyperammonemia (HA) produced by three i.p. administrations of ammonium acetate, where the biochemical and pathophysiological symptoms resembled those noted in HE (30). Further we sought to account for one other important fact that recurs in many of the other chapters: Hyperammonemia influences an array of metabolic processes outside– and within the brain and therefore its intracerebral effects cannot be considered as equivalent to a direct action of ammonia. Therefore, we also used an in vitro model, in which the mitochondrial fractions were preincubated with 3 mM ammonium chloride for 10 min, immediately before the enzyme assays.

2.3 Results and Discussion

Table 1 summarizes the results of the tests which comprised the key enzymes of the scheme outlined in Fig. 1. Below we recapitulate in some detail the present views on the role of each enzyme activity in the metabolism of neurotransmitter GLU and discuss the results obtained with regard to the possible implications of the HE– and HA–induced changes for energy metabolism and glutamatergic neurotransmission:
– **Pyruvate carboxylase** (PC). This is an astroglia–specific enzyme which is essential for de novo synthesis of TCA constituents (31–33). As mentioned above, a number of these TCA constituents appear to be shuttled to the nerve cells and become precursors of the neurotransmitter pool of GLU (18–21). PC activity was exclusively present in the nonsynaptic mitochondria, demonstrating the enrichment of this fraction in astrocytic mitochondria. Both HE and HA, but also in vitro treatment with ammonia suppressed this enzyme, which is likely

Table 1. Effects of thioacetamide–induced hepatic encephalpathy (HE), ammonium acetate–induced hyperammonemia (HA) and in vitro treatment with 3 mM ammonium chloride (IN VITRO) on the activities of enzymes coupling energy metabolism to the synthesis and metabolism of neurotransmitter GLU in nonsynaptic and synaptic mitochondria – a summary.

ENZYME ACTIVITY (CHANGES VS. CONTROL)							
ENZYME	NONSYNAPTIC MITOCHONDRIA			SYNAPTIC MITOCHONDRIA			REF
	HE	HA	IN VITRO	HE	HA	IN VITRO	
PC	−30	−53	−20	tr	tr	tr	(40)
AAT	nch	+30	−27	−26	−30	nch	(40)
MDH	nch	nch	−16	−50	−45	nch	(40)
OGDH: V_{max}	nch	+33	−30	+12	+28	nch	(41)
K_m	−19	+19	−60	nch	+21	nch	
OGDH– E1: V_{max}	nch	+35	−21	+84	+110	nch	(42)
K_m	nch	+30	−35	+38	+30	nch	
OGDH– E3:	nch	nch	nch	+20	·+20	nch	(42)
GLDH–NAD: specific	nch	nch	nch	+81	+92	nch	(43)
V_{max}	nt	nt	nt	+102	+105	nch	
K_m	nt	nt	nt	nch	nch	nch	
GLDH– NADH: specific	+33	+49	–	−21	−28	–	(43)
V_{max}	nt	nt	–	−22	−29	–	
K_m	nt	nt	–	−29	−43	–	

nch – not changed, nt – not tested, tr – traces.

to result in a depletion of astroglia–derived precursors of synaptic GLU. An earlier study with whole brain homogenate revealed an almost perfect correlation between the changes of PC activity and 2–OG content at different stages of thioacetamide–induced HE (29).

– **The malate–aspartate shuttle enzymes:** aspartate aminotransferase (AAT) and malate dehydrogenase (MDH). As mentioned above, these two enzymes are thought to participate in the conversion of GLN to the neurotransmitter pool of GLU (22,23). The response to ammonia added in vitro (a decrease of both enzyme activities) was observed only in nonsynaptic mitochondria. By contrast, HE and HA markedly decreased both enzyme activities in the synaptic compartment. Suppression of AAT may be expected to lower the production of aspartate. In turn, suppression of MDH would result in the accumulation of malate and would limit the formation of oxaloacetate available for transamination of GLU.

– **2–oxoglutarate dehydrogenase** (OGDH), which is considered to be the rate–limiting enzyme of TCA (34). OGDH is a multienzyme complex, and we have dealt with two of its components: E1 (2–oxoglutarate dehydrogenase), which is rate–limiting and accounts for the catalytic properties of the complex, and E3 (lipoamide dehydrogenase), which is believed to serve as a regulator for all the complex. Except for the absence of change in nonsynaptic mitochondria after HE, both in vivo conditions stimulated the whole complex or E1 activity (increased its V_{max}) in both synaptic and nonsynaptic mitochondria. HE and HA increased E3 activity in synaptic mitochondria. Stimulation of both OGDH components in the synaptic compartment may cooperatively lead to increased utilization of 2–OG in TCA at the expense of its transaminations and, subsequently, synthesis of neurotransmitter GLU. Here again, the effect of ammonia in vitro was quite different from the effects of HE or HA; ammonia decreased E1 activity in nonsynaptic mitochondria.

– **Glutamate dehydrogenase** (GlDH), which is abundant in both nerve and glial cells (35) and carries out the interconversion of 2–OG and GLU. We have measured the enzyme activity both in the thermodynamically more favored direction of reductive amination of 2–OG (GlDH–NADH) and in the direction of GLU oxidation (GlDH–NAD) which appears to prevail in both physiological (36) and hyperammonemic conditions (37–39). In nonsynaptic mitochondria, HE and HA stimulated GlDH–NADH. This could lead to increased conversion of 2–OG to the metabolic (nonsynaptic pool) of GLU, decreasing the amount of 2–OG normally serving as a precursor of neurotransmitter GLU. In synaptic mitochondria, HE and HA stimulated GlDH–NAD. This could result in increased consumption of GLU which in consequence would decrease the amount of this amino acid available for neural transmission.

2.4 Conclusions

The results taken together show that HE and HA produce changes in the synaptic and nonsynaptic mitochondrial enzymes that may cooperatively lead to the decrease of the neurotransmitter pools of GLU. As such, the results add metabolic arguments in favor of the long held hypothesis that depletion of the releasable pools of GLU is one of the ways in which hyperammonemic conditions depress excitatory, glutamatergic neurotransmission (44–47). Each of the two cerebral compartments studied appears to contribute in a distinct way to the final negative outcome. Changes in the nonsynaptic (astrocytic?) compartment may be held responsible for the decreased availability of GLU precursors to be transported to the nerve endings: inhibition of PC would lead to decreased synthesis of TCA cycle constituents, whereas stimulation of GlDH–NADH and OGDH would jointly result in increased "intracompartmental" (astrocytic?) consumption of 2–OG. In turn, changes in the synaptic compartment would act towards increased intrasynaptic utilization of GLU in the TCA cycle (stimulation of GlDH–NAD) and decreased synthesis of the neurotransmitter pools of GLU (inhibition of GlDH–NADH, AAT and MDH). Notably, in both compartments the responses to HA and HE were always identical in their direction and often similar in magnitude, which emphasizes the predominant contribution of increased blood ammonia as compared to other toxins, to the changes accompanying HE, at least regarding the metabolic reactions under study. However, all the effects of in vitro treatment with ammonia (inhibition of PC excepted) were different from those found in the in vivo models, reflecting the complexity of the in vivo response (see below). Interpreting the described effects of HE and HA as partly reflecting an impaired cross–talk between astrocytes and adjacent nerve endings, we remain fully aware that nonsynaptic mitochondria are only partly equivalent to astrocytic mitochondria: we tried to document our awareness of this methodological limitation by using the term "astrocytic" in brackets and with a question mark behind. However, no satisfactory preparation that would adequately represent the astrocytic compartment of adult brain is technically feasible at this moment. Murthy group measured the effects of acute hyperammonemia in vivo on some of the mitochondrial enzymes in bulk isolated cerebral cortical astrocytes and obtained results identical to ours with regard to AAT, but conflicting with regard to GlDH–NAD (48). Interestingly, the responses in astrocytes isolated from cerebellum appeared to be exactly opposite (49). However, these results have to be interpreted with caution, as bulk–isolated CNS cell preparations have been repeatedly criticized for impaired cell integrity (50, and references therein).

3. Effects of HE and Ammonia on the Uptake of Ions and Neurotransmitters by Astrocytes

It has been repeatedly demonstrated that astrocytes possess transport systems for a variety of ions and neurotransmitters and as such are thought to play an important role in fine–tuning the extracellular and perisynaptic milieu in the CNS (for recent review see ref. [51]). Considering the significance of these astrocytic functions, amazingly little attention has been devoted to their response to hyperammonemic conditions. Thioacetamide–induced HE in the early, precomatose stage stimulated GABA transport and Na/K ATPase activity in bulk isolated astrocytes (52), but this stimulatory effect disappeared at more advanced stages of HE (29). A stage–dependent response was also noted with regard to the astrocytic uptake of the nonmetabolizable GLU analogue D–ASP, which was not affected in early HE but was inhibited in advanced HE (29). Advanced HE was also accompanied by decreased potassium–stimulated Ca^{2+} uptake in bulk–isolated astrocytes (53). Notably, all the effects turned out to be astroglia–specific: no such changes were observed in the nerve endings (synaptosomes) isolated from HE rats. A similar biphasic response (early stimulation followed by inhibition) with regard to GLU and GABA uptake and Na/K–ATPase activity was noted by Norenberg group in cultured astrocytes treated with low millimolar concentrations of ammonia (54). Long–term treatment of cultured astrocytes with ammonia also resulted in a marked reduction of Ca^{2+} influx (55). These studies indicate in most general terms that the basic "milieu–buffering" functions of astrocytes are compromised by HE and ammonia. Further studies will have to account for regional heterogeneity of astrocytes with regard to the amino acid uptake systems (56), but also for the uptake of other neuroactive compounds. Insofar, HE was observed to remain without effect on the astrocytic transport of histamine (57).

4. Ammonia–Induced Release of Taurine from Glia: Stimulation of Glial Transmission, Osmoregulatory (Osmosensory) Response, or Unwanted Side Effect?

Astrocytes have been shown to release neuroactive amino acids in response to a variety of stimuli, including changes in the ionic composition or tonicity of the medium, activation of cell membrane receptors, heavy metals etc. (for an exhaustive review see ref. [58]). However, for most of the compounds, the functional meaning of their release remains obscure. A sulphur amino acid taurine (TAU) might be a positive exception to this rule. TAU is more abundant in astrocytes than any other amino acid (59,60), and is very actively released from these cells in response to environmental stimuli that tend to increase cell volume (61, 62). Because by physicochemical criteria TAU appears to be an ideal osmolyte, its release has been suggested to subserve an osmoregulatory or osmosensory function (reviewed in ref. [63]). Since TAU is also known to act as an inhibitory neuromodulator, astroglia–derived TAU has been postulated to act as a gliotransmitter (63,64).

The concept that ammonia may act as a trigger of TAU release from astrocytes was derived from the observations by others that hyperammonemic conditions produce astrocytic swelling (65,66). However, our studies revealed vivid TAU release from cultured rabbit Müller cells treated briefly with ammonia at relatively low (< 1mM) concentrations that are unlikely to produce cell swelling (67). We speculated that ammonium ions may activate a (hypothetical) intracellular osmosensor to trigger TAU release and that, the outward driven–TAU could counteract ammonia–induced neuronal disinhibition. If this is true, TAU would serve a programmed, neuroprotective, gliotransmitter role. In another recent study, however, we noted that long–term treatment of cultured cerebellar astrocytes with 1 mM ammonium chloride increased unstimulated release of newly taken up radiolabelled TAU and, accordingly, caused a significant loss of endogenous TAU from the cells (68). However, this enhanced release turned out to merely reflect ammonia–induced cell damage. Firstly, unlike the release from osmoregulating or osmosensing astrocytes, that induced by ammonium chloride was not suppressed in a hypertonic medium. Secondly, the so treated astrocytes lost the ability to release additional TAU in response to high potassium ions, indicating an intrinsic loss of osmosensation (68). In vivo, such an unprogrammed increase of TAU leakage from astrocytes would be unwanted. Considering that TAU acts as an inhibitory neuromodulator, this would favor inhibitory neurotransmission – a generally considered contributor to hyperammonemic coma.

Obviously, the outlined sequence of events will remain a speculation until we acquire technical means with which to identify the neuronal targets of TAU released from astrocytes. However, a breakthrough appears to be not too far away. Most recently, Ottersen group has successfully used quantative electron–microscopic immunocytochemistry to demonstrate a redistribution of TAU from cerebellar Purkinje cells to neighboring glia in rats during hypoosmotic stress (69). This technique may be used to study the fluxes of TAU and other neuroactive compounds in hyperammonemic rats.

5. Summary and Perspectives

In general terms, it is now clear that HE compromises several aspects of metabolism and transport functions of astrocytes directly pertaining to their role in neural transmission and that, ammonia acts as a major trigger of these changes. It has also become apparent that, as is the case with the metabolism of neurotransmitter GLU (Section 2), changes in the neuronal compartment cooperatively contribute to the final outcome. However, more specific questions, such as the role of a particular astrocytic dysfunction in the onset and progression of a particular HE symptom remain to be addressed. With regard to the astrocytic functions sofar studied, our progress has been hampered by the lack of appropriate techniques. As already mentioned, the poor quality of the subcellular and cell–enriched fractions obtained with the available methods, makes their properties a far cry from their "native", in situ counterparts. On the other hand, astrocytes in culture are separated "at birth" from their native milieu, and as such miss the properties that normally develop in contact with other cell components of the CNS. This problem may be partly overcome by using astrocytic–neuronal "sandwich" cocultures, which were successfully employed in basic studies on GLU metabolism and transport (14, 70). Further studies will have to account for the regional heterogeneity of astrocytes (cf. Section 3), which will inevitably direct the research efforts to the as yet unexplored issue of the role of astrocytes in the HE–induced disturbances of non–amino acid neurotransmitter systems.

The sofar conducted studies have almost bypassed one property of astrocytes with a potential neuromodulatory function: the presence on astrocytic cell membranes of receptors for virtually all neurotransmitters and neuromodulators (for the most recent review see ref. [71]). In the only study on this subject that we are aware of, Ducis et al. demonstrated a decrease of the binding affinity of the peripheral BZD receptor in ammonia–treated astrocytes in culture (72). Insofar, the prevailing skepticism of HE explorers to get involved in the astrocytic receptors appears to be justified: their role in the astrocytic–neuronal interactions remains obscure.

References

1. Von Hösslin, C., and Alzheimer, A., 1912, Ein Beitrag zur Klinik und pathologischen Anatomie der Westphal Strumpellschen Pseudosklerose, Z. Ges. Neurol. Psychiatirie. 8:183–209.

2. Adams, R. D., and Foley, J. M., 1953, The neuroglial disorder associated with liver discase, Res. Publ. Assoc. Res. Nerv. Ment. Dis. 32:198–237.

3. Diemer, N. H., 1978, Glial and neuronal changes in experimental hepatic encephalopathy, Acta Neurol. Scand. 58:1–144 (Suppl. 71).

4. Norenberg, M. D., 1986, Hepatic encephalopathy: A disorder of astrocytes, IN: S. Fedoroff, and A. Vernadakis (Eds.),Astrocytes: Cell biology and pathology of Astrocytes,Vol. 3, Academic Press, New York, pp. 425–460.

5. Berl, S., Tokagaki, G., Clarke, D. D., Waelsch, H., 1962, Metabolic compartments in vivo. Ammonia and glutamic acid metabolism in brain and liver, J. Biol. Chem. 237:2562–2569.

6. Clarke, D. D., and Waelsch, H., 1962, Carbon dioxide fixation in the brain, J. Biol. Chem.**237**:2570–2573.

7. Farrow, N. A., Kanamori, K., Ross, R. D., and Parivar, F., 1990, A 15-n.m.r. study of cerebral, hepatic and renal nitrogen metabolism in hyperammonemic rats, Biochem. J. **270**:473–481.

8. Martinez–Hernandez A., Bell K. P., Norenberg M. D. 1977. Glutamine synthetase: glial localization in brain. Science **195**:1356–1358.

9. Norenberg, M. D., Martinez–Hernandez, A., 1979, Fine structural localization of glutamine synthetase in astrocytes of rat brain, Brain Res. **161**:303–310.

10. Hamberger, A., Chiang, G. H., Nylen, E. S., Scheff, S. W., Cotman, C W., 1979, Glutamate as a CNS transmitter. I. Evaluation of glucose and glutamine as precursors for the synthesis of preferentially released glutamate, Brain Res. **168**:513–530.

11. Waniewski, R. A., and Martin, D. L., 1986, Exogenous glutamate is metabolized to glutamine and exported by rat primary astrocytic cultures, J. Neurochem. **47**:304–313.

12. Waniewski, R. A., 1992. Physiological levels of ammonia regulate glutamine synthesis from extracellular glutamate in astrocyte cultures, J. Neurochem. **58**:167–174.

13. Farinelli, S. E., and Nicklas, W. J., 1992, Glutamate metabolism in rat cortical astrocyte cultures, J. Neurochem. **58**:1905–1915.

14. Sonnenwald, U., Westergaard, N., Schousboe, A., Svendsen, J. S., Unsgard, G., and Petersen, S. B., 1993, Direct demonstration by [^{13}C]NMR spectroscopy that glutamine from astrocytes is a precursor for GABA synthesis in neurons, Neurochem. Int. **22**:19–29.

15. Hawkins, R. A., Jessy, J., Mans, A. M., and De Joseph, M. R., 1993, Effect of reducing brain glutamine synthesis on metabolic symptoms of hepatic encephalopathy, J. Neurochem. **60**:1000–1006.

16. Norenberg, M. D., 1987, The role of astrocytes in hepatic encephalopathy, Neurochem. Pathol. **6**:13–33.

17. Norenberg, M. D., Neary, A. S., Bender, A. S., and Dombro, R. S., 1992, Hepatic encephalopathy: a disorder in glial–neuronal communication, In: A. C. H. Yu, L. Hertz, M. D. Norenberg, E. Sykova, and S. G. Waxman (Eds.), Progress in Brain Research, Vol. **94**:261–269, Elsevier Science Publishers B. V.

18. Shank, R. P., Campbell, G. L., 1984, α–ketoglutarate and malate uptake and metabolism by synaptosomes: Further evidence for an astrocyte–to–neuron metabolic shuttle, J. Neurochem. **42**:1153–1161.

19. Carter, C. J., Savasta, M., Fage, D., Scatton, B., 1986, 2–oxo–[^{14}C] glutarate is taken up by glutamatergic nerve terminals in the rat striatum, Neurosci. Lett. **72**:227–231.

20. Shank, R. P., and Bennett, D. J., 1993, 2–oxoglutarate transport: a potential mechanism for regulating glutamate and tricarboxylic acid cycle intermediates in neurons, Neurochem. Res. **18**:401–410.

21. Sonnewald, U., Westergaard, N., Krane, J., Unsgard, G., Petersen, S. B., Schousboe, A., 1991, First direct demonstration of preferential release of citrate from astrocytes using [^{13}C]NMR spectroscopy of cultured neurons and astrocytes, Neurosci. Lett. **128**:235–239.

22. Palaiologos, G., Hertz, L., Schousboe, A., 1989, Role of aspartate aminotransferase and mitochondrial dicarboxylate transport for release of endogenously and exogenously supplied neurotransmitter in glutamatergic neurons, Neurochem. Res. **14**:359–366.

23. Peng, L., Schousboe, A., Hertz, L., 1991, Utilization of alpha-ketoglutarate as a precursor for transmitter glutamate in cultured cerebellar granule cells, Neurochem. Res. **16**: 29–34.

24. Clark, J. B., and Nicklas, W. J., 1970, The metabolism of rat brain mitochondria, J. Biol. Chem. **245**: 4724–4731.

25. Dennis, S. C., and Clark, J. B., 1978, The synthesis of glutamate by rat brain mitochondria, J. Neurochem. **31**:673–680.

26. Zieve, L., 1987, Pathogenesis of hepatic encephalopathy, Metab. Brain Dis, **2**:147–165.

27. Albrecht, J., Hilgier, W., 1984, Brain carbonic anhydrase activity in rats in experimental hepatogenic encephalopathy, Neurosci. Lett. **45**:7–10.

28. Pluta, R., Albrecht, J., 1984, Thioacetamide-induced hepatic encephalopathy in the rat, Clinical observations. Neuropat. Pol. **22**:379–385.

29. Albrecht, J., Hilgier, W., Lazarewicz, J.W., Rafalowska, U., Wysmyk–Cybula U., 1988, Astrocytes in acute hepatic encephalopathy: Metabolic properties and transport function, In: Norenberg,

M. D., Hertz, L., and A., Schousboe (Eds.), Biochemical Pathology of Astrocytes 465–476, Alan R Liss, New York.

30. Hilgier, W. ,Albrecht, J., Lisy, V., Stastny, F., 1990, The effect of acute and repeated hyperammonemia on γ–glutamyl–transpeptidase in homogenates and capillaries of various rat brain regions, Mol Chem Neuropathol. 13:47–45.

31. Yu, A. C. H., Drejer, J., Hertz, L., Schousboe, A., 1983, Pyruvate carboxylase activity in primary cultures of astrocytes and neurons, J. Neurochem. 41: 1484–1487.

32. Shank, R. P., Bennett, G. S., Freytag, S. O., Campbell, G. L., 1985, Pyruvate carboxylase: An astrocyte–specific enzyme implicated in the replenishment of amino acid neurotransmitter pools, Brain Res. 329: 364–367.

33. Kaufman, E. E., Driscol, B. F., 1992, CO_2 fixation in neuronal and astroglial cells in culture, J. Neurochem. 58:258–162.

34. Lai, J. C. K., Cooper, J. L., 1986, Brain α–ketoglutarate dehydrogenase complex: kinetic properties, regional distribution, and effect of inhibitors, J. Neurochem 47:1376–1386.

35. Aoki, C., Milner, T. A., Sheu, K.–F. R., Blass, J. P., Pickel, V. M., 1987, Regional distribution of astrocytes with intense immunoreactivity for glutamate dehydrogenase in rat brain: implications for neuron–glia interactions in glutamate transmission, J. Neurosci. 7:2214–2231.

36. Yudkoff, M., Nissim, I., and Hertz, L., Precursors of glutamic acid nitrogen im primary neuronal cultures: studies with 15N, Neurochem. Res. 15:1191–1196.

37. Cooper, A. J. L., Mora, S. N., Cruz, N. F., Gelbard, A. S., 1985, Cerebral ammonia metabolism in hyperammonemic rats, J. Neurochem. 44:1716–1723.

38. Kanamori, K., Ross, B. D., Farrow, N. A., and Parivar, F. A., 1991, A 15N–NMR study of isolated brain in portacaval–shunted rats after acute hyperammonemia, Biochim. Biophys. Acta 1096:270–276.

39. Lai, J. C. K., Murthy, Ch. R. K., Cooper, A. J. L., Hertz, E., Hertz L., 1989, Differential effects of ammonia and β–methylene–DL–aspartate on the metabolism of glutamate and related amino acids by astrocytes and neurones in primary cultures, Neurochem. Res. 14:377–389.

40. Faff–Michalak, L., and Albrecht, J., 1991, Aspartate aminotransferase, malate dehydrogenase, and pyruvate carboxylase activities in rat cerebral synaptic and nonsynaptic mitochondria: Effects of in vitro treatment with ammonia, hyperammonemia and hepatic encephalopathy, Metab. Brain Dis. 6:187–197.

41. Faff–Michalak, L., Wysmyk–Cybula, U., and Albrecht, J., 1991, Different responses of rat cerebral mitochondrial 2–oxoglutarate activity to ammonia and hepatic encephalopathy in synaptic and nonsynaptic mitochondria, Neurochem. Int. 19:573–579.

42. Faff–Michalak, L., and Albrecht, J., 1993, The two catalytic components of the 2–oxoglutarate dehydrogenase complex in rat cerebral synaptic and nonsynaptic mitochondria: Comparison of the response to in vitro treatment with ammonia, hyperammonemia, and hepatic encephalopathy, Neurochem. Res. 18:119–123.

43. Faff–Michalak, L., Albrecht, J., 1993, Hyperammonemia and hepatic encephalopathy stimulate rat cerebral synaptic mitochondrial glutamate dehydrogenase activity specifically in the direction of glutamate oxidation, Brain Res. 618:299–302.

44. Hamberger, A. C., Hedquist, B., Nystrom, B., 1979, Ammonium ion inhibition of evoked release of endogenous glutamate from hippocampal slices, J. Neurochem. 33:1295–1302.

45. Theoret, Y., and Bossu, J. L., 1985, Effects of ammonium salts on synaptic transmission in hippocampal CA1 and CA3 pyramidal cells in vivo, Neuroscience 14: 807–821.

46. Theoret, Y., Davies, M. F., Esplin, B., and Capek, R., 1985, Effects of ammonium chloride on synaptic transmission in the rat hippocampal slice, Neuroscience 14: 798–806.

47. Hilgier, W., Haugvicova, R., Albrecht, J., 1991, Decreased potassium–stimulated release of [³H] D–aspartate from hippocampal slices distinguishes encephalopathy related to acute liver failure from that induced by simple hyperammonemia, Brain Res. 567:165–168.

48. Subbalakshmi, G. Y. C. V., Murthy, Ch. R. K., 1983, Acute metabolic effects of ammonia on the enzymes of glutamate metabolism in isolated astroglial cells, Neurochem. Int. 5:593–597.

49. Rao, V. L. R., Murthy, Ch. R. K., 1991, Hyperammonemic alterations in the uptake and release of glutamate and aspartate by rat cerebellar preparations, Neurosci. Lett. 130:49–52.

50. Albrecht, J., Hilgier, W., Ulas, J., and Wysmyk–Cybula, U., 1982, Some properties of a "crude" fraction of astrocytes prepared with trypsin, Neurochem. Res. 7:513–517.

53

51. Kimelberg, H. K., Jalonen, T., and Walz, W., 1993, Regulation of the brain microenvironment: Transmitters and ions, In: S. Murthy (Ed.), Astrocytes. Pharmacology and function, Academic Press, INC, pp. 193–228.

52. Albrecht, J., Wysmyk–Cybula, U., and Rafalowska, U., 1985, Na+/K+–ATPase activity and GABA uptake in astroglial cell–enriched fractions and synaptosomes derived from rats in the early stage of experimental hepatogenic encephalopathy, Acta Neurol. Scand. 72:317–320.

53. Albrecht, J., and Lazarewicz J., 1990, Acute hepatic encephalopathy decreases potassium–evoked calcium uptake in astrocytes but not in synaptosomes of the rat, Neurosci. Lett. 111:321–324.

54. Norenberg, M. D., Mozez, L. W., Papendick, R. E., and Norenberg, L. O. B., 1985, Effect of ammonia on glutamate, GABA, and rubidium uptake by astrocytes, Ann. Neurol. 18:149.

55. Norenberg, M. D., 1981, The astrocyte in liver disease, In: S. Fedoroff and L. Hertz (Eds.), The biochemical pathology of astrocytes, Alan R. Liss, New York, pp.451–464.

56. Amundson, R. H., Goderie, S. K., and Kimelberg, H. K., 1992, Uptake of [3H]serotonin and [3H]glutamate by primary astrocyte cultures II. Differences in cultures prepared from different brain regions, Glia 6:9–18.

57. Albrecht, J., and Rafalowska, U., 1987, Enhanced potassium–stimulated γ–aminobutyric acid release by astrocytes derived from rats with early hepatogenic encephalopathy, J. Neurochem. 49:9–11.

58. Dutton, G. R., 1993, Astrocyte amino acids: Evidence for release and possible interactions with neurons, In: S. Murthy (Ed.), Astrocytes. Pharmacology and function, Academic Press, INC, pp. 173–191.

59. Holopainen, I., Oja, S. S., Marnela, K.–M., and Kontro, P., 1986, Free amino acids of rat astrocytes in primary culture: Changes during cell maturation, Int. J. Dev. Neurosci. 4:493–496.

60. Brookes, N., 1992, Effects of pH on glutamine content derived from exogenous glutamate in astrocytes, J. Neurochem. 59:1017–1023.

61. Kimelberg, H. K., Goderie, S. K., Higman, S., Pang, S., and Waniewski, R. A., 1990, Swelling–induced release of glutamate, aspartate and taurine from astrocyte cultures, J. Neurosci. 10:1583–1589.

62. Pasantes–Morales, H., and Schousboe, A., 1988, Volume regulation in astrocytes: a role of taurine as osmoeffector, J. Neurosci. 20:505–509.

63. Martin, D. L., 1992, Synthesis and release of neuroactive substances by glial cells, Glia 5:81–94.

64. Walz, W., 1989, Role of glial cells in the regulation of the brain ion microenvironment, Prog. Neurobiol. 33:309–333.

65. Norenberg, M. D., Baker, L., Norenberg, L. O. B., Blicharska, J., Bruce–Gregorios, J. H., and Neary, J. T., 1991, Ammonia–induced astrocyte swelling in primary culture, Neurochem. Res. 16:833–836.

66. Traber, P. G., Dal Canto, M., Ganger, D., and Blei, A. T., 1987, Electron microscopic evaluation of brain edema in rabbits with galactosamine–inuced fulminant hepatic failure, Hepatology 7:1257–1261.

67. Faff–Michalak, L., Reichenbach, A., Dettmer, D., Kellner, K., and Albrecht, J., 1994, K+–, Hypoosmolarity–, and NH+–induced taurine release from cultured rabbit Muller cells: Role o|f Na+ and Cl- ions and relation to cell volume changes, Glia 10:114–120.

68. Wysmyk, U., Oja, S. S., Saransaari, P., and Albrecht, J., 1994, Long–term treatment with ammonia differently affects the content and release of taurine in cultured cerebellar astrocytes and granule neurons, Neurochem. Int. 24:317–322.

69. Nagelhus, E. A., Lehmann, A., and Ottersen, O. P., 1993, Neuronal–glial exchange of taurine during hypo–osmotic stress: a combined immunocytochemical and biochemical analysis in rat cerebellar cortex, Neurosci. 54:615–631.

70. Schousboe, A., Westergaard, N., Sonnewald, U., Petersen, S. B., Yu, A. C. H., and Hertz, L., 1992, Regulatory role of astrocytes for neuronal biosynthesis and homeosthasis of glutamate and GABA, In: A. C. H. Yu, L. Hertz, M. D. Norenberg, E. Sykova, and S. G. Waxman (Eds.), Progress in Brain Research, Vol. 94:199–211, Elsevier Science Publishers B. V.

71. Hösli, E., and Hösli, L., 1993, Receptors for neurotransmitters on astrocytes in the mammalian central nervous system, Prog. Neurobiol. 40:477–506.

72. Ducis, I., Norenberg, L. O. B., and Norenberg, M. D., 1989, Effect of ammonium chloride on the astrocyte benzodiazepine receptor, Brain Res. 493:362–365.

Spinal Seizures in Ammonia Intoxication

W. Raabe

1. Introduction

Ammonia intoxication is well known to produce seizures (1). These seizures may be cortical or spinal in origin (1,2,3,4,5). Because ammonia predominantly increases the excitability of the spinal cord (1,2), most seizures are probably spinal in origin. The pathophysiology of cortical and spinal seizures induced by ammonia intoxication is not well understood. In addition, it has not been investigated when these spinal seizures occur during the course of ammonia intoxication. This study attempts to elucidate these little understood issues.

2. Spinal and Cortical Seizures

Experiments were conducted in pentobarbital anesthetized cats paralyzed with gallamine triethiodide and artificially respirated as described elsewhere in detail (6). In brief, pentobarbital sodium 50–90 mg/kg i.v. was given every 4–8 h to suppress monosynaptic reflex discharges. The monosynaptic motoneuron pool population excitatory postsynaptic potential (EPSP) was recorded at the ventral root L_7 or S_1 (VR–EPSP, L_7VR, S_1VR) (7). The monosynaptic focal synaptic potential (FSP) was recorded with an extracellular electrode in a motoneuron nucleus (8). An electrode at the dorsal root L_7 or S_1 (L_7DR, S_1DR) entry into the spinal cord recorded the dorsal root action potential. The nerves to the posterior biceps and semitendinous muscles (PBST), medial and lateral gastrocnemius muscles (MG, LG) or the common peroneal nerve (Per) were stimulated at 1.5xT to excite Ia–afferent fibers (9). Spontaneous activity on extracellular and ventral root electrodes was recorded with a band pass of 0.1 KHz to 10 KHz. Evoked potentials at dorsal root, extracellular and ventral root electrodes were recorded with a band pass of 0.5–5 Hz to 10 KHz. An EEG, bandpass 5 Hz to 300 Hz, was recorded via a gold pin (1 mm $\varnothing$) inserted into the skull over the left cruciate gyrus.

In control conditions, the ventral root (VR) showed no spontaneous discharges. With infusion of ammonium acetate (AA), action potentials appeared spontaneously at irregular intervals in the VR (spontaneous discharges, SDs) (N=18), Figure 1, AA 6.33 mmol/kg, and Figure 2 A. Further infusion of AA produced spontaneous bursts of action potentials in the VR in addition to the irregular action potential discharges, Figure 1, AA 6.65 mmol/kg. These action potential bursts were distinct from SDs because action potentials occurred for a prolonged period of time. Action potential bursts were arbitrarily defined as spinal seizures (SZs) when they lasted for more than 50 ms, Figure 2. The action potential bursts underlying SZs were not stereotyped and changed with each SZ. The SZs could be of the crescendo type, Figure 1, the decrescendo type, Figure 2 B, the spindle type, Figure 2 C, or consist of

Neurology, VA Medical Center, Depts. Neurology and Physiology, University of Minnesota, Minneapolis, 55417

Hepatic Encephalopathy, Hyperammonemia, and Ammonia Toxicity
Edited by V. Felipo and S. Grisolia, Plenum Press, New York, 1994

55

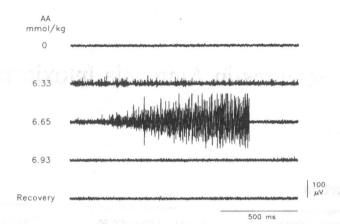

Figure 1. Effects of increasing doses of AA on spontaneous action potential discharges in VR. AA 0 mmol/kg – absence of spontaneous action potentials before AA. AA 6.33 mmol/kg – spontaneous action potential discharges (SDs) in S₁VR. AA 6.65 mmol/kg – SDs and SZs in S₁VR. AA, 6.93 mmol/kg – absence of spontaneous discharges in S₁VR. Recovery – absence of spontaneous discharges in S₁VR 15 min after end of AA. In this and all subsequent figures electronegativity is upwards.

repetitive bursts, Figure 2 D. When infusion of AA was continued beyond the appearance of SZs, all action potential activity in the VR ceased, Figure 1, AA 6.93 mmol/kg. During and after recovery from AA infusion, the VR showed no SDs or SZs, Figure 1, Recovery.

The dose of AA necessary to initiate SDs was 4.66±0.60 mmol/kg (mean±S.E.M., N=9, first AA infusions only). In four animals, SDs were followed by SZs. In these four animals, SDs occurred at 4.54±1.09 mmol/kg of AA (mean±S.E.M., N=4), and SZs occurred at 5.72±0.96 mmol/kg of AA (mean±S.E.M., N=4). The AA dose to initiate SZs was significantly higher (p<0.05) than the dose necessary to initiate SDs. The AA dose to terminate all discharges in the VR, SDs and SZs, was 6.36 mmol/kg±1.00 (mean±S.E.M., N=3).

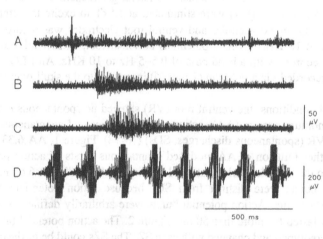

Figure 2. Patterns of spontaneous action potential activity in VR produced by AA. A – irregular spontaneous action potential discharges and randomly occurring action potential bursts lasting <50 ms, i.e. SDs. B – spontaneous action potential burst >50 ms duration, i.e., SZ, of decrescendo type. C – SZ of spindle type. D – repetitive SZs. Records from S₁VR. A, B and C from same experiment.

The extracellular electrode in the ventral horn never reflected SDs or SZs recorded at the VR electrode, Figure 3 A. This observation could be potentially explained by an exclusion of the particular motoneuron nucleus recorded from the hyperexcitation underlying SDs and SZs. However, the lack of all signs of hyperexcitation including action potentials at the extracellular electrode during numerous seizures in five different experiments made this explanation unlikely. The extracellular space acts as low–pass filter. Long duration voltage transients like synaptic potentials give rise to a greater extracellular potential than do short duration and large amplitude transients like action potentials (10). Accordingly, when AA initiated a reflex discharge superimposed on a VR–EPSP, no reflex discharge was superimposed on the simultaneously recorded FSP, Figure 3 B.

As a rule, the occurrence of SDs and SZs was not associated with signs of altered excitability of the cerebral cortex, e.g., high voltage sharp waves in the EEG as signs of cerebral cortical seizures, Figure 4. Only in one of nine experiments, the occurrence of SZs was associated with the appearance of high voltage sharp waves in the EEG. These high voltage sharp waves were seen only during the period that SDs and SZs occurred, Figure 5 asterisk.

In summary, a systemic ammonia intoxication not only initiates spinal seizures but also terminates these seizures. Because of low–pass filter properties of the spinal cord tissue, extracellular electrodes in the ventral horn do not show seizure discharges. Only rarely, spinal seizures are associated with seizure discharges in the EEG. When ammonia intoxication is discontinued as soon as seizures occur, the animal can recover completely from the effects of NH_4^+.

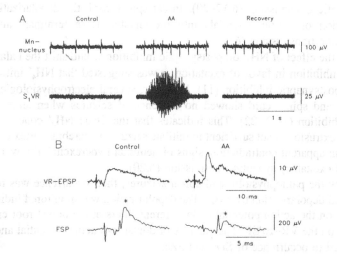

Figure 3. A – SZs recorded from VR are not reflected in simultaneous extracellular record from motoneuron nucleus. Control – absence of spontaneous discharges in extracellular record from motoneuron nucleus (Mn–nucleus) and at S_1VR before AA. AA – AA, 7.68 mmol/kg i.v., produces SZ in S_1VR without change of electrical activity in motoneuron nucleus. Recovery – absence of spontaneous discharges at 14 min after termination of AA i.v. Record from motoneuron nucleus contaminated by EKG. B – Action potentials generated by motoneurons show in record from VR but not in record from motoneuron nucleus. Control – PBST stimulation elicits VR–EPSP at S_1VR and FSP in PBST motoneuron nucleus. AA – AA i.v. elicits a reflex discharge from VR–EPSP; arrow indicates origin of reflex discharge from VR–EPSP, which is decreased in amplitude. Reflex discharge has no correlate in simultaneous extracellular record from PBST motoneuron nucleus, i.e., FSP. Asterisks mark FSP. FSP decreased by AA i.v. Negative spike preceding FSP is afferent fiber spike (ref. 6).

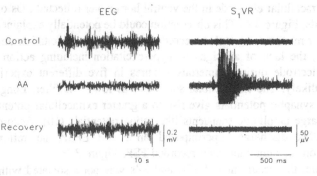

Figure 4. EEG during spinal seizures. Simultaneous records of EEG and S_1VR. Control EEG and S_1VR records before AA infusion. AA – after AA, 4.44 mmol/kg, EEG is of low voltage and shows no correlate to SDs and SZ in S_1VR. Recovery – 20 min after termination of AA i.v., the EEG and VR resemble control records.

3. Pathogenesis of Spinal Seizures

NH_4^+ has two known effects on the function of neurons. These effects depend on the concentration of NH_4^+. The extrusion of Cl^- from neurons is inactivated by about 1.0 mM NH_4^+ (11–16). The inactivation of Cl^-–extrusion shifts the equilibrium potential of the IPSP to the resting membrane potential, abolishes the hyperpolarizing action of postsynaptic inhibition and impairs the efficacy of postsynaptic inhibition to suppress neuronal excitation (14). NH_4^+, >1.5–2 mM, depolarizes the resting membrane potential (6,16,17) and decreases excitatory synaptic transmission (6,17–20). In cat spinal cord, the depolarization by NH_4^+ blocks conduction of action potentials into presynaptic nerve terminals and decreases excitatory synaptic transmission (6).

Because the effect of NH_4^+ on postsynaptic inhibition would shift the balance between excitation and inhibition in favor of excitation, it was suggested that NH_4^+ initiates seizures by decreasing postsynaptic inhibition (11). However, several electrophysiological studies in cerebral cortex and spinal cord showed no evidence of seizures when ammonia affected postsynaptic inhibition (14,21,22). This indicates that the tissue NH_4^+ concentration which inactivates Cl^-–extrusion is not sufficient to inititate seizures in cerebral cortex or spinal cord. In contrast, in an apparent contradiction, signs of neuronal hyperexcitability were seen when NH_4^+ decreased excitatory synaptic transmission (6,20).

To clarify the pathophysiology of spinal seizures, their occurrence was related to the signs of neuronal depolarization by NH_4^+. The depolarization was monitored indirectly by the effects of NH_4^+ on the action potential of Ia–afferent fibers at the dorsal root entry into the spinal cord and on the VR–EPSP. The changes of dorsal root action potential and VR–EPSP were then related to occurrence of SDs and SZs.

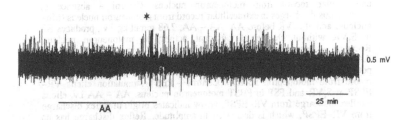
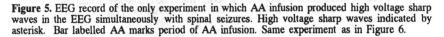

Figure 5. EEG record of the only experiment in which AA infusion produced high voltage sharp waves in the EEG simultaneously with spinal seizures. High voltage sharp waves indicated by asterisk. Bar labelled AA marks period of AA infusion. Same experiment as in Figure 6.

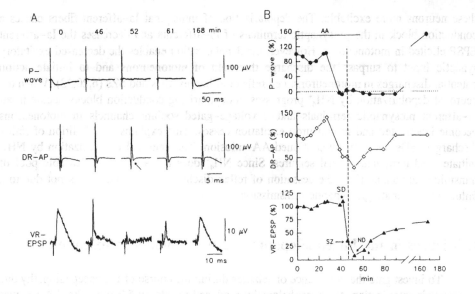

Figure 6. SDs and SZs in relation to effects of AA on excitatory synaptic transmission from low threshold muscle afferents. A – P-wave, dorsal root action potential (DR-AP) and VR-EPSP elicited by PBST stimulation. Numbers above tracings indicate time in minutes after begin of AA infusion. AA i.v. 6.88 mmol/kg in 59 min. Arrow points to decreased second positive phase of DR-AP after AA. Decreased VR-EPSPs trigger reflex discharges at min 46 and 61. Records from S_1DR and S_1VR. B – Plots of amplitudes of P-wave (●), second positive phase of DR-AP (◊) and VR-EPSP (▲). Asterisks indicate estimated VR-EPSP amplitudes because reflex discharges obscured peak of VR-EPSP. Bar labelled AA indicates period of AA infusion. "SD" and "SZ" indicate occurrences of SDs and SZs. "ND" indicates no spontaneous discharges in VR. Cat, pentobarbital anesthesia, cf. ref. 6.

AA infusion decreased and eventually abolished the VR-EPSP indicating a decrease of monosynaptic excitatory synaptic transmission (6), Figure 6. AA regularly initiated reflex discharges from the VR-EPSP in spite of a significant decrease in amplitude of the VR-EPSP, Figure 6 A, VR-EPSP, 46 and 61 min. The decrease of the VR-EPSP was associated with decreases of the second positive phase of the triphasic afferent spike recorded from the DR-electrode and the P-wave, a sign of presynaptic inhibition, Figure 6. The P-wave decreased slightly earlier and recovered later than the VR-EPSP from the effects of AA, Figure 6 B.

The decrease of the second positive phase of the afferent fiber spike is a sign of a depolarizing conduction block for action potentials in presynaptic terminals of Ia-afferents (6). Decrease of VR-EPSP is caused by this conduction block which decreases excitatory synaptic transmission from Ia-afferents to motoneurons (6). Initiation of reflex discharges by a decreased VR-EPSP is indicative of a depolarization of motoneurons. Thus, the depolarization by NH_4^+ has two sequelae on excitatory synaptic transmission from Ia-afferents to motoneurons: (i) excitatory synaptic transmission decreases due to a depolarizing conduction block in intraspinal presynaptic terminals of Ia-afferent fibers, and (ii) the depolarization enables decreased synaptic excitation of motoneurons to surpass the motoneuron discharge threshold.

SDs and SZs occurred only when AA initiated a reflex discharge from the VR-EPSP. While SDs could be seen when an unchanged or mildly decreased VR-EPSP triggered a reflex discharge, SZs were only seen when the VR-EPSP had decreased to <50% of control. SDs and SZs ceased when AA-infusion decreased the VR-EPSP to <10% of control and could be considered abolished, Figure 6 B. SDs or SZs were never seen during the recovery from AA infusion.

These data show that ammonia intoxication produces SDs and SZs when NH_4^+ exerts a depolarizing action on neurons. This depolarization affects motoneurons and the intraspinal terminals of Ia-afferent fibers in the spinal cord. The depolarization of motoneurons makes these neurons more excitable. The depolarization of intraspinal Ia–afferent fibers causes a conduction block in the presynaptic terminals of Ia–afferents and decreases the Ia–afferent EPSP elicited in motoneurons. However, the depolarization enables the decreased excitatory synaptic input to surpass the discharge threshold of motoneurons and to initiate action potential discharges in motoneurons, i.e., reflex discharges, SDs and SZs (6,20,23). When the neuronal depolarization by NH_4^+ progresses, a depolarizing conduction blocks occurs in all Ia–afferent presynaptic terminals and/or voltage–gated sodium channels in motoneurons become inactivated and motoneuron excitation ceases. This explains the abolition of reflex discharges, SDs and SZs by continued AA–infusion. The neuronal depolarization by NH_4^+ initiates and terminates spinal seizures. Since NH_4^+ does not affect the releasable pool of transmitter glutamate (24), the cessation of reflex discharges, SDs and SZs is not due to a failure of glutamatergic synaptic transmission.

4. Seizures in the Encephalopathy due to Ammonia Intoxication

To investigate the occurrence of seizures during the course of the encephalopathy due to ammonia intoxication, the encephalopathy produced in rats by 5.2 mmol/kg AA i.p. was subdivided into different stages. The encephalopathy was graded according to the following criteria: (i) hyperventilation, (ii) loss of motor activity in response to pull on a limb (motor response), (iii) loss of the righting reflex, and (vi) loss of a whole body jerk in response to a loud hand clap (startle response) (25), see Table 1. Animals with grade 4 encephalopathy laid motionless on their side and did not respond to sensory stimuli, i.e, were in coma.

The occurrence of seizures was related to encephalopathy grade. Clonic movements or tonic extremity extremity movements or tonic body extension were taken as signs of seizures. In addition, seizures were characterized as to their type, partial or generalized. Clonic jerks always involved a whole extremity and, therefore, were counted as partial clonic seizures. The electrical activity of the cerebral cortex (EEG), spinal cord or nerve trunks was not monitored. Therefore, non–convulsive, i.e., electrical seizures, if they occurred, were not recorded.

The mean encephalopathy grade of all animals (N=28) is shown in Figure 7 A. Three animals each reached only Grade 2 and Grade 3 encephalopathy, respectively. Twenty–two animals reached encephalopathy grade 4. The highest encephalopathy grade for all animals was 3.54±0.17 (mean±S.E., N=28) at min 24–26 after AA i.p. Grade 4 encephalopathy was reached at 22±1 (mean±S.E., N=22, range: 16–38) minutes after AA i.p. Grade 4 encephalopathy lasted for 23.05±3.25 (mean±S.E., N=22, range: 6–50) minutes. Two animals died during grade 4 encephalopathy.

Table 1. Grading system to stage the encephalopathy due to ammonia intoxication.

Encephalopathy Grade	Respiration	Motor Response	Righting Reflex	Startle Response
0	Normal	+	+	+
1	HV	+	+	+
2	HV	–	+	+
3	HV	–	–	+
4	HV	–	–	–

HV – hyperventilation, (+) – present, (–) – absent. From ref. 25.

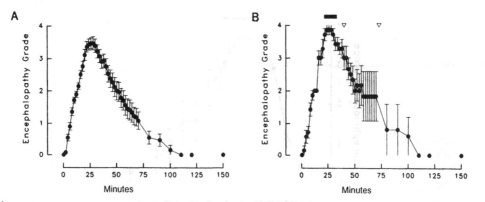

Figure 7. Encephalopathy in rat due to AA 5.2 mmol/kg bodyweight i.p. A – Plot of encephalopathy grade (mean±S.E.) of all animals (N=∞) vs. time after AA i.p. B – Plot of encephalopathy grade (mean±S.E.) of those animals which developed seizures (N=7) vs. time after AA i.p. Occurrence of partial or generalized clonic seizures is indicated by bar. Occurrence of tonic extensor seizures with subsequent death of the animal is indicated by inverted triangles.

Fifteen animals reached grade 4 encephalopathy, i.e., were in coma, and never had seizures. Seizures were observed in only seven animals and only after the onset of grade 4 encephalopathy. Five animals had partial or generalized clonic seizures. In these animals the duration of seizure activity was less than the duration of grade 4 encephalopathy. All five animals with partial or generalized clonic seizures recovered fully from the encephalopathy due to AA i.p., see Table 2 and Figure 7 B.

Two animals had seizures characterized by tonic extension of all four extremities. Both animals died within 30–60 seconds after onset of these seizures. The onset of grade 4 encephalopathy in one of these two animals was with 38 minutes significantly later than in all other animals. This late onset of grade 4 encephalopathy produced a statistically significant difference between the onset of grade 4 encephalopathy in animals without seizures and the two animals with tonic seizures.

Seizures occured only in animals which reached the highest grade of encephalopathy, grade 4, the equivalent of coma. Only a minority of the animals with grade 4 encephalopathy developed seizures. No animal had seizures without reaching grade 4 encephalopathy. Therefore, it may be inferred that the development of seizures indicates a more severe grade of encephalopathy than grade 4 encephalopathy (coma). This encephalopathy grade may be called grade 5 encephalopathy (coma + seizures).

The type of seizures seen had a certain prognostic value. Tonic extensor seizures were always followed by death within about one minute. Partial or generalized clonic seizures were compatible with survival and complete recovery of the animal from the effects of AA.

Table 2. Grade 4 Encephalopathy (Coma), Seizures and Death in the Encephalopathy due to Ammonia Intoxication.

Encephalopathy	Seizures	N	Death (N)	Onset Grade 4 (min)	Onset Seizures (min)	Duration Grade 4 (min)	Duration Seizures (min)
Grade 4 (Coma)	–	15	0	21.5±0.9* (18–28)	–	26.3±4.3 (6–50)	–
Grade 4 (Coma)	Clonic	5	0	20.4±2.5 (16–24)	22.2±1.8 (17–27)	12.4±1.9 (10–20)	10.8±1.7 (6–15)
Grade 4 (Coma)	Tonic	2	2	30.0±8.0* (22–38)	56.0±16.5 (39.5–72.5)	25.5±9.5 (16–25)	<1

Data are mean±S.E.; numbers in parentheses give the range of observations.
* p<0.05; all other comparisons are NS.

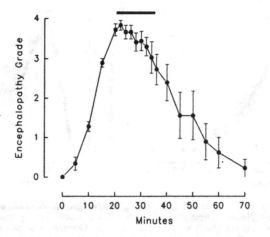

Figure 8. H–reflex in the encephalopathy due to ammonia intoxication (rat, 5.2 mmol/kg AA i.p.). Plot of encephalopathy grade (mean±S.E.) vs. time after AA i.p. All animals (N=9) lost the H–reflex and eventually recovered from the encephalopathy. Solid bar marks average period of disappearance of H–reflex. Modified from ref. 25.

These observations correspond to those by other investigators on the effects of 5.0–5.2 mmol/kg of AA i.p. in rats and mice (26–29). In particular, Hindfeldt and Siesjö (28) McCandless and Schenker (29) described that ammonia intoxication produced unresponsiveness before the occurrence of seizures.

The occurrence of seizures in unanesthetized rats correlates well with signs of neuronal depolarization by NH_4^+. The H–reflex disappears as a sign of neuronal depolarization by NH_4^+ (20,25). Neuronal depolarization by NH_4^+ decreases excitatory synaptic transmission so that EPSPs in motoneurons do not surpass the discharge threshold for action potentials. The H–reflex disappears at the transition from grade 3 to grade 4 encephalopathy or during grade 4 encephalopathy, Figure 8. This time of disappearance of the H–reflex corresponds well to the period when seizures occur, cf. Figure 7 B. Thus, also in unanesthetized rats seizures occur only when signs of neuronal depolarization by NH_4^+ can be detected.

5. Conclusions

Ammonia intoxication produces seizures in experimental animals. The seizures are almost exclusively spinal in origin. A pathogenesis of seizures due to ammonia intoxication can be suggested. Although ammonia intoxication inactivates Cl^--extrusion from neurons and impairs neuronal postsynaptic inhibition, inefficacy of neuronal inhibition in cerebral cortex and spinal cord is not associated with seizures. Seizures occur only when a progressive ammonia intoxication is continued beyond the stage that impairs inhibition and signs of neuronal depolarization occur. Neuronal depolarization partially decreases excitatory synaptic transmission due to conduction block for action potentials in presynaptic terminals. However, depolarization of the resting membrane potential permits the remaining synaptic excitation to exceed the discharge threshold and to initiate abnormal action potential discharges, i.e., reflex discharges as well as spontaneous discharges in the form of SDs and SZs. Progressive ammonia intoxication continued beyond the occurrence of seizures terminates the seizures. Excessive neuronal depolarization by NH_4^+ blocks all synaptic transmission and/or renders neurons inexcitable.

In the encephalopathy induced by moderate doses of AA, seizures occur only in animals which are already severely encphalopathic and are in coma, i.e., totally unresponsive to all sensory stimuli. This observation contradicts the belief that ammonia intoxication produces seizures before coma, and that ammonia induced coma represents postictal coma (30,31). The occurrence of seizures represents a grade of encephalopathy more advanced than coma. Although most animals recover readily from ammonia induced seizures, some animals may die during or after the occurrence of seizures. The occurrence of seizures in the encephalopathy due to ammonia intoxication indicates that the animal reached a stage of encephalopathy which is on the verge of being irreversible and may result in death (23).

Acknowledgements: This research was supported by grants from the Department of Veterans Affairs.

References

1. Trendelenburg, P., 1923, Ammoniak and Ammoniumsalze. In: HANDBUCH DER EXPERIMENTELLEN PHARMAKOLOGIE, A. Heefter, W. Heubner, O. Eichler and A. Farah (Eds.), Berlin, Springer, Vol. 1, pp. 470–503.
2. Ajmone-Marsan, C., Fuortes, M.G.F. and Marossero, F., 1949, Influence of ammonium chloride on the electrical activity of the brain and spinal cord, Electroenceph. Clin. Neurophysiol. 1:291–298.
3. Torda, C., 1953, Ammonium ion content and electrical activity of the brain during the preconvulsive and convulsive phases induced by various convulsants, J. Pharmacol. Exp. Ther. 107:197–203.
4. Tews, J.K., Carter, S.H., Roa, P.D. and Stone, W.E., 1963, Free amino acids and related compounds in dog brain: post-mortem and anoxic changes, effects of ammonium chloride infusion, and levels during seizures induced by picrotoxin and pentylenetetrazol, J. Neurochem. 10:641–653.
5. Gastaut, H., Saier, J., Mano, T., Santos, D. and Lyagoubi, S., 1968, Generalized epileptic seizures, induced by "non-convulsant" substances. Part 2. Experimental study with special reference to ammonium chloride, Epilepsia 9:317–327.
6. Raabe, W., 1989, Ammonia decrease excitatory synaptic transmission in cat spinal cord in vivo, J. Neurophysiol. 62:1461–1473.
7. Eccles, J.C., 1946, Synaptic potentials of motoneurones, J. Neurophysiol. 9:87–120.
8. Brooks, McC. and Eccles, J.C., 1947, Electrical investigation of the monosynaptic pathway through the spinal cord, J. Neurophysiol. 10:251–274.
9. Bradley, K. and Eccles, J.C., 1953, Analysis of fast afferent impulses from thigh muscles, J. Physiol. Lond. 122:462–473.
10. Humphrey, D.R., 1968, Re-analysis of the antidromic cortical response. II. On the contribution of cell discharge and PSPs to the evoked potentials, Electroenceph. Clin. Neurophysiol. 25:421–442.
11. Lux, H.D., Loracher, C. and Neher, E., 1970, The action of ammonium on postsynaptic inhibition of cat spinal motoneurons, Exp. Brain Res. 11:431–447.
12. Lux, H.D., 1971, Ammonium and chloride extrusion: hyperpolarising synaptic inhibition in spinal motoneurones, Science Wash. DC 173:555–557.
13. Llinas, R., Baker, R. and Precht, W., 1974, Blockade of inhibition by ammonium acetate action on chloride pump in cat trochlear motoneurons, J. Neurophysiol. 37:522–533.
14. Raabe, W. and Gumnit, R.J., 1975, Disinhibition in cat motor cortex by ammonia, J. Neurophysiol. 38:347–355.
15. Raabe, W. and Lin, S., 1984, Ammonia, postsynaptic inhibition and CNS-energy state, Brain Res. 303:67–76.
16. Nicoll, R.A., 1978, The blockade of GABA mediated responses in the frog spinal cord by ammonium ions and furosemide, J. Physiol. Lond. 283:121–132.
17. Alger, B.E. and Nicoll, R., 1984, Ammonia does not selectively block IPSPs in rat hippocampal cells, J. Neurophysiol. 49:1381–1392.
18. Théoret, Y., Davies, M.F., Esplin, B. and Capek, R., 1985, Effects of ammonium chloride on synaptic transmission in the rat hippocampal slice, Neuroscience 14:798–806.

19. Théoret, Y. and Bossu, J.-L., 1985, Effects of ammonium salts on synaptic transmission to hippocampal CA1 and CA3 pyramidal cells in vivo, Neuroscience 14:807–821.
20. Raabe, W., 1990, Effects of NH_4^+ on reflexes in cat spinal cord, J. Neurophysiol. 64:565–574.
21. Raabe, W. and Lin, S., 1985, Pathophysiology of ammonia intoxication, Exp. Neurol. 87:519–532.
22. Lin, S. and Raabe, W., 1985, Ammonia intoxication: Effects on cerebral cortex and spinal cord, J. Neurochem. 44:1252–1258.
23. Raabe, W., 1991, Effects of NH_4^+ on the function of the CNS, Adv. Exp. Med. Biol. 272:89–98.
24. Raabe, W., 1992, Ammonium ions abolish excitatory synaptic transmission between cerebellar neurons in primary dissociated tissue culture, J. Neurophysiol. 68:93–99.
25. Raabe W., 1987, The H-reflex in the encephalopathy due to ammonia intoxication, Exp. Neurol. 96:601–611.
26. Hindfeldt, B., Plum, F. and Duffy, T.E., 1977, Effect of acute ammonia intoxication on cerebral metabolism in rats with portacaval shunts, J. Clin. Invest. 59:386–396.
27. Ehrlich, M., Plum, F. and Duffy, T.E., 1980, Blood and brain ammonia concentrations after portacaval anastomosis. Effects of acute ammonia, J. Neurochem. 34:1538–1542.
28. Hindfeldt, B., Siesjö, B.K., 1971, Cerebral effects of acute ammonia intoxication. I. The influence on intracellular and extracellular acid–base parameters, Scand J. clin. Lab. Invest. 28:353–364.
29. McCandless, D.W. and Schenker, S., 1981, Effect of acute ammonia intoxication on energy stores in the cerebral reticular activating system, Exp. Brain Res. 44:325–330.
30. Ferenci, P., Pappas, S.C., Munson, P.J. and Jones, E.A., 1984, Changes in glutamate receptors on synaptic membranes associated with hepatic encephalopathy or hyperammonemia in the rabbit, HEPATOLOGY 4:25–29.
31. Ferenci, P., 1992, Current concepts in the pathophysiology of hepatic encephalopathy, Eur. J. Clin. Invest. 22:573–581.

Molecular Mechanism of Acute Ammonia Toxicity and of its Prevention by L-Carnitine

Vicente Felipo, Elena Kosenko, María-Dolores Miñana, Goizane Marcaida and Santiago Grisolía

1. Introduction

One of the more remarkable consequences of liver failure (fulminant hepatic failure, liver cirrhosis, etc) and of deficiencies in the enzymes of the urea cycle is the defective elimination of ammonia and the increase of ammonia levels in blood. Hyperammonemia seems to be one of the main factors contributing to the pathogenesis of hepatic encephalopathy and, probably, to the development of hepatic coma.

Ammonia is a product of the metabolism of proteins and other compounds and it is also required for the synthesis of essential compounds for the cells. However, when it is in excess, ammonia is a toxic compound. A five- to ten-fold increase of the normal ammonia levels in blood induces toxic effects in most animal species, with alterations in the function of the central nervous system.

Ammonia toxicity was reported one century ago by Hahn et al (1). They subjected dogs to an Eck's fistula, excluding the liver from the circulation, and found that when these animals were fed meat, they developed hyperammonemia, which was associated with coma and death of the dogs. It is also well known that injection of large doses of ammonium salts causes the death in many animal species. During the last century a lot of work has been done trying to unveil the mechanism involved in acute ammonia toxicity; however, this mechanism still remains unclear.

To study the effects of hyperammonemia and of hepatic failure a number of different animal models have been used (see chapter from Dr. Mullen in this book). Animal models of hepatic failure produce, in addition to hyperammonemia, other alterations which make difficult to discern which effects are produced by hyperammonemia and which are mediated by other factors. Also, the levels of hyperammonemia usually reached with these models are not enough to induce per se the death of the animal. Therefore these animal models, which can be good models of hepatic failure and/or hepatic encephalopathy, are not suitable to study the molecular mechanism of acute ammonia toxicity.

In this chapter we will discuss the molecular mechanism involved in the mediation of the toxicity of a large amount of an ammonium salt injected to a normal animal.

Instituto de Investigaciones Citológicas de la Fundación Valenciana de Investigaciones Biomédicas. Amadeo de Saboya, 4. 46010 Valencia. Spain

Hepatic Encephalopathy, Hyperammonemia, and Ammonia Toxicity
Edited by V. Felipo and S. Grisolia, Plenum Press, New York, 1994

65

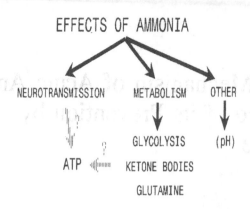

Figure 1. Some parameters which are affected by ammonia in brain.

Acute ammonia toxicity affetcs many parameters in brain, including metabolism, neurotransmission and possibly others like pH (Figure 1).

Injection of large doses of ammonia into animals is associated with marked alterations in brain energy metabolites, including increased lactate, pyruvate, glucose and mitochondrial $[NAD^+]/[NADH]$ and decreased glycogen, ketone bodies, cytosolic $[NAD^+]/[NADH]$ and, in a later step, decreased ATP content (2-7).

Ammonia intoxication also affects markedly the brain content of ammonia metabolites, with a remarkable increase in glutamine and decreased content of glutamate (3,4,6,7). Bessman and Bessman (8) found that, in hyperammonemia, the brain removes ammonia from the blood and suggested that incorporation of ammonia into glutamate and glutamine would deplete α-ketoglutarate, thus interfering the function of the Krebs cycle and leading to depletion of ATP. It has been later shown that, for the whole brain, ammonia toxicity induces depletion of ATP without affecting the content of α-ketoglutarate. It has also been suggested that ATP depletion could be a consequence of the increased synthesis of glutamine, since glutamine synthetase consumes ATP.

In spite of much work, it is not clear which is the mechanism by which ammonia leads to ATP depletion and to the death of the animals. It is also unclear which of the above alterations are directly related to ATP depletion and animal death and which are not.

We have shown that acute ammonia toxicity is prevented by MK-801, a selective antagonist of the NMDA type of glutamate receptors (9), suggesting that activation of these receptors mediates ammonia toxicity. We then decided to use MK-801 as a tool to discern which of the above effects of ammonia are directly involved in ammonia toxicity and ATP depletion and which are not. Since MK-801 prevents ammonia-induced death of the animals, changes in those parameters directly related to the death would be prevented by MK-801 and the ammonia-induced alterations which are not prevented by MK-801 should not play a role in the mediation of ammonia toxicity.

2. Molecular Mechanism of Ammonia-Induced Depletion of Brain ATP and of Ammonia Toxicity

2.1 Ammonia-Induced Depletion of Brain ATP is Mediated by Activation of the NMDA Receptor

We first assessed whether depletion of ATP induced by injection of large doses of ammonia is mediated by activation of the NMDA receptor. To test this possibility we injected

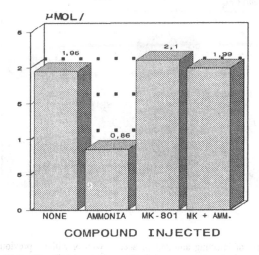

Figure 2. MK–801 prevents depletion of brain ATP induced by ammonium injection. Groups of 12 rats were injected intraperitoneally with 7 mmol/Kg of ammonium acetate with or without previous injection of 2 mg/Kg of MK–801 (i.p., 15 min before ammonia). Rats were killed 15 min after ammonium injection, brains were taken immediately and ATP content was measured. Data from (42).

rats i.p. with 7 mmol/kg of ammonium acetate with or without previous injection of MK–801, a selective antagonist of the NMDA receptor.

As shown in Fig. 2, 15 min after injection of 7 mmol/kg of ammonium acetate, the content of ATP in brain decreased by 56%. This depletion of ATP is completely prevented by previous injection of MK–801. This suggests that activation of the NMDA receptor mediates ammonia–induced ATP depletion.

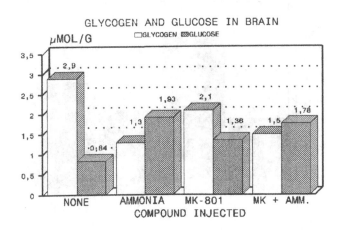

Figure 3. Effects of injecting ammonium acetate with or without previous injection of MK–801 on the brain levels of glycogen and glucose. Experiments were carried out exactly as in Fig. 1. Data from (42).

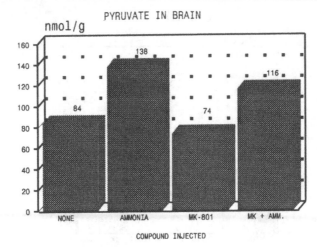

PYRUVATE IN BRAIN

Figure 4. Effects of injecting ammonium acetate with or without previous injecti on of MK–801 on the brain content of pyruvate. Experiments were carried out as in Fig. 1. Data from (42).

2.2 The Effects of Acute Ammonia Intoxication on Other Brain Energy Metabolites are not Mediated by Activation of the NMDA Receptor

Injection of ammonia induces a remarkable decrease in brain glycogen (57%) and an increase in free glucose (230% of control). As shown in Fig. 3, previous injection of MK–801 did not prevent at all these changes, indicating that they are not mediated by activation of the NMDA receptor.

Ammonium injection also induces an increase in the brain content of pyruvate (64%) and lactate (126%). These effects are only slightly prevented by injection of MK–801 (Figs 4 and 5).

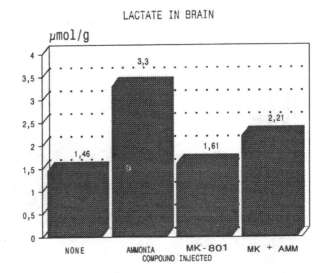

LACTATE IN BRAIN

Figure 5. Effects of injecting ammonium acetate with or without previous injecti on of MK–801 on the brain content of lactate. Experiments were carried out as in Fig. 1. Data from (42).

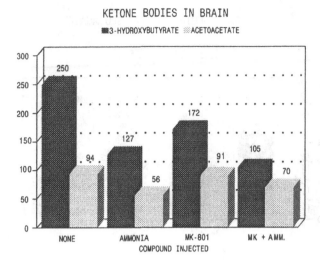

Figure 6. Effects of injecting ammonium acetate with or without previous injection of MK–801 on the brain content of ketone bodies. Experiments were carried out as in Fig. 1. Data from (42).

Acute ammonia intoxication also induces a depletion of ketone bodies in brain. 3–Hydroxybutyrate decreases by 50% and acetoacetate by 40%. As shown in Fig. 6, these changes are not prevented at all by previous injection of MK–801.

These results indicate that the effects of ammonium injection on energy metabolites other than ATP are not mediated by activation of the NMDA receptor. The effects on these compounds are the same in animals injected with ammonia alone and in those previously injected with MK–801; however, animals in the first group die while those injected previously with the antagonist of the NMDA receptor survive. This indicates that changes in these compounds are not directly related with the death of the animal. Also, ATP content decreases in animals injected with ammonia alone but not in those previously injected with MK–801; this indicates that changes in the above compounds are not directly involved in the ammonia–induced depletion of ATP.

2.3 Ammonia–Induced Changes in Brain Glutamine and Glutamate are not Prevented by MK–801

Glutamine content in brain increased by 147% 15 min after injection of 7 mmol/kg of ammonium acetate while glutamate content decreased by 38%. Injection of MK–801 alone also induced a slight increase of glutamine (39%) and a slight decrease of glutamate (21%). In animals injected with both MK–801 and ammonia, glutamine increase (218%) and glutamate decrease (48%) were greater than in rats injected with ammonia alone (Fig. 7). These results show that blocking the NMDA receptor did not prevent but further estimulate ammonia–induced changes in glutamine and glutamate. This indicates that alterations of these metabolites do not play a direct role in ammonia toxicity. Also, in rats injected with ammonia alone (with ATP depletion) glutamine reached 9.4 μmol/g and in those injected with both MK–801 and ammonia (without ATP depletion) glutamine reached 12.1 μmol/g. This indicates that ATP depletion is not a consequence of accumulation of glutamine.

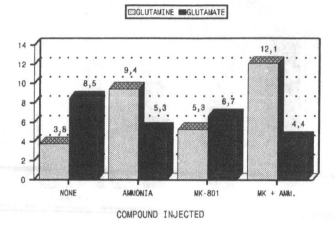

Figure 7. Effects of injecting ammonium acetate with or without previous injecti on of MK–801 on the brain content of glutamine and glutamate. Experiments were carried out as in Fig. 1. Data from (42).

2.4 Ammonium Injection Induces an NMDA Receptor–Mediated Activation of Brain Na⁺/K⁺–ATPase

The fact that MK–801, a selective antagonist of the NMDA receptor, completely prevents ammonia–induced ATP depletion (Fig. 2), suggests that activation of this receptor is involved in the increased consumption of ATP. Activation of the NMDA receptor leads to the opening of the associated ion channel, allowing the entry into the neuron of Ca^{2+} and Na^+. To maintain Na^+ homeostasis, the excess of Na^+ entering through the ion channel must be extruded and this work is mainly carried out by Na^+/K^+–ATPase. We therefore supposed that activation of the NMDA receptor following ammonium injection should be associated with increased activity of the ATPase, which in turn could be responsible for depletion of ATP. To test this possibility we measured Na^+/K^+–ATPase activity in brains of rats injected or not with ammonium acetate with or without previous injection of MK–801. As shown in Fig. 8, the activity of the ATPase increased by 78% 15 min after injection of 7 mmol/kg of ammonium acetate. It is also shown that MK–801 completely prevents activation of the ATPase, indicating that this is mediated by activation of the NMDA receptor.

2.5 Ammonia–Induced Activation of Na⁺/K⁺–ATPase is Due to Decreased Protein Kinase C–Dependent Phosphorylation of the ATPase

The fact that ammonia–induced activation of the ATPase can be measured in vitro after preparation of brain homogenates suggests that this activation is a consequence of a covalent modification of the enzyme. It is well known that Na^+/K^+–ATPase is a substrate for protein kinase C (10) and that phosphorylation of the ATPase by PKC decreases its activity (11–13). We have previously shown that hyperammonemia decreases PKC–mediated phosphorylation of the microtubule–associated protein MAP–2 (14). It is therefore possible that increased activity of the ATPase in ammonia–injected animals could be due to decreased

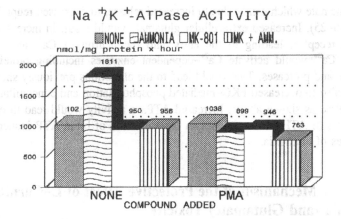

Figure 8. Brain Na⁺/K⁺-ATPase activity is increased after ammonium injection and the increase is prevented by MK-801 and reversed by addition of PMA in vitro. Groups of 8 rats were injected and killed exactly as in Fig. 1 and Na⁺/K⁺-ATPase activity was determined. To test whether ammonia-induced activation of the ATPase is due to decreased PKC-mediated phosphorylation, the ATPase activity was determined in the absence or the presence of 150 nM PMA, an activator of PKC. Data from (42).

phosphorylation by PKC. We tested this possibility by measuring Na⁺/K⁺-ATPase activity in the same homogenates in the presence of PMA, an activator of PKC. As shown in Fig. 8, under these conditions, the increase in the activity of the ATPase in samples from ammonia-injected rats is completely reversed, thus confirming that activation is due to decreased PKC-mediated phosphorylation of the ATPase. As shown above, this effect is mediated by activation of the NMDA receptor and can be due to decreased activity of PKC or to increased activity of a phosphatase that dephosphorylates residues phosphorylated by PKC.

2.6 Sequence of Events Involved in Ammonia–Induced ATP Depletion and in the Molecular Mechanism of Ammonia Toxicity

The results shown above and other previously reported (15) are summarized in the scheme shown in Fig. 9. High ammonia levels would induce an increase in the extracellular

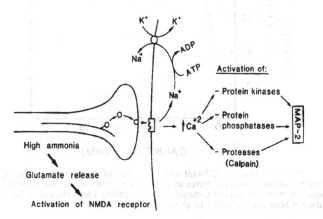

Figure 9. Proposed sequence of events involved in ammonia–induced ATP depletion and in the molecular mechanism of acute ammonia toxicity. See text for details. Modified from (15).

level of glutamate which can be due to increased release, to decreased reuptake or both (see references 16–25). Increased extracellular glutamate would result in increased activation of the NMDA receptor, leading to the entry into the neuron of Ca^{2+} and Na^+. Increased intracellular Ca^{2+} would activate Ca^{2+}-dependent enzymes including protein kinases and phosphatases and proteases. This would lead to the alterations previously shown in MAP-2 (14,15) and also to decreased PKC–mediated phosphorylation and concomitant activation of Na^+/K^+–ATPase as shown above. Increased ATPase activity would lead to consumption of larger amounts of ATP and could explain the depletion of brain ATP induced by injection of large doses of ammonia.

3. Molecular Mechanism of the Protective Effect of L–Carnitine Against Ammonia (and Glutamate) Toxicity

3.1 L–Carnitine Prevents Glutamate Neurotoxicity in Primary Cultures of Cerebellar Neurons

It is well known that L–carnitine prevents ammonia toxicity (26–35). As discussed above, we propose that acute ammonia toxicity is mediated by activation of the NMDA type of glutamate receptors. We then decided to test whether L–carnitine prevents ammonia toxicity because it prevents glutamate toxicity.

To assess this hypothesis we used primary cultures of cerebellar neurons. Incubation of these cells with 1 mM glutamate lead to the death of ≈ 80% of the neurons. However when cells were preincubated with L–carnitine, glutamate toxicity was prevented. The protective effect of different doses of carnitine is shown in Fig. 10. Protection was complete when neurons were preincubated with 3 mM carnitine. The high concentration of carnitine required is in agreement with the large amounts of carnitine required to prevent ammonia toxicity in animals.

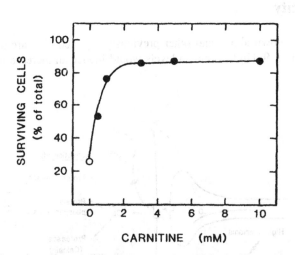

Figure 10. Protective effect of different concentrations of L–carnitine against glutamate-induced neuronal death. Primary cultures of cerebellar neurons were preincubated for 15 min with the indicated concentrations of L–carnitine before adding 1 mM glutamate. Neuronal death was quantified 4 hour after addition of glutamate. From (43).

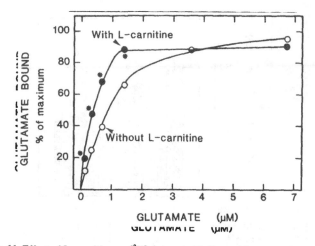

Figure 11. Effect of L–carnitine on [³H]glutamate binding to hippocampal synaptic membranes. Synaptic membranes were incubated with the indicated concentrations of [³H]glutamate in the absence or the presence of 10 mM L–carnitine. Specific binding is shown. Values which are significantly different from controls are indicated by asterisks. From (43).

3.2 Carnitine Increases the Affinity of Glutamate for the Quisqualate Type of Glutamate Receptors

We tested the possibility that the protective effect of L–carnitine against glutamate neurotoxicity could be due to an alteration of the binding of glutamate to its receptors. As shown in Fig. 11, carnitine increases the affinity of glutamate for its receptors in hippocampal synatic membranes. We then studied the effect of carnitine on the binding to different types of glutamate receptors. As shown in Fig. 12, carnitine increases the affinity of glutamate for the quisqualate type but not for the NMDA or kainate types of glutamate receptors.

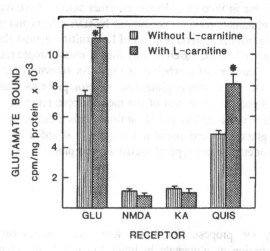

Figure 12. Effect of L–carnitine on glutamate binding to different types of glutamate receptors. Synaptic membranes were incubated with 360 nM [³H]glutamate. The specific binding to glutamate (GLU), N–methyl–D–aspartate (NMDA), kainate (KA) and quisqualate (QUIS) receptors are shown. Values which are significantly different from controls are indicated by asterisks. From (43).

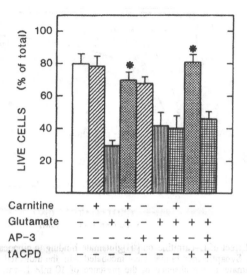

Figure 13. AP–3 prevents the protective effect of L–carnitine and of trans–ACPD against glutamate neurotoxicity. Primary cultures of cerebellar neurons were treated with 1 mM glutamate after preincubation with the indicated compounds. Preincubations with carnitine (5 mM) or with trans–ACPD (100 μM) were for 15 min. Pretreatments with AP–3 (0.2 mM) were for 40 min. Neuronal death was determined 4 hours after addition of glutamate. From (43).

3.3 The Protective Effect of L–Carnitine Against Glutamate Toxicity Seems to be Mediated by Activation of the Metabotropic Glutamate Receptor

It has been reported that activation of the metabotropic glutamate receptor by trans–ACPD, a selective agonist, attenuates NMDA neurotoxicity in cortical and cerebellar cultures (36–38) and in rat retina in vivo (39). However, other authors have reported that activation of the metabotropic glutamate receptor potentiates NMDA effects and neurotoxicity (40,41). It is therefore possible that the protective effect of L–carnitine against glutamate neurotoxicity could be a consequence of the increased affinity for the metabotropic receptor. We tested this possibility in primary cultures of cerebellar neurons. As shown in Fig. 13, trans–ACPD, a selective agonist of the metabotropic glutamate receptor prevents glutamate neurotoxicity. Moreover, AP–3, a selective antagonist of the metabotropic receptor is able to prevent the protective effect of both trans–ACPD and of carnitine. This indicates that the protective effect of carnitine against glutamate (and ammonia) toxicity is afforded by increasing the affinity of glutamate for the metabotropic type of glutamate receptors.

4. Summary

In summary, we propose that acute ammonia intoxication leads to increased extracellular concentration of glutamate in brain and results in activation of the NMDA receptor. Activation of this receptor mediates ATP depletion and ammonia toxicity since blocking the NMDA receptor with MK–801 prevents both phenomena. Ammonia–induced metabolic alterations (in glycogen, glucose, pyruvate, lactate, glutamine, glutamate, etc) are not prevented by MK–801 and, therefore, it seems that they do not play a direct role in ammonia–induced ATP depletion nor in the molecular mechanism of acute ammonia toxicity. The above results suggest that ammonia–induced ATP depletion is due to activation of Na^+/K^+–ATPase, which, in turn, is a consequence of decreased phosphorylation by protein kinase C. This can be due to decreased activity of PKC or to increased activity of a protein phosphatase.

We also show that L–carnitine prevents glutamate toxicity in primary neuronal cultures. The results shown indicate that carnitine increases the affinity of glutamate for the quisqualate type (including metabotropic) of glutamate receptors. Also, blocking the metabotropic receptor with AP–3 prevents the protective effect of L–carnitine, indicating that activation of this receptor mediates the protective effect of carnitine.

We suggest that the protective effect of carnitine against acute ammonia toxicity in animals is due to the protection against glutamate neurotoxicity according to the above mechanisms.

Acknowledgments: Supported in part by grant 93/0187 of the Fondo de Investigaciones Sanitarias of Spain and grant GV–1002/93 from the Conselleria de Educación y Ciencia de la Generalitat Valenciana. E. Kosenko received a sabatical grant from the Comisión Interministerial de Ciencia y Tecnología and G. Marcaida a fellowship from the Consellería de Cultura de la Generalitat Valenciana.

References

1. Hahn, M., Massen, O., Nencki, M. and Pavlov, I. (1893) Die Eck's Fistel zwischen der unteren hohlvene und der pfortader und ihre folgen für den organisms. Arch. Experiment. Pathol. Pharmakol. **32**:161–210.
2. Hindfelt, B. and Siesjo, B. K. (1971) Cerebral effects of acute ammonia intoxication. The effect upon energy metabolism. Scand. J. Clin. Lab. Invest. **28**:365–374.
3. Hawkins, R. A., Miller, A. L., Nielsen, R. C. and Veech, R. L. (1973) The acute action of ammonia on rat brain metabolism in vivo. Biochem. J. **134**:1001–1008.
4. Hindfelt, B., Plum, F. and Duffy, T. E. (1977) Effect of acute ammonia intoxication on cerebral metabolism in rats with portacaval shunts. J. Clin. Invest. **59**:386–396.
5. McCandless, D. W. and Schenker, S. (1981) Effect od acute ammonia intoxication on energy stores in the cerebral reticular activating system. Exp. Brain Res. **44**:325–330.
6. Lin, S. and Raabe, W. (1985) Ammonia intoxication: Effects on cerebral cortex and spinal cord. J. Neurochem. **44**:1252–1258.
7. Kosenko, E., Kaminsky, Y. G., Felipo, V., Miñana, M. D. and Grisolía, S. (1993) Chronic hyperammonemia prevents changes in brain energy and ammonia metabolites induced by acute ammonium intoxication. Biochim. Biophys. Acta **1180**:321–326.
8. Bessman, S. P. and Bessman, A. N. (1955) The cerebral and peripheral uptake of ammonia in liver disease with an hypothesis for the mechanism of hepatic coma. J. Clin. Invest. **34**:622–628.
9. Marcaida, G., Felipo, V., Hermenegildo, C. Miñana, M. D. and Grisolía, S. (1992) Acute ammonia toxicity is mediated by the NMDA type of glutamate receptors. FEBS Lett. **296**:67–68.
10. Lowndes, J. M., Hokin–Neaverson, M. and Berties, P. (1990) Kinetics of phosphorylation of Na^+/K^+–ATPase by protein kinase C. Biochim. Biophys. Acta **52**:143–151.
11. Bertorello, A. M., Aperia, A., Walaas, I., Nairn, A. C. and Greengard, P. (1991) Phosphorylation of the catalytic subunit of Na^+/K^+–ATPase inhibits the activity of the enzyme. Proc. Natl. Acad. Sci. USA **88**:11359–11362.
12. Hermenegildo, C., Felipo, V., Miñana, M. D. and Grisolía, S. (1992) Inhibition of protein kinase C restores Na^+/K^+–ATPase activity in sciatic nerve of diabetic mice. J. Neurochem. **58**:1246–1249.

13. Hermenegildo, C., Felipo, V., Miñana, M. D., Romero, F. J. and Grisolía, S. (1993) Sustained recovery of Na⁺/K⁺-ATPase activity in sciatic nerve of diabetic mice by administration of H7 or calphostin C, inhibitors of PKC. Diabetes **42**:257–262.

14. Felipo, V., Grau, E., Miñana, M. D. and Grisolía, S. (1993) Hyperammonemia decreases protein kinase C-dependent phosphorylation of microtubule-associated protein 2 and increases its binding to tubulin. Eur. J. Biochem. **214**:243–249.

15. Felipo, V., Grau, E., Miñana, M. D. and Grisolía, S. (1993) Ammonium injection induces an N-methyl-D-aspartate receptor-mediated proteolysis of the microtubule-associated protein MAP-2. J. Neurochem. **60**:1626–1630.

16. Moroni, F., Lombardi, G., Moneti, G. and Cortesini, C. (1983) The release and neosynthesis of glutamic acid are increased in experimental models of hepatic encephalopathy. J. Neurochem. **40**:850–854.

17. Mena, E. E. and Cotman, C. W. (1985) Pathologic concentrations of ammonium ions block L-glutamate uptake. Exp. Neurol. **89**:259–263.

18. Schmidt, W., Wolf, G., Grüngreif, K., Meier, M. and Reum, T. (1990) Hepatic encephalopathy influences high-affinity uptake of transmitter glutamate and aspartate into the hippocampal formation. Metabol. Brain Dis. **5**:19–31.

19. Rao, V. L. R. and Murthy, C. R. K. (1991) Hyperammonemic alterations in the uptake and release of glutamate and aspartate by rat cerebellar preparations. Neurosci. Lett. **130**:49–52.

20. Butterworth, R. F., Le, O., Lavoie, J. and Szerb, J. C. (1991) Effect of portacaval anastomosis on electrically stimulated release of glutamate from rat hippocampal slices. J. Neurochem. **56**:1481–1484.

21. Hilgier, W., Haugvicova, R. and Albrecht, J. (1991) Decreased potassium-stimulated release of [³H]D-aspartate from hippocampal slices distinguishes encephalopathy related to acute liver failure from that induced by simple hyperammonemia. Brain res. **567**:165–168.

22. Rao, V. L. R., Murthy, C. R. K. and Butterworth, R. F. (1992) Glutamatergic synaptic dysfunction in hyperammonemic syndromes. Metab. Brain Dis. **7**:1–20.

23. Bosman, D. K., Deutz, N. E. P., Maas, M. A. W., van Eijk, H. M. H., Smit, J. J. H., de Haan, J. G. abd Chamuleau, R. A. F. M. (1992) Amino acid release from cerrebral cortex in experimental acute liver failure, studied by in vivo cerebral cortex microdialysis. J. Neurochem. **59**:591–599.

24. Butterworth, R. F. (1992) Evidence that hepatic encephalopathy results from a defect of glutamatergic synatic regulation. Mol. Neuropharmacol. **2**:229–232.

25. Schmidt, W., Wolf, G., Grüngreiff, K. and Linke, K. (1993) Adenosine influences the high-affinity uptake of transmitter glutamate and aspartate under conditions of hepatic encephalopathy. Metabol. Brain Dis. **8**:73–80.

26. O'Connor, J. E., Costell, M. and Grisolía, S. (1984) Protective effect of L-carnitine on hyperammonemia. FEBS Lett. **166**:331–334.

27. O'Connor, J. E., Costell, M. and Grisolía, S. (1984) Prevention of ammonia toxicity by L-carnitine: Metabolic changes in brain. Neurochem. Res. **9**:563–570.

28. Costell, M., O'Connor, J. E., Miguez, M. P. and Grisolía, S. (1984) Effects of L-carnitine on urea synthesis following acute ammonia intoxication in mice. Biochem. Biophys. Res. Commun. **120**:726–733.

29. O'Connor, J. E., Costell, M., Miguez, M. P., Portolés, M. and Grisolía, S. (1987) Effect of L-carnitine on ketone bodies, redox state and free amino acids in the liver of hyperammonemia mice. Biochem. Pharmacol. **36**:3169–3173.

30. O'Connor, J. E., Costell, M. and Grisolía, S. (1987) The potentiation of ammonia toxicity by sodium benzoate is prevented by L-carnitine. Biochem. Biophys. Res. Commun. **145**:817–824.

31. Ohtsuka, Y. and griffith, O. W. (1991) L-carnitine protection in ammonia intoxication. Effect of aminocarnitine on carnitine-dependent metabolism and acute ammonia toxicity. Biochem. Pharmacol. **41**:1957–1961.

32. Matsuoka, M., Igisu, H., Kohriyama, K. and Inoue, N. (1991) Suppresion of neurotoxicity of ammonia by L-carnitine. Brain res. **567**:328–331.

33. Tremblay, G. C. and Bradley, T. M. (1992) L-carnitine protects fish against acute ammonia toxicity. Comp. Biochem. Physiol. **101** C:349–351.

34. Matsuoka, M. and Igisu, H. (1993) Comparison of the effects of L-carnitine, D-carnitine and acetyl-L-carnitine on the neurotoxicity of ammonia. Biochem. Pharmacol. **46**:159–164.

35. Ratnakumari, L., Qureshi, I. A. and Butterworth, R. F. (1993) Effect of L–carnitine on cerebral and hepatic energy metabolites in congenitally hyperammonemic Sparse–Fur mice and its role during benzoate therapy. Metabolism **42:**1039–1046.

36. Koh, J. Y., Palmer, E. and Cotman, C. W. (1991) Activation of the metabotropic glutamate receptor attenuates N–methyl–D–aspartate neurotoxicity in cortical cultures. Proc. natl. Acad. Sci. USA **88:**9431–9435.

37. Courtney, M. J. and Nicholls, D. G. (1992) Interactions between phospholipase C–coupled and N–methyl–D–aspartate receptors in cultured cerebellar granule cells: Protein kinase C mediated inhibition of N–methyl–D–aspartate responses. J. Neurochem. **59:**983–992.

38. Pizzi, M., Fallacara, C., Arrighi, V., Memo, M. and Spano, P. F. 81993) Attenuation of excitatory amino acid toxicity by metabotropic glutamate receptor agonists and aniracetam in primary cultures of cerebellar granule cells. J. Neurochem. **61:**683–689.

39. Siliprandi, R., Lipartiti, M., Fadda, E., Sautter, J. and Manev, H. (1992) Activation of the glutamate metabotropic receptor protects retina against N–methyl–D–aspartate toxicity. Eur. J. Pharmacol. **219:**173–174.

40. McDonald, J. W. and Schoepp, D. D. (1992) The metabotropic excitatory amino acid receptor agonist 1S,3R–ACPD selectively potentiates N–methyl–D–aspartate–induced brain injury. Eur. J. Pharmacol. **215:**353–354.

41. Kinney, G. A. and Slater, N. T. (1993) Potentiation of NMDA receptor–mediated transmission in turtle cerebellar granule cells by activation of metabotropic glutamate receptors. J. Neurophysiol. **69:**585–594.

42. Kosenko, E., Kaminsky, Y., Grau, E., Miñana, M. D., Marcaida, G., Grisolía, S. and Felipo, V. (1994) Brain ATP depletion induced by acute ammonia intoxication in rats is mediated by activation of the NMDA receptor and of Na^+/K^+–ATPase. J. Neurochem. (in press).

43. Felipo, V., Miñana, M. D., Cabedo, H. and Grisolía, S. (1994) L–carnitine increases the affinity of glutamate for quisqualate receptors and prevents glutamate neurotoxicity. Neurochem. Res. **19:**373–377.

Portal–Systemic Encephalopathy: a Disorder of Multiple Neurotransmitter Systems

Roger F. Butterworth

1. Introduction

Portal–Systemic Encephalopathy (PSE) is a serious complication of chronic liver disease; portal–systemic shunting rather than hepatic dysfunction appears to be the primary abnormality in PSE.

Cerebral metabolic rates for both oxygen and glucose are significantly reduced in PSE. Such reductions parallel the onset of clinical symptoms and are further reduced as neurologic status worsens. Decreased brain glucose utilization is most likely a consequence, rather than the cause of PSE; reduced neuronal activity resulting from PSE leads to decreased energy requirements and, hence, reduced fuel (glucose) requirements. Studies in portacaval shunted rats administered ammonium salts to precipitate severe encephalopathy demonstrate that brain ATP levels are maintained until terminal stages of PSE (l). Studies using IH–NMR give similar results (2). Such findings have led to the suggestion that neurotransmission failure rather than primary energy failure is the major cause of PSE.

Several neurotransmitter–related mechanisms have been proposed to explain the spectrum of neurological and neuropsychiatric symptoms of PSE (Table 1).

2. Ammonia (NH_4^+): Direct Effects on Inhibitory and Excitatory Neurotransmission

Ammonia neurotoxicity remains the leading candidate implicated in the pathogenesis of PSE. The association between PSE and ammonia dates back over a century to the pioneering work of Eck in which he and subsequent investigators described the effects of the first portacaval anastomoses (the so-called "Eck Fistula") in dogs. Feeding of meat to these animals resulted in loss of coordination, stupor and coma (3). Similar findings are reported following the administration of ammonium salts to portacaval shunted dogs (4) and rats (5).

Both direct neurotoxic effects of ammonia per se as well as neurotoxic effects mediated via ammonia metabolism have been described.

Results of electrophysiologic studies demonstrate that ammonia (NH_4^+), in concentrations equivalent to those reported in brain in experimental PSE, directly affects the neuronal membrane by blocking the extrusion of chloride (Cl^-) ions (6) suggesting that the resulting loss of inhibitory synaptic mechanisms could contribute to the CNS consequences of hyperammonemia.

Neuroscience Research Unit. Hôpital Saint-Luc (University of Montreal). Montreal, Ouebec, Canada H2X 3J4

Hepatic Encephalopathy, Hyperammonemia, and Ammonia Toxicity
Edited by V. Felipo and S. Grisolia, Plenum Press, New York, 1994

Table 1. Neurotransmission failure in PSE: candidate systems

1. Ammonia (NH_4^+): Direct effects on inhibitory and excitatory neurotransmission.

2. The glutamate system.

3. The Serotonin system (and related neuroactive/neurotoxic metabolites of L-tryptophan).

4. The Dopamine system.

5. The GABA system.

In a series of experiments by Raabe and coworkers (6), the effects of ammonia intoxication on postsynaptic inhibition in the cerebral cortex were examined before and after portacaval anastomosis. Electrophysiologic studies were combined with the measurement of ammonia and of its detoxification product glutamine in the tissue. Normal cats required 2.43 mmol/kg of ammonium acetate (IV) to significantly affect postsynaptic inhibition whereas in portacaval–shunted animals, only 0.77 mmol/kg ammonium acetate was required to cause similar disinhibition (6). Concentrations of ammonia in the brains of shunted animals, in which disinhibition was evident, were increased 2–fold compared to ammonia–treated normal animals suggesting a limitation in the removal of ammonia following portacaval shunting. Further direct biochemical evidence for a reduced capacity of brain for the removal of blood–borne ammonia following portacaval shunting in the rat, has been presented (7).

In addition to its effects on postsynaptic inhibition, there is evidence to suggest that the ammonium ion (NH_4^+) in millimolar concentrations, adversely affects postsynaptic glutamatergic synaptic function (8). Synaptic transmission from Schaffer collaterals to CA–1, pyramidal cells in hippocampus is reversibly depressed by 1 mM NH_4^+ (9). In addition, it was shown that the firing of CA–1, pyramidal cells, which are known to use glutamate as neurotransmitter, evoked by iontophoretic application of glutamate, is inhibited by NH_4^+ in the 2 to 5 mM range, reinforcing the notion that NH_4^+ decrease excitatory neurotransmission by a direct postsynaptic action.

3. The Glutamate System in PSE

In addition to effects of NH_4^+ on postsynaptic glutamatergic function and its role in the CNS consequences of hyperammonic conditions including PSE, there is strong suggestive evidence for alterations of glutamatergic synaptic regulation in these disorders.

Glutamate released into the synapse is inactivated mainly by reuptake into perineuronal astrocytes. These astrocytes possess the requisite high affinity, high capacity uptake system for glutamate and, following entry into the astrocyte, glutamate is transformed into glutamine by action of the enzyme glutamine synthetase (GS).

$$\text{glutamate} + NH_3 \xrightarrow{\text{GS}} \text{glutamine}$$

In conditions of chronic hyperammonia, in which the GS system becomes overwhelmed in its attempts to remove blood–borne ammonia, the glutamate–glutamine cycle ceases to function in an optimal fashion resulting in glutamatergic synaptic dysregulation.

Evidence in favour of this hypothesis may be summarized as follows:

(i)   Cultured astrocytes exposed for 4 days to 2 mM ammonia demonstrate a diminished capacity for glutamate uptake (10). Similar deleterious effects of exposure of synaptosomal preparations to millimolar concentrations of ammonia have also been reported (11).

(ii)   In a study with clinical correlates to the observations in (i), it was demonstrated that blood extracts from patients with varying degrees of PSE and of hyperammonemia, inhibit, in a dose–dependent fashion, the uptake of D–aspartate into rat hippocampal slices (12). D–aspartate is a non–metabolizable analog of L–glutamate used for the study of the high affinity glutamate carrier system. The relative potency of inhibition of D–aspartate uptake in these studies correlated with the blood ammonia concentrations in these PSE patients.

(iii)   Both K^+ –evoked and electrically–stimulated release of glutamate (i.e: release from the nerve terminal compartment) from superfused rat hippocampal slices from portacaval shunted rats is increased compared to that from sham–operated controls (13). Similarly, glutamate release has been shown to be significantly increased following portacaval shunting, using in vivo release techniques (14,15). This apparent increased release of glutamate following portacaval anastomosis is likely the result of decreased astrocytic (and neuronal) reuptake resulting from ammonia–related mechanisms outlined in (i) and (ii).

(iv)   High affinity binding sites for glutamate are reportedly decreased in density in brain in both PSE (16) and in experimental chronic hyperammonemic syndromes (17). In both cases, a selective loss of the N–methyl–D–aspartate (NMDA) subclass of glutamate receptors is lost (Figure l). Loss of NMDA–displaceable glutamate receptors in experimental PSE could result from "downregulation" of these sites following exposure to increased concentrations of endogenous ligands. As detailed in section (iii), there is evidence to suggest that extracellular glutamate concentrations are increased following portacaval anastomosis (13). In addition, there is evidence to suggest that a second endogenous ligand for the NMDA receptor, quinolinic acid, is increased in concentration in the brains of animals following portacaval anastomosis (18). These findings are particularly interesting in view of the recent report that the NMDA antagonist MK801 attenuates, to some extent, the neurotoxic effects of ammonia (19). Further studies of the role of NMDA receptors in the pathogenesis of the neurotoxic effects of ammonia are clearly warranted.

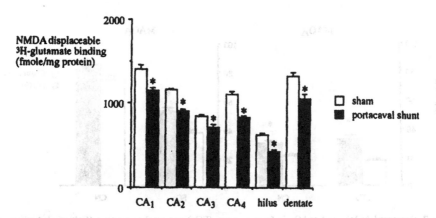

Figure 1. Loss of NMDA–displaceable ^{3}H–glutamate binding sites from hippocampal structures following portacaval anastomosis. Values significantly different from controls indicated by *p<0.05 by Analysis of Variance (Data from Peterson et al., 1990).

4. The Serotonin System (and other Neuroactive/Neurotoxic Metabolites of Tryptophan)

CSF concentrations of tryptophan are increased in hepatic coma (20). Since tryptophan is the precursor of the monoamine neurotransmitter serotonin (5HT) and since tryptophan hydroxylation (the rate–limiting step in brain 5HT synthesis) is not fully saturated at normal blood and brain concentrations of tryptophan, increased availability of the precursor has the potential to increase brain 5HT synthesis. There is a growing body of evidence to suggest that 5HT synthesis and, consequently, serotoninergic function may be compromised in PSE. For example:

(i)   A report of increased monoamine oxidase MAO_A in autopsied brain tissue from cirrhotic patients who died in hepatic coma (Figure 2) (25). In human brain, MAO_A is responsible for the oxidative metabolism of 5HT; concentrations of the 5HT metabolite, 5HIAA, were increased in the same material.

(ii)   Densities of the postsynaptic 5HT receptor ligand ^{3}H–ketanserin were found to be significantly increased in hippocampus of cirrhotic patients who died in hepatic coma (26). These findings, taken in conjunction with the increased 5HIAA concentrations and the increased activity of the degradative enzyme (MAO_A) suggest a 5HT synaptic deficit in human PSE. Further evidence consistent with this possibility is provided by reports of a clinical study in which cirrhotic patients with portal hypertension were treated with ketanserin; although beneficial effects on portal pressure were noted, severe encephalopathy was precipitated in 25% of patients (27). Taken together, these findings suggest that 5HT hypofunction could contribute to the pathologic mechanisms responsible for PSE.

As already mentioned, portacaval anastomosis results in increased brain concentrations of quinolinic acid (QUIN). QUIN levels are also increased in the CSF and brains of patients who died in hepatic coma (18) as well as in patients with congenital hyperammonemia (28).

Using CSF concentrations of Indoleacetic Acid IAA, as an index of tryptamine turnover, it has been reported that patients in hepatic coma had increased tryptamine turnover rates compared to non–comatose patients (29). Furthermore, the grade of coma was directly

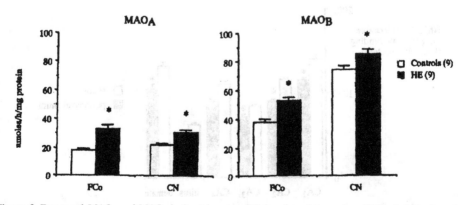

Figure 2. Decreased MAO_A and MAO_B in frontal cortex (FCo) and caudate nucleus (CN) of cirrhotic patients who died in hepatic coma. Values significantly different from controls indicated by *p<0.05 by Student's t test (Data from Reghavendra Rao et al., 1993).

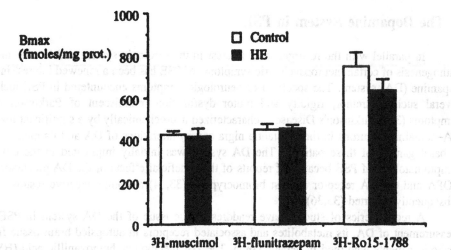

Figure 3. Densities of high affinity binding sites for the GABA-A receptor ligand ^{3}H-muscimol and GABA-related benzodiazepine receptor ligands ^{3}H-flunitrazepam and ^{3}H-Ro15-1788 are unchanged in autopsied frontal cortex from cirrhotic patients who died in hepatic coma (Data from Butterworth et al., 1988).

proportional to CSF IAA concentrations in these patients. A recent series of studies have characterized the tryptamine receptor of human brain (30,31) and have gone on to demonstrate that high affinity binding sites for ^{3}H-tryptamine are reduced by 40-60% in autopsied brain tissue from cirrhotic patients who died in hepatic coma. It was suggested that these findings demonstrate a role for this neuroactive amine in the pathogenesis of early neuropsychiatric manifestations of chronic liver failure (31).

Table 2. Alterations of monoaminergic systems in PSE: a review of recent evidence

Monoaminergic system		Reference
5HT system		
Increased 5HIAA in CSF	Human PSE	20
Increased 5HIAA in brain	Human PSE	21
	Portacaval shunted rat	22
	Portacaval Shuntad rat	24
Increased MAO$_A$ in brain	Human PSE	25
Increased 5HT$_2$ binding sites	Human PSE	26
Decreased 5HT$_{1A}$ binding sites	Human PSE	26
Tryptamine system		
Increased IAA in CSF	Human PSE	29
Loss of ^{3}H-tryptamine binding sites	Human PSE	21
Dopamine system		
Increased HVA in brain	Human PSE	21
Increased MAO$_A$, MAO$_B$ in brain	Human PSE	25
Loss of pallidal D$_2$ binding sites	Human PSE	37

5. The Dopamine System in PSE

In parallel with the resurgence of interest in the serotonin system and its role in the pathogenesis of certain neuropsychiatric symptoms of PSE has been a renewed interest in the dopamine (DA) system. The spectrum of neurologic symptoms encountered in PSE include several such as tremor, rigidity and motor dysfunction reminiscent of Parkinson–type symptoms (32). Parkinson's Disease is characterized neurochemically by a significant loss of DA–containing neurons in the substantia nigra and by alterations of DA and its metabolites in basal ganglia of these patients. The DA system was initially implicated in the clinical symptomatology of PSE because of reports of the beneficial effects of the DA precursor L–DOPA and the DA receptor agonist bromocriptine (33,34) although negative results were subsequently reported (35,36).

A recent series of studies have readdressed the issue of the DA system in PSE by measurement of DA, its metabolites and associated receptors in autopsied brain tissue from cirrhotic patients who died in hepatic coma. The DA metabolites homovanillic acid (HVA) and 3–methoxytyramine (3MT) were significantly increased (21) and activities of the DA–metabolizing enymes Monoamine Oxidase (MAO_A and MAO_B) were likewise found to be significantly increased (Figure 3) (25). Studies of DA receptors revealed a significant loss of postsynaptic D_2 receptor densities in globus pallidus of PSE patients (37). It was suggested that this loss of pallidal D_2 sites could be responsible for the motor dysfunction consistently reported in human PSE.

6. The GABA System in HE

In 1982, it was proposed that the inhibitory amino acid γ–aminobutyric acid (GABA) was generated, in liver failure, in increased quantities in the gut, after which it crossed the blood–brain barrier and caused the neural inhibition characteristic of hepatic encephalopathy (38). Evidence in support of this theory came mainly from studies in experimental animal models of acute liver failure. In dogs with experimental PSE, both significant alterations of GABA parameters (39) as well as no significant changes (40) were reported. In a series of studies of GABA concentrations (41), GABA–related enzymes (42) and postsynaptic GABA receptors (43) in autopsied brain tissue from cirrhotic patients with PSE, no significant alterations were observed suggesting that PSE in humans does not result from modifications of the GABA system per se.

On the other hand, substances that competitively bind to benzodiazepine receptors (which themselves form part of the so–called "GABA–benzodiazepine receptor complex") have been identified in PSE. Increased concentrations of such substances as diazepam and N,N–desmethyldiazepam have been reported in serum and CSF of a subgroup of PSE patients (44). It was suggested that increased concentrations of these "endogenous ligands" for the GABA–related benzodiazepine receptor could contribute to the pathogenesis of PSE by facilitation of GABAergic neurotransmission. It should be noted, however, that the benzodiazepine receptors themselves are not modified in experimental (45) or human (43) PSE (Figure 3).

The finding of increased benzodiazepine–like material in human PSE resulted in clinical assessments of the potential use of benzodiazepine receptor antagonists in the treatment of PSE. The best known antagonist, flumazenil (Ro15–1788) was found to be efficacious in the treatment of a small subgroup of patients with PSE in both uncontrolled and controlled clinical trials (46–49, Table 3). It still remains unclear, however, whether the presence of benzodiazepines in these patients is the result of previous exposure to benzodiazepine mediation or result from their synthesis in situ. The former possibility would render flumazenil useful in the reversal of benzodiazepine–induced coma in cirrhotic patients (a not infrequent occurrence). It should be borne in mind, however, that the majority of PSE

Table 3. Controlled clinical trials of flumazenil in PSE

Trial	No. of patients	Outcome	Reference
Rotterdam	9	No improvement in any of 9 patients	48
Montreal	13	Improvement in 5 patients	49
Multinational (Roche)	28	Improvement in 7 patients	52

patients do not have increased blood or CSF concentrations of benzodiazepines, nor do they respond favorably to flumazenil.

7. Prevention and Treatment of PSE

Approaches to the treatment of PSE still rely heavily on the reduction of blood–borne ammonia. Two such approaches are generally used:

a) The use of oral antibiotics such as neomycin to control urea–hydrolyzing bacteria in the gut.
b) Administration of lactulose to increase nitrogen trapping in the gut.

Recent studies by Grisolia and colleagues have suggested a third approach, namely that of the administration of L–carnitine. Carnitine levels are reduced in the serum of patients with liver disease (50). Portacaval shunted rats have significantly depressed total as well as free carnitine levels in blood compared to sham–operated controls (51). The hypocarnitinemia but not the hyperammonemia was normalized by oral administration of carnitine. It was suggested that the protective effect of carnitine in acute ammonia toxicity was due mainly to peripheral mechanisms.

The recent findings of modifications of glutamatergic and monoaminergic neurotransmitter systems in human PSE suggest that modulation of these systems could ultimately afford a second "downstream" series of therapeutic approaches. In favour of such a possibility, administration of MK 801, a potent antagonist of NMDA receptors, offers protection against the neurotoxic effects of ammonia (19) and dopamine receptor agonists such as bromocriptine have, on occasion, been found to be useful in the treatment of PSE in humans (34).

Controlled clinical trials with the benzodiazepine receptor antagonists Ro 15–1788 (flumazenil) have yielded results suggesting that a subgroup of PSE patients may benefit from this approach. Of a total of 50 patients so far treated, under controlled clinical trial conditions, 12 (24%) have shown transient improvement. It remains unclear, however, to what extent the improvement is mediated by the action of flumazenil on previously administered benzodiazepine medication.

References

1. Hindfelt B., Plum F., Duffy T.E., 1977, Effects of acute ammonia intoxication on cerebral metabolism in rats with portacaval shunts, J. Clin. Invest. **59**:386–396.
2. Fitzpatrick S.M., Behar K.L. and Shulman R.G., 1989, In vivo NMR spectroscopy studies of cerebral metabolism in rats after portacaval shunting. In "Hepatic Encephalopathy: Pathophysiology and Treatment" (R.F. Butterworth and G. Pomier Layrargues, eds.), Humana Press, pp. 177–187.

3. Hahn M., Massen O., Nencki M., Pavlov J., 1893, Die Ecksche Fistel zwischen der unteren Hohlvene und der Pfortader und ihre Folgen für den Organismus, Arch. Exp. Path. Pharmakol. **32**:161–170.

4. Matthews S.W., 1922, Ammonia, a causative factor in meat poisoning in Eck fistula dogs, Am. J. Physiol. **59**:459–460.

5. Giguère J.F. and Butterworth R.F., 1984, Amino acid changes in regions of the CNS in relation to function in experimental portal–systemic encephalopathy, Neurochem. Res. **9**:1309–1321.

6. Raabe W., 1987, Synaptic transmission in ammonia intoxication, Neurochem. Pathol. **6**:145–166.

7. Butterworth R.F., Girard G., Giguère J.F., 1988, Regional difference in the capacity of ammonia removal by brain following portacaval anastomosis, J. Neurochem. **51**:486–490.

8. Szerb J.C. and Butterworth R.F., 1992, Effect of ammonium ions on synaptic transmission in the mammalian central nervous system, Prog. Neurobiol. **39**:135–153.

9. Fan P., Lavoie J., Le N.L.O., Szerb J.C., Butterworth R.F., 1990, Neurochemical and electrophysiological studies on the inhibitory effect ol ammonium ions on synaptic transmission in slices of rat hippocampus: evidence for a postsynaptic action, Neurosci. **37**:327–324.

10. Norenberg M.D., Mozes L.W., Papendick R.E., Norenberg L.0.B., 1985, Effect of ammonia on glutamate, GABA and rubidium uptake by astrocytes, Ann. Neurol. **18**:149.

11. Mena E.E. and Cotman C.W., 1985, Pathologic concentrations of ammonium ions block L–glutamatc uptake. Exp. Neurol. **59**:259– 263.

12. Schmidt W., Wolf G., Grungreiff K., Meier M., Reum T., 1990, Hepatic encephalopathy influences high–affinity uptake of transmitter glutamate and aspartate into the hippocampal formation, Metab. Brain Dis. **5**:19–31.

13. Butterworth R.F., Le O., Lavoie J., Szerb J.C., 1991, Effect of portacaval anastomosis on electrically–stimulated release of glutamate from rat hippocampal slices. J. Neurochem. **56**:1481–1484.

14. Moroni F., Lombardi G., Moneti G., Cortesini C., 1983, The release and neosynthesis of glutamic acid are increased in experimental models of hepatic encephalopathy, J. Neurochem. **40**:850–854.

15. Tossman U., Delin A., Eriksson L.S., Ungerstedt U., 1987, Brain cortical amino acids measured by intracerebral dialysis in portacaval shunted rats, Neurochem. Res. **12**:265–269.

16. Peterson C., Giguère J.F., Cotman C.W., Butterworth R.F., 1990, Selective loss of N–methyl–D–aspartate–sensitive L–^{3}H–glutamate binding sites in rat brain following portacaval anastomosis, J. Neurochem. **55**:386–390

17. Rao V.L.R., Murthy C.R.K., Butterworth R.F., 1992, Glutamatergic synaptic dysfunction in hyperammonemic syndromes, Metab. Brain Dis. **7**:1–20.

18. Moroni E, Lombardi G., Carla V., Pellegrini D., Carassale O.L., Cortesini C., 1986, Content of quinolinic acid and other tryptophan metabolites increases in brain regions of rats used as experimental models of hepatic encephalopathy, J. Neurochem. **46**:869–874.

19. Marcaida G, Felipo V, Hermenegildo C, Minana M–D, and Grisolia S., 1992, Acute ammonia toxicity is mediated by the NMDA type of glutamate receptors. FEBS Lett, **296**:67–68.

20. Young S.N., Lal S., Feldmuller F., Aranoff A., Martin J.B., 1975, Relationships between tryptophan in serum and CSF and 5–hydroxyindoleacetic acid in CSF of man: effects of cirrhosis of the liver and probenecid administration, J. Neurol. Neurosurg. Psychiat. **38**:322–330.

21. Bergeron M., Reader T.A., Pomier Layrargues G., Butterworth R.E, 1989, Monoamines and metabolites in autopsied brain tissue from cirrhotic patients with hepatic encephalopathy, Neurochem. Res. **14**:853– 849.

22. Bergeron M., Swain MS., Reader T.A., Grondin L., Butterworth R.F., 1990, Effect of ammonia on brain serotonin metabolism in relation to function in the portacaval shunted rat, J. Neurochem. **55**:222–229.

23. Bachmann C. and Colombo JP., 1984, Increase of trytophan and 5–hydroxyindoleacetic acid in the brain in ornithine carbamoyl transferase deficient sparse–fur mice. Pediat. Res. **18**:372–375.

24. Bengtsson F., Bugge M., Johansen K.H., Butterworth R.F., 1991, Brain tryptophan hydroxylation in the portacaval shunted rat: a hypothesis for the regulation of serotonin turnover in vivo, J. Neurochem. **56**:1069–1074.

25. W. Raghavendra Rao V.L., Giguère J.-F., Pomier Layrargues G., Butterworth R.F., 1993, Increased activities of MAO$_A$ and MAO$_B$ in autopsied brain tissue from cirrhotic patients with hepatic encephalopathy, Brain Res. **621**:349-352.

26. Raghavendra Rao V.L. and Butterworth R.F., 1994, Alterations of ^{3}H-8H-DPAT and ^{3}H-ketanserin binding sites in autopsied brain tissue from cirrhotic patients with hepatic encephalopathy, Neurosci. Lett. (in press).

27. Vorobioff J., Garcia-Tsao G., Groszmann R., Aceves G., Picabea E., Villavicencio R., Hernandez-Ortiz, J., 1988, Long-term hemodynamic effects of ketanserin, a 5-hydroxytryptamine blocker, in portal hypertensive patients, Hepatology **9**:88-91.

28. Batshaw M.L., Heyes M., Diali S., Rorke L. and Robinson M.B., 1990, Tryptophan (Trp), Quinolinate (Quin) and serotonin (5HT): 1. Alterations in children with hyperammonemia, Soc. Neurosci. Abs.

29. Young S.N. and Lal S., 1980, CNS tryptamine metabolism in hepatic coma, J. Neural. Transm. **47**:153-161.

30. Mousseau D.D., 1993, Tryptamine, a metabolic of tryptophan implicated in various neuropyschiatric disorders, Metab. Brain Dis., **8**:1-44.

31. Mousseau D.D., 1994, Region-selective decreases in densities of ^{3}H-tryptamine binding sites in autopsied brain tissue from cirrhotic patients witb hepatic encephalopathy, J. Neurochem. (in press)

32. Conn H.O., 1988, The hepatic encephalopathies. In: Conn HO, Bircher J., Eds. Hepatic Encephalopathy: Management with Lactulose and Related Carbohydrates. East-Lansing MI: Medi-Press, pp 3-14.

33. Lunzer M., James I.M., Weinman J., Sherlock S., 1974, Treatment of chronic hepatic encephalopathy with levodopa, Gut **15**:555-561.

34. Morgan M.Y., Jakobovits A.W., James I.M., Sherlock S., 1980, Successful use of bromocriptine in the treatment of chronic hepatic encephalopathy, Gastroenterology **78**:663-670.

35. Uribe M., Farca A., Marquez M.A., Garcia-Ramos G., Guevara L., 1979, Treatment of chronic portal systemic encephalopathy with bromocriptine, Gastroenterology **76**:1347-1351.

36. Michel H., Solere M., Granier P., Cauvet G., Bali J.P., Bellet-Hermann H., 1980, Treatment of cirrhotic hepatic encephalopathy with L-DOPA. A controlled trial, Gastroenterology **79**:207-211.

37. Mousseau D.D., Perney P., Pomier Layrargues G., Butterworth R.P., 1993, Selective loss of pallidal dopamine D$_2$ receptor density in hepatic encephalopathy, Neurosci. Lett. **162**:192-196.

38. Schafer D.F. and Jones E.A., 1982, Hepatic encephalopathy and the γ-aminobutyric acid system, Lancet **1**:18-20

39. Baraldi M, Zeneroli M.L, Ventura E., Penne A., Pinelli G., Ricci P., Santi M., 1984, Supersensitivity of benzodiazepine receptors in hepatic encephalopathy due to fulminant hepatic failure in thet rat: reversal by a benzodiazepine antagonist, Clin. Sci. **61**:167-175.

40. Roy S., Pomier Layrargues G., Butterworth R.F., Huet P.M, 1988, Hepatic encephalopathy in cirrhotic and portacaval shunted dogs: lack of changes in brain GABA uptake, brain GABA levels and brain glutamic acid decarboxylase activity aad brain postsynaptic GABA receptors, Hepatology **8**:845-849.

41. Lavoie J., Giguère J.F., Pomier Layrargues G., Butterworth R.F., 1987, Amino acid changes in autopsied brain tissue from cirrhotic patients with hepatic encephalopathy, J. Neurochem. **49**:692-697.

42. Lavoie J., Giguère J.F., Pomier Layrargues G., Butterworth R.F., 1987, Activities of neuronal and astrocytic marker enymes in autopsied brain tissue from cirrhotic patients with hepatic encephalopathy, Metab. Brain Dis. **2**:283-290.

43. Butterworth R.F., Lavoie J., Giguère J.F., Pomier Layrargues G., 1988, Affinities and densities of GABA-A receptors and of central benzodiazepine˙ receptors are unchanged in autopsied brain tissue from cirrhotic patients with hepatic encephalopathy, Hepatology **8**:1084-1088.

44. Olasmaa M., Rothstein J.D., Guidotti A., Weber R.J., Paul S.M., Spector S., Zeneroli M.L., Baraldi M., Costa E., 1990, Endogenous benzodiazepine receptor ligands in human and animal hepatic encephalopathy, J. Neurochem. **55**:2015-2023.

45. Mans A.M., Kukulka K.M., McAvoy K.J. and Rokosz N.C., 1992, Regional distribution and kinetics of three sites on the GABA$_A$ receptor: lack of effect of portacaval shunting, J. Cerebr. Blood Flow and Metab.**12**:334-3461.

46. Bansky G., Meier P.J., Riedere E., Walser H., Ziegler W.H., Schmid M., 1989, Effects of the benzodiazepine receptor antagonist flumazenil in hepatic encephalopathy in humans, Gastroenterology **97**:744–750.

47. Klotz U. and Walker S., 1989, Flumazenil and hepatic encephalopathy, Lancet **1**:155–156.

48. Van der Rijt C.C.D., Schalm S.W., Meulstee J., Stijnen T., 1989, Flumazenil therapy for hepatic encephalopathy: a double-blind cross-over study, Hepatology **10**:590 (abstract).

49. Pomier Layrargues G., Giguère J.F., Lavoie J., Gagnon S., D'Amour M., Caillé G., Wells J. and Butterworth R.F., 1994, Efficacy of Ro15-1788 in cirrhotic patients with hepatic coma: results of a randomized double-blind placebo-controlled crossover trial, Hepatology **19**:32–37.

50. Rudman D., Sewell C.W. and Ansley J.D.,1977, Deficiency of carnitine in cachectic cirrhotic patients, J. Clin. Invest. **60**:716–623.

51. Hearn T.J., Coleman A.E., Lai J.C.K., Griffith O.W. and Cooper A.J.L., 1989, Effect of orally administered L-carnitine on blood ammonia and L-carnitine concentrations in portacaval shunted rats, Hepatology **10**:822–828.

The GABA Hypothesis – State of the Art

E. Anthony Jones[1], Cihan Yurdaydin[2], Anthony S. Basile[3]

Before the gamma–aminobutyric acid (GABA) hypothesis was proposed more than a decade ago there had been increasing awareness that the hypotheses of the pathogenesis of hepatic encephalopathy (HE) then in vogue did not adequately account for all of the manifestations of this syndrome. A particular deficiency of those hypotheses was their failure to account for the manifestations of the syndrome in terms of abnormal neural mechanisms (1). Although GABA had been included in lists of substances that had been considered in relation to HE (2), the possibility of an involvement of the GABA neurotransmitter system in its pathogenesis had not been seriously assessed.

1. Origin of the Hypothesis

In 1979, to facilitate research on HE, Schafer recorded visual evoked responses (VERs) from the rabbit model of galactosamine–induced fulminant hepatic failure (FHF) in an attempt to quantitate the magnitude of overall neurophysiological disturbance (3). He found that HE in this model was associated with highly distinctive and reproducible changes in the VER waveform (3,4). Having characterised these changes, further experiments were conducted to determine whether similar changes could be induced in normal rabbits by the administration of a drug that induces encephalopathy and coma. Preliminary experiments revealed that many of the changes in VERs associated with HE could be reproduced by administering pentobarbital (4,5). Pentobarbital was known to inhibit neuronal activity as a consequence of binding to the chloride ionophore of the GABA/benzodiazepine (BZ) receptor complex. This binding leads to increased flux of chloride through the ionophore into the neuron and consequently leads to hyperpolarization of the neuronal surface membrane (6). Accordingly, the question arose whether increased inhibitory neurotransmission mediated by the GABA/BZ receptor complex was implicated in the pathogenesis of HE.

2. The Hypothesis

Increased GABAergic tone contributes to the pathogenesis of HE.

3. Formulation of the Hypothesis

The article in which the hypothesis was originally proposed (7) was entitled "Hepatic encephalopathy and the gamma–aminobutyric acid neurotransmitter system." The hypothesis

Department of Health, London[1]; Department of Gastroenterology, University of Ankara, Ankara[2]; Laboratory of Neuroscience, NIDDK, National Institutes of Health, Bethesda, Maryland[3]

Hepatic Encephalopathy, Hyperammonemia, and Ammonia Toxicity
Edited by V. Felipo and S. Grisolia, Plenum Press, New York, 1994

89

is implicit in this title. Manifestations of both HE and increased neurotransmission mediated by the GABA neurotransmitter system include impaired motor function and decreased consciousness (8,9). It follows that if changes in the functional status of the GABA neurotransmitter system are related to some of the manifestations of HE the nature of the relationship would be that increased GABAergic tone contributes to HE.

In retrospect the article appears to have been deficient in at least three respects. First, the hypothesis may not have been stated unambiguously. The second deficiency was the lack of a clear statement of the important questions that are attendant to the hypothesis and which have dominated all subsequent research in relation to the hypothesis: (i) is GABAergic tone increased in HE?; and (ii) if it is, what mechanisms are involved? At the time, the only findings relevant to answering the first question were observations that VER waveforms in the rabbit model of HE and normal rabbits with barbiturate or BZ-induced encephalopathies were similar to each other, yet different from those in ether-induced coma (5). All of the other findings cited in the article could be interpreted as being potentially relevant to the second question, i.e. the presence in HE of a GABA-like factor in plasma (10,11), evidence that gut bacteria are a source of GABA (12), the ability of an analogue of GABA to cross the blood-brain-barrier (BBB) in acute liver failure (13) and data which suggested that the densities of receptors for GABA and BZs in the brain might be increased in HE (14). It is clear, therefore, that most of the experimental findings included in the original article related to the feasibility of certain specific mechanisms for increased GABAergic tone in HE rather than to the demonstration that GABAergic tone is increased in HE. The third deficiency of the original article was the failure to clearly distinguish between the primary hypothesis, as defined above, and secondary hypotheses that were proposed to stimulate research and were relevant to answering the second question. These secondary hypotheses involved three concepts (7). (i) Gut-derived GABA might gain access to the brain in liver failure. The attractiveness of this possibility was the known association of HE with gut factors (2). (ii) The possibility of gut-derived GABA inducing GABA receptors in the brain was entertained as a potential explanation of the apparent increase in GABA receptors in the brain in HE (14), which, if confirmed, could be an explanation of increased GABA-ergic tone by rendering the brain more sensitive to prevailing amounts of GABA in synaptic clefts. However, this notion of upregulation of GABA receptors was contrary to conventional concepts of the regulation of neurotransmitter receptors in the CNS (15). (iii) The apparent increase in the density of BZ receptors in HE afforded a potential mechanism for the observed increased sensitivity of patients with cirrhosis to the neuroinhibitory effects of BZs (16).

As the technology to test primary and secondary hypotheses has matured, new secondary hypotheses have been proposed. Some experimental findings have disproved some of the secondary hypotheses, while other experimental findings have provided support for the primary hypothesis as well as some of the secondary hypotheses. The validity of the primary hypothesis is not dependent on the validity of any single secondary hypothesis. However, more than one of the secondary hypotheses may be correct. Furthermore, the testing of secondary hypotheses is proving valuable in ascertaining the relative importance of different mechanisms mediating increased GABAergic tone in HE.

4. Issues Responsible for Controversy

4.1. Plasma Levels of GABA Receptor Ligands

As gut factors are known to be implicated in hepatic encephalopathy (2), an attractive hypothesis to test was that an accumulation of GABA in plasma might contribute to increased GABAergic tone in HE. The application of a radioreceptor assay for GABA indicated that levels of material which inhibited the binding of radiolabelled GABA to GABA receptors were increased in an animal model of FHF (10,11) and in patients with decompensated chronic liver disease, particularly after a gastrointestinal haemorrhage (17). Support for the concept that the gut might be a source of this GABA–like activity in plasma in liver failure came from the demonstration that the gut is a source of GABA (12, 18). The subsequent demonstration that GABA does not account for all of this activity in liver failure (19), some of it being attributable to taurine (20), was incorrectly considered to be evidence against the GABA hypothesis. However, on balance the available evidence indicates that plasma levels of true GABA (as measured by HPLC or gas liquid chromatography) do increase in liver failure (21,22). Moreover, taurine is a GABA receptor agonist. Nevertheless, increased levels of plasma GABA would not necessarily increase GABAergic neurotransmission in the absence of increased plasma–to–brain transfer of GABA. Finally, potential mechanisms existed for increasing GABAergic tone in HE without requiring elevated levels of plasma GABA (23,24).

4.2. Blood–Brain–Barrier Permeability

A crucial issue in any consideration of a potential role of plasma GABA in HE is whether GABA can cross the BBB in liver failure. GABA, being a polar compound, does not cross a normal BBB (25). If the permeability of the BBB is not increased in liver failure it seems unlikely that plasma GABA would contribute to the pathogenesis of HE. However, as the properties of the BBB have been shown to change in models of liver failure (26), studies of the plasma–to–brain transfer of GABA in models of HE were of interest. In two such studies, which employed satisfactory methodology, no increase in plasma–to–brain transfer of GABA was detected (27,28), but the model used, the rat with galactosamine–induced FHF, has shortcomings (29). In other studies, in which the extensively characterised rabbit model (29–32) was used, increased plasma–to–brain transfer of an analogue of GABA (alpha–aminoisobutyric acid) (13) and GABA itself (33) was convincingly demonstrated. Thus, it is possible that plasma GABA could contribute to HE in acute liver failure if it reaches GABA$_A$ receptors before undergoing degradation or neuronal uptake (34). This concept is supported by the similarity between HE and encephalopathy precipitated by increasing GABA levels in brain extracellular fluid (e.g. by administering gamma–vinyl GABA) (9). Whether plasma GABA gains access to brain extracellular fluid in chronic liver failure is uncertain.

4.3. Brain and CSF GABA Levels

Observations that GABA levels in whole brain from models of HE (35,36) and in the CSF of humans with HE (37) were not increased have also been interpreted as evidence that the GABA neurotransmitter system does not play a role in HE. However, increased GABA levels are not a prerequisite for increased GABA–ergic tone. A change in the status of the GABA/BZ receptor complex or the presence of an agonist ligand (other than GABA) for a component of the GABA/BZ receptor complex, which potentiates the action of GABA, could be responsible for increased GABA–ergic tone. Alternatively, if increased GABA–ergic tone is due to increased GABA levels in synaptic clefts, such increased levels would not necessarily be reflected in detectable changes in GABA levels in either whole brain or CSF. Most brain GABA is located in synaptosomes in neurons (34). GABA in brain extracellular fluid can be measured by applying the technique of brain microdialysis (38).

4.4. GABA$_A$ and Benzodiazepine Receptor Status

When the VER data originally suggested that the GABA neurotransmitter system might be involved in HE (4,5), methods for studying this system further were sought. One approach being applied at that time was a radioligand–receptor binding assay to estimate the densities of GABA$_A$ and BZ receptors and the affinities of ligands for these receptors (39). In original applications of this approach to study HE, the apparent binding of radioligands to brain GABA and BZ receptors appeared to be greater in models of HE than in control animals (14,40). The most logical interpretation of these findings at the time seemed to be that the densities of GABA$_A$ and BZ receptors were increased in HE. Many workers appear to have believed that the validity of the GABA hypothesis depended on an ability to reproduce these early findings, even though the findings only suggested one possible mechanism for increased GABAergic tone in HE (i.e. increased responsiveness of the brain to prevailing levels of GABA in synaptic clefts). The methodology originally used for assessing the status of brain GABA and BZ receptors was state-of-the-art at the time. However, radioligand–receptor binding assays were subsequently refined and numerous additional studies of the status of GABA and BZ receptors in HE were undertaken with conspicuously inconsistent results. Some studies appeared to confirm the original findings, whereas others completely failed to reproduce them (41,42). It seemed likely that the reason for the apparently conflicting results from many carefully conducted studies would provide a valuable clue relating to a mechanism of increased GABA–ergic tone in HE. Eventually, this important issue was addressed and partially resolved. It was recognised that in some, but not all, of the relevant studies detergent was used to facilitate radioligand access to receptors on plasma membranes and that exposure to detergent caused a loss of receptors from neuronal membranes. The relevant new finding was that the magnitude of this loss was relatively greater for control membranes than for membranes from an animal model of HE (43). Thus, the relatively greater binding of radioligands to membranes from models of HE than control membranes observed in some studies could have been attributable to differential detergent solubilization of membrane receptors rather than an increase in the densities of receptors on membranes in HE (43). In addition, this study raised the intruiging possibility that the physicochemical change in brain membranes in HE responsible for decreased receptor solubility might be related to a mechanism of increased GABA–ergic tone (42). One such possibility would be increased binding of endogenous ligands to brain membranes in HE (e.g. BZ receptor ligands) (44,45).

5. Evidence for Increased GABA–ergic Tone in HE

Currently, four lines of evidence support the concept that increased GABA–ergic tone contributes to the pathogenesis of HE.

5.1. Patterns of Visual Evoked Responses

The abnormal patterns of VERs of HE resemble those in animals with encephalopathies induced by drugs which augment GABA-mediated neurotransmission (e.g. pentobarbital, diazepam or the GABA agonist, muscimol), but differ from those induced by drugs which induce encephalopathies by mechanisms that do not appear to depend primarily on stimulation of the GABA/BZ receptor complex (4,46,47).

5.2. Resistance to Drugs which Decrease GABA–ergic Tone

If GABA–ergic tone is reduced to a sufficient extent a convulsion will occur (34). In models of HE increased resistance to bicuculline (9) or (intraventricularly– administered) mercaptopropionic acid (48)–induced convulsions has been demonstrated. Bicuculline is a GABA$_A$ receptor antagonist, whereas mercaptopropionic acid reduces the synthesis of GABA by inhibiting glutamate decarboxylase (49). Available reports on the effects of these two compounds in models of HE lack adequate control data.

5.3. Sensitivity of Neurons to GABA and BZ Receptor Agonists

Purkinje neurons in cerebellar slices from a model of HE exhibit increased sensitivity to the neuroinhibitory effects of a GABA agonist (muscimol) and a BZ agonist (flunitrazepam) (50). In contrast to the abnormal patterns of VERs in models of HE which reflect electrophysiological changes in large groups of neurons, the data obtained using Purkinje neurons indicate functional changes at the single neuron level in HE. The Purkinje neuron data are consistent with the VER data in HE and indicate that the observed alterations in the activity of single neurons can account for the overall changes in CNS electrical activity in HE as reflected in the VER changes.

5.4. Pharmacological Antagonism of GABA/BZ Receptor Complex Components

In animal models of HE behavioural and electrophysiological ameliorations of encephalopathy have been induced by bicuculline (9), by flumazenil (9,51) (a benzodiazepine receptor antagonist with weak partial agonist properties (49,50)) and by Ro 15-3505 and Ro 15-4513 (51-53) (benzodiazepine antagonists with weak partial inverse agonist properties (54,55)). All of these observations are compatible with improvements in HE being attributable to the normalisation of GABA-ergic tone. However, the mechanisms by which the drugs used in these studies decrease GABA-ergic tone differ. Bicuculline directly antagonises the action of GABA (9). Flumazenil displaces endogenous ligands responsible for potentiating the action of GABA from the central BZ receptor (e.g. BZ agonist ligands such as 1,4-BZs) (49). Ro 15-3505 and Ro 15-4513 may have a similar mode of action to that of flumazenil, but in addition they may also reduce GABA-ergic tone as a consequence of their intrinsic (partial inverse agonist) action at the BZ receptor, independent of their ability to displace ligands from it (54-56).

The most extensively studied BZ antagonist in patients with HE has been flumazenil (49). This drug has been reported to induce ameliorations of HE in a majority of patients with FHF or cirrhosis (57-59) and in a single patient with chronic intractable portal-systemic encephalopathy (60). These observations indicate that increased GABA-ergic tone can contribute to some of the manifestations of HE in man.

6. Mechanisms of Increased GABA-Ergic Tone in HE

Theoretically, increased GABA-ergic neurotransmission could occur as a consequence of non-humoral factors, such as functionally significant changes in the status of the GABA/BZ receptor complex, or humoral factors, such as increased availability of agonist ligands for the GABA/BZ receptor complex.

6.1. Non-humoral Factors

(i) **Functional status of the chloride ionophore**. A GABA agonist (muscimol) stimulated $^{36}Cl^-$ uptake into cerebral cortical synaptoneurosomes from rats with HE due to thioacetamide-induced FHF and from control rats to a similar extent. Furthermore, potentiation of this phenomenon by a BZ agonist (diazepam) was equivalent in both experimental groups (61). These findings indicate that chloride ionophore function is not significantly altered in this model of HE.

(ii) **Status of GABA and BZ receptors**. Recent studies, using appropriate modern methodologies for assaying radioligand–receptor binding, provide no evidence for a change in density of GABA or BZ receptors or in the affinities of ligands for these receptors in models of HE (44,45,62,63).

6.2. Humoral Factors

(i) **GABA receptor agonists**. Potential sources of GABA at $GABA_A$ receptors in liver failure include plasma, astrocytes and neurons. The finding of increased plasma–to–brain transfer of GABA in the rabbit model (33) (mentioned above) is consistent with (but does not prove) that increased availability of plasma–derived GABA may contribute to increased GABA–ergic tone in HE due to acute liver failure. In addition, recent findings in rats with HE due to thioacetamide–induced FHF provide evidence consistent with increased release of GABA from astrocytes and/or neurons (23,64,65). Furthermore, a substantial loss of $GABA_B$ receptors has been reported in this model and has been related to increased GABA release (66). The potential of increased availability of GABA at $GABA_A$ receptors as a mechanism of increased GABA–ergic tone in HE has been inadequately investigated, particularly during the last few years when it has become apparent that agonist ligands of the BZ receptor of the GABA/BZ receptor complex accumulate in liver failure (59) (see below). Increased GABA–ergic tone due to increased availability of GABA at $GABA_A$ receptors may not only itself be responsible for some of the manifestations of HE, but this phenomenon may also be responsible for potentiating the neuroinhibitory effects of BZ receptor agonist ligands and hence the contribution of such ligands to HE (59).

(ii) **Benzodiazepine receptor agonist ligands**. BZ agonists, such as diazepam, mediate their neuroinhibitory effects by potentiating the action of GABA (34,49,59). The GABA hypothesis was the basis for the suggestion that increased availability of BZ receptor agonist ligands might contribute to some of the manifestations of HE by augmenting GABA–mediated neurotransmission and its corollary that a BZ antagonist might ameliorate some of the manifestations of HE (67,68).

Although CGS 8216 was the first BZ antagonist to be reported to induce a transient behavioral amelioration of encephalopathy and an improvement in VER abnormalities when administered to a model of HE (69), the feasibility of these predictions did not become fully apparent until the BZ antagonist flumazenil was found to induce behavioural and electrophysiological ameliorations of HE in the rabbit model (70) and, anecdotally, in humans with FHF or cirrhosis (68,71). The animal observations were confirmed (9) and the ability of flumazenil to ameliorate HE was shown to be neither species nor model specific (51). However, flumazenil failed to induce detectable ameliorations of HE in some models (52,53,72). Uncontrolled observations in humans suggest that flumazenil induces ameliorations of HE in about 60% of patients with acute or chronic liver failure (57–59). As flumazenil is a BZ receptor antagonist with weak agonist properties (49,50), flumazenil–induced ameliorations of HE cannot be explained by the intrinsic activity of the drug. The most logical explanation for such ameliorations is a normalisation of increased GABAergic tone as a consequence of neuronal disinhibition due to the displacement of agonist ligands from central BZ receptors. Flumazenil has been reported to induce transient anxiety in a patient with chronic portal–systemic encephalopathy (60). This observation also cannot be explained by the intrinsic activity of the drug; it seems likely to be due to the decrease in GABA–ergic neurotransmission precipitated by the displacement of agonist ligands from BZ receptors.

Thus, flumazenil–precipitated anxiety in a patient with HE probably implies the presence of BZ receptor agonist ligands in the brain.

Indirect evidence of increased levels of BZ receptor ligands in HE has been supplemented by unequivocal direct evidence for their presence. In particular, increased levels of BZ receptor ligands in the CSF (73) and brain (44,45) of animal models of HE have been demonstrated using neuropharmacolgical, neurochemical and autoradiographic techniques. Furthermore, several substances with elution profiles similar to those of known 1,4–BZs have been demonstrated in the brains of animal models of HE (63,74,75). In addition, in animal models of HE the total brain concentrations of BZ receptor ligands (expressed as diazepam equivalents) and brain concentrations of diazepam and N–desmethyl diazepam were significantly greater than corresponding concentrations in control brains (63,75). Increased levels of BZ receptor ligands, including 1,4–BZs, have been reported in plasma and urine of patients with HE due to decompensated cirrhosis (76) and in the brain of a majority of patients dying from FHF (77). Brain levels of BZ receptor ligands in an animal model of FHF (78) and plasma levels of BZ receptor ligands in humans with FHF (79) or decompensated cirrhosis (76) have been shown to correlate with the degree of encephalopathy.

While some of the BZ receptor–binding material present in the brain in HE has been shown to be due to 1,4–BZs, the chemical and functional nature of a large proportion of this material is currently unknown (59,75). The brain levels of these BZ receptor ligands, when expressed in units of diazepam equivalents, would appear to be sufficient to account for mild sedation (59). However, the distribution of BZ receptor ligands in the brain has been shown to be heterogeneous in an animal model of HE (45) and their neuroinhibitory action may be substantially potentiated if increased availability of GABA at GABA$_A$ receptors is also contributing to increased GABAergic tone (59).

Recently, the BZ receptor ligands Ro 15–4513 and Ro 15–3505 have been shown to be more efficacious than flumazenil in inducing behavioural and electrophysiological ameliorations of HE in animal models (51–53). These ligands are not only BZ receptor antagonists but also BZ receptor partial inverse agonists (54–56). Thus, they have the potential of decreasing GABA–ergic tone not only by displacing agonist ligands from the BZ receptor, but also as a consequence of their intrinsic action at the BZ receptor. Irrespective of the relative contribution of these two mechanisms to the actions of Ro 15–4513 and Ro 15–3505 in HE, ameliorations of HE induced by either of these ligands imply that some of the manifestations of HE can be reversed by normalising increased GABA–ergic tone.

It is evident that much further work needs to be undertaken to fully explore which mechanisms are responsible for increased GABA–mediated neurotransmission in HE.

7. Milestones in Development of GABA Concept

1982 Suggestion that GABA–mediated inhibitory neurotransmission may contribute to manifestations of HE (7).

1984 Abnormal patterns of VERs similar in a model of HE and in animals with encephalopathies induced by drugs which augment GABAergic neurotransmission (4). Hypothesis that BZ antagonists may ameliorate HE (67).

1985 First reports of ameliorations of HE associated with the administration of a BZ antagonist in patients with cirrhosis and FHF (68,71).

1987 HE in a model of FHF ameliorated by pharmacological antagonism of components of GABA/BZ receptor complex and associated with increased resistance to the convulsive properties of a GABA antagonist (9).

1988 Differential responsiveness of individual Purkinje neurons to GABA$_A$ and BZ receptor ligands in a model of HE (50). Hypothesis that increased levels of BZ receptor agonist ligands may be a mechanism of increased GABAergic tone in HE (80).

1989 Increased levels of BZ-like activity in CSF of a model of HE (73). Characterisation of pharmacological nature of this material (44). Case report of sustained remission of chronic intractable portal-systemic encephalopathy induced by oral administration of a BZ antagonist (60).

1990 Behavioural and electrophysiological ameliorations of HE in FHF induced by BZ antagonists neither species nor model dependent (51). Increased plasma-to-brain transfer of GABA in a model of FHF (33). Increased levels of 1,4-BZs in brain of a model of HE (75) and increased levels of BZ activity in plasma and urine of patients with decompensated cirrhosis (76).

1991 Increased levels of 1,4-BZs in brains of patients dying from FHF (77). Certain BZ receptor ligands with antagonist and partial inverse agonist properties particularly efficacious in ameliorating HE in models of FHF (52,53).

8. Current Perspectives

1. The hypothesis that increased GABAergic tone contributes to HE has stimulated research activity into HE as a neuropsychiatric disorder and has focused attention on the role of specific neurochemical mechanisms in this syndrome.

2. Two important questions have inevitably been raised by the hypothesis: (i) Is GABAergic tone increased in HE? (ii) If it is, what mechanisms are involved?

3. Four lines of evidence support the hypothesis. (i) The abnormal pattern of VERs in HE is similar to that induced by drugs that cause encephalopathy by increasing GABAergic tone (4,46,47). (ii) In HE there is increased resistance to the induction of seizures by drugs which decrease GABAergic tone (9,48). (iii) CNS neurons from a model of HE exhibit increased sensitivity to a GABA agonist and a BZ agonist (50). (iv) Ameliorations of HE can be induced by drugs that pharmacologically antagonise components of the GABA/BZ receptor complex (9,51-53,57-60). All of the relevant evidence has been obtained in animal models of FHF, except for reports of ameliorations of HE in humans with FHF or cirrhosis induced by the BZ antagonist flumazenil (57-60).

4. Potential mechanisms for increased GABAergic tone in HE have been tested experimentally. The lack of HE-associated changes in the structure or functional status of the GABA/BZ receptor complex (44,45,61-63) has suggested that humoral mechanisms might be important. Potential humoral factors would include $GABA_A$ and BZ receptor agonists.

5. That $GABA_A$ receptor agonists may contribute to HE has not been excluded and has been inadequately tested. The observations of increased plasma-to-brain transfer of GABA (33) and increased release of GABA from astrocytes and/or neurons (23,64,65) in models of FHF are consistent with this possibility.

6. Evidence is accumulating that increased brain levels of BZ receptor ligands with agonist properties contribute to HE by potentiating the action of GABA (59). Such evidence has arisen as a direct result of testing potential mechanisms of increased GABAergic tone in HE and this evidence provides strong support for the GABA hypothesis (56). The presence of increased levels of BZ agonists may be only one of several mechanisms responsible for increased GABAergic tone in HE.

7. The GABA hypothesis implies that therapeutic modalities that normalise increased GABAergic tone should ameliorate some of the manifestations HE. $GABA_A$ and BZ receptor ligands that decrease GABAergic tone ameliorate HE in animal models (9,51-53). However, $GABA_A$ receptor antagonists and BZ receptor full inverse agonists are potent convulsants (9,51). In contrast, BZ antagonists with minimal or no inverse agonist properties may reduce GABAergic tone in HE with a clinically acceptable risk/benefit ratio (56).

8. Flumazenil is a BZ antagonist with weak partial agonist properties (50) and an acceptable safety profile (49). This drug is commercially available for clinical use and may have several applications in the management of HE. The response to flumazenil may be of

value in the differential diagnosis of encephalopathies and may provide a prognostic index in HE. Continuous administration of flumazenil may facilitate optimization of the mental status of a patient with liver failure. Finally, orally–administered flumazenil may reduce protein intolerance in chronic portal–systemic encephalopathy (42,49,59,81). However, flumazenil may not be the ideal BZ antagonist for administration to patients with HE and flumazenil–induced ameliorations of HE are not a requirement of the GABA hypothesis.

9. In animal models other BZ receptor ligands, e.g. Ro 15–3505, have been shown to be more efficacious than flumazenil in ameliorating HE (52,53). However, data on their safety profile is absent or sparse, in particular assessments of their convulsive potential.

10. The GABA hypothesis has opened up new therapeutic horizons for the treatment of HE by indicating that HE can be ameliorated by subtly decreasing GABAergic tone via the central BZ receptor (56). This therapeutic approach is appropriate irrespective of whether BZ receptor ligands are responsible for increased GABAergic tone in HE and may only be fully realised after the properties of a wide spectrum of BZ receptor ligands have been assessed.

References

1. Schafer, D.F., and Jones, E.A., 1982, Potential neural mechanisms in the pathogenesis of hepatic encephalopathy, in: Progress in Liver Diseases, volume VII, Popper, H. and Schaffner, F. (Eds.), Grune and Stratton, New York, 615–627.
2. Conn, H.O. and Lieberthal, M.M., 1978, The Hepatic Coma Syndromes and Lactulose, Williams and Wilkins, Baltimore, 1978.
3. Schafer, D.F., Brody, L.E. and Jones, E.A., 1979, Visual evoked potentials: an objective measurement of hepatic encephalopathy in the rabbit, Gastroenterology 77:A38.
4. Schafer, D.F., Pappas, S.C., Brody, L.E., Jacobs, R. and Jones EA, 1984, Visual evoked potentials in a rabbit model of hepatic encephalopathy. I. Sequential changes and comparisons with drug–induced comas, Gastroenterology 86:540–545.
5. Schafer, D.F., Fowler, J.M., Brody, L.E., and Jones, E.A., 1980, Hepatic coma and inhibitory neurotransmission: the enteric bacterial flora as a source of gamma–aminobutyric acid, Gastroenterology 79:1052.
6. Paul, S.M., Marangos, P.J., and Skolnick, P., 1981, The benzodiazepine–GABA–chloride ionophore receptor complex: common site of minor tranquiliser action, Biol. Psych. 16:213–229.
7. Schafer, D.F., and Jones, E.A., 1982, Hepatic encephalopathy and the gamma–aminobutyric–acid neutotransmitter system, Lancet i:18–19.
8. Smialowski, A., 1978, The effect of intrahippocampal administration of gamma–aminobutyric acid (GABA), in: Amino Acids as Chemical Transmitters, Fonnum, F. (Ed.), Plenum Press, New York, 1977–1980.
9. Bassett, M.L., Mullen, K.D., Skolnick, P., and Jones, E.A., 1987, Amelioration of hepatic encephalopathy by pharmacological antagonism of the GABA$_A$–benzodiazepine receptor complex in a rabbit model of fulminant hepatic failure, Gastroenterology 93:1069–1077.
10. Schafer, D.F., Waggoner, J.G., and Jones, E.A., 1980, Sera from rabbits in acute hepatic coma inhibit the binding of [^{3}H] gamma–aminobutyric acid to neural membranes, Gastroenterology 78:1320.
11. Schafer, D.F., Thakur, A.K., and Jones, E.A., 1980, Acute hepatic coma and inhibitory neurotransmission: increase in gamma–aminobutyric acid levels in plasma and receptors in brain, Gastroenterology 79:1123.
12. Schafer, D.F., Fowler, J.M., and Jones, E.A., 1981, Colonic bacteria: a source of gamma–aminobutyric acid in blood, Proc. Soc. Exp. Biol. Med. 167:301–303.
13. Horowitz, M.E., Schafer, D.F., Molnar, P., Jones, E.A., Blasberg, R.G., Patlak, C.S., Waggoner, J., and Fenstermacher, J.D., 1983, Increased blood–brain transfer in a rabbit model of acute liver failure, Gastroenterology 84:1003–1011.
14. Schafer, D.F., Fowler, J.M., Munson, P.J., Thakur, A.K., Waggoner, J.G., and Jones, E.A., 1983, Gamma–aminobutyric acid and benzodiazepine receptors in an animal model of fulminant hepatic failure, J. Lab. Clin. Med. 102:870–880.

15. Lefkowitz, R.J., Caron, M.G., Stiles, G.L, 1984, Mechanisms of membrane receptor regulation, N. Engl. J. Med. **310**:1570–1579.

16. Bakti, G., Fisch, H.U., Karlaganis, G., Minder,C., and Bircher, J., 1987, Mechanism of the excessive sedative response of cirrhotics to benzodiazepines: model experiments with triazolam, Hepatology **7**:629–638.

17. Ferenci, P., Schafer, D.F., Kleinberger, G., Hoofnagle, J.H., and Jones, E.A., 1983, Serum levels of gamma–aminobutyric–acid–like activity in acute and chronic hepatocellular disease, Lancet ii:811–814.

18. van Berlo, C.L.H., de Jonge, H.R., van den Bogaard, A.E.J.M., Janssen, M.A., van Eijk, H.M.H., van der Heijden, M.A.H., and Soeters, P.B., 1987, Gamma–aminobutyric acid production in small and large intestine of normal and germ–free Wistar rats. Influence of food intake and intestinal flora, Gastroenterology **93**:472–479.

19. Ferenci, P., Ebner, J., Zimmermann, C., Kikuta, C., Roth, E., and Hausinger, D., 1988, Overestimation of serum concentrations of gamma–aminobutyric acid in patients with hepatic encephalopathy by the gamma–aminobutyric acid–radioreceptor assay, Hepatology **8**:69–72.

20. Maddison, J.E., Leong, D.K., Dodd, P.R., and Johnson, G.A.R., 1990, Plasma GABA–like activity in rats with hepatic encephalopathy is due to GABA and taurine, Hepatology **11**:105–110.

21. Minuk, G.Y., Winder, A., Burgess, E.D., and Sargeant, E.J., 1985, Serum gamma–aminobutyric acid (GABA) levels in patients with hepatic encephalopathy, Hepatogastroenterology **32**:171–174.

22. Levy, L.J., Leek, J., and Losowsky, M.S., 1987, Evidence for gamma–aminobutyric acid as the inhibitor of gamma–aminobutyric acid binding in the plasma of humans with liver disease and hepatic encephalopathy, Clin. Sci. **73**:531–534.

23. Albrecht, J., and Rafalowska, U., 1987, Enhanced potassium–stimulated gamma–aminobutyric acid release by astrocytes derived from rats with early hepatic encephalopathy, J. Neurochem. **49**:9–11.

24. Jones, E.A., Gammal, S.H., Basile, A.S., Mullen, K.D., Bassett, M.L., Schafer, D.F., and Skolnick, P., 1988, Hepatic encephalopathy and benzodiazepine receptor ligands, in: Hepatic Encephalopathy. Pathophysiology and Treatment, Butterworth, R.F., and Layrargues, G.P. (Eds.), Humana Press, Clifton, New Jersey, 273–286.

25. Oldendorf, W.H., 1971, Brain uptake of radiolabeled amino acids, amines and hexoses after arterial injection, Am. J. Physiol. **221**:1629–1639.

26. Goldstein, G.W., 1984, The role of brain capillaries in the pathogenesis of hepatic encephalopathy, Hepatology **4**:565–567.

27. Lo, W.D., Ennis, S.R., Goldstein, G.W., McNeely, D.L., and Betz, A.L., 1987, The effects of galactosamine–induced hepatic failure upon blood–brain barrier permeability, Hepatology **7**:452–456.

28. Knudsen, G.M., Poulsen, H.E., Paulsen, O.B., 1988, Blood–brain barrier permeability in galactosamine–induced hepatic encephalopathy. No evidence for increased GABA transport, J. Hepatol. **6**:187–192.

29. Mullen, K.D., Schafer, D.F., Cuchi, P., Rossle, M., Maynard, T.F., and Jones, E.A., 1988, Evaluation of the suitability of galactodamine–induced fulminant hepatic failure as a model of hepatic encephalopathy in the rat and the rabbit, in: Advances in Ammonia Metabolism and Hepatic Encephalopathy, Soeters, P.B., Wilson, J.H.P., Meijer, A.J., and Holm, E. (Eds.), Elsevier Science Publishers, Amsterdam, 205–212.

30. Blitzer, B.L., Waggoner, J.G., Jones, E.A., Gralnick, H., Towne, D., Butler, J., Weise, V., Kopin, I., Walters, I., Teychenne, P.F., Goodmam, D.G., and Berk, P.D., 1978, A model of fulminant hepatic failure in the rabbit, Gastroenterology **74**:664–671.

31. Traber, P.G., Ganger, G.R., and Blei, A.T., 1986, Brain edema in rabbits with galactosamine–induced fulminant hepatitis: regional differences and effects on intracranial pressure, Gastroenterology **91**:1347–1356.

32. Traber, P.G., DelCanto, M.D., Ganger, D.R., and Blei, A.T., 1987, Electronmicroscopic evaluation of brain edema in rabbits with galactosamine–induced fulminant hepatic failure: ultrastructure and integrity of the blood–brain barrier, Hepatology **7**:1272–1277.

33. Bassett, M.L., Mullen, K.D., Scholz, B., Fenstermacher, J.D., and Jones, E.A., 1990, Increased brain uptake of gamma–aminobutyric acid in a rabbit model of hepatic encephalopathy, Gastroenterology **98**:747–757.

34. Cooper, J.R., Bloom, F.E., Roth, R.H., 1991, The Biochemical Basis of Neuropharmacology, Oxford University Press, New York, 1991.

35. Wysmyk-Cybula, U., Dabrowiecki, Z., and Albrecht, J., 1986, Changes in the metabolism and binding of GABA in the rat brain in thioacetamide-induced hepatogenic encephalopathy, Biomed. Biochim. Acta 45:413-419.

36. Zimmermann, C., Ferenci, P., Pifl, C., Yurdaydin, C., Ebner, J., Lassman, H., Roth, E., and Hortnagl, H., 1989, Hepatic encephalopathy in thioacetamide-induced acute liver failure: characterization of an improved model and study of amino acid-ergic neurotransmission, Hepatology 9:594-601.

37. Moroni, F., Riggio, O., Carla, V., Festuccia, V., Ghinelli, F., Marino, I.R., Merli, M., Natali, L., Pedretti, G., Fiaccadori, F., and Capocaccia, L., 1987, Hepatic encephalopathy: lack of changes of gamma-aminobutyric acid content in plasma and cerebrospinal fluid, Hepatology 7:816-820.

38. Ungerstedt, U., 1984, Measurement of neurotransmitter release by intracranial dialysis, in: Measurement of Neurotransmitter Release, Marsden, C.A. (Ed.), John Wiley and Sons, New York, 81-105.

39. Enna, S.J., and Snyder, S.H., 1977, Influence of ions, enzymes, and detergents on gamma-aminobutyric acid receptor binding in synaptic membranes of rat brain, Mol. Pharmacol. 13:442-453.

40. Baraldi, M., and Zeneroli, M.L., 1982, Experimental hepatic encephalopathy: changes in the binding of gamma-aminobutyric acid, Science 216:427-428.

41. Schenker, S., and Brady III, C.E., 1988, Pathogenesis of hepatic encephalopathy, in: Hepatic Encephalopathy: Management with Lactulose and Related Carbohydrates, Conn, H.O., and Bircher, J. (Eds.), Medi-Ed Press, East Lansing, Michigan, 15-30.

42. Jones, E.A., and Skolnick, P., 1990, Benzodiazepine receptor ligands and the syndrome of hepatic encephalopathy, in: Progress in Liver Diseases, volume IX, Popper, H., and Schaffner, F. (Eds.), W.B. Saunders, Philadelphia, 345-370.

43. Rossle, M., Mullen, K.D., and Jones, E.A., 1989, Cortical benzodiazepine receptor binding in a rabbit model of hepatic encephalopathy: the effect of Triton X-100 on receptor solubilization, Metabolic Brain Dis. 4:203-212.

44. Basile, A.S., Gammal, S.H., Jones, E.A., and Skolnick, P., 1989, GABA_A receptor complex in an experimental model of hepatic encephalopathy: evidence for elevated levels of an endogenous benzodiazepine receptor ligand, J. Neurochem. 53:1057-1063.

45. Basile, A.S., Ostrowski, N.L., Gammal, S.H., Jones, E.A., and Skolnick, P., 1990, The GABA_A receptor complex in hepatic encephalopathy. Autoradiographic evidence for the presence of elevated levels of a benzodiazepine receptor ligand, Neuropsychopharmacol 3:61-71.

46. Pappas, S.C., Ferenci, P., Schafer, D.F., and Jones, E.A., 1984, Visual evoked potentials in a rabbit model of hepatic encephalopathy. II. Comparison of hyperammonemic encephalopathy, postictal coma and coma induced by synergistic neurotoxins, Gastroenterology 86:546-551.

47. Jones, D.B., Mullen, K.D., Roessle, M., Maynard, T., and Jones, E.A., 1987, Hepatic encephalopathy: application of visual evoked responses to test hypotheses of its pathogenesis in rats, J. Hepatol. 4:118-126.

48. Ferreira, M.R., Gammal, S.H., and Jones, E.A., 1988, Hepatic encephalopathy: evidence of increased GABA-mediated neurotransmission in a rat model of fulminant hepatic failure, Gastroenterology 94:A616.

49. Jones, E.A., Basile, A.S., Mullen, K.D., and Gammal, S.H., 1990, Flumazenil: potential implications for hepatic encephalopathy, Pharmac. Ther. 45:331-343.

50. Basile, A.S., Gammal, S.H., Mullen, K.D., Jones, E.A., and Skolnick, P., 1988, Differential responsiveness of cerebellar Purkinje neurons to GABA and benzodiazepine receptor ligands in an animal model of hepatic encephalopathy, J. Neurosci. 8:2414-2421.

51. Gammal, S.H., Basile, A.S., Geller, D., Skolnick, P., and Jones, E.A., 1990, Reversal of the behavioral and electrophysiological abnormalities of an animal model of hepatic encephalopathy by benzodiazepine receptor ligands, Hepatology 11:371-378.

52. Bosman, D.K., van der Buijs, C.A.C.G., de Haan, J.G., Maas, M.A.W., and Chamuleau, R.A.F.M., 1991, The effects of benzodiazepine receptor antagonists and partial inverse agonists in acute hepatic encephalopathy in the rat, Gastroenterology 101:772-781.

53. Steindl, P., Puspok, A., Druml, W., and Ferenci, P., 1991, Beneficial effect of pharmacological modulation of the GABA$_A$-benzodiazepine receptor on hepatic encephalopathy in the rat: comparison with uremic encephalopathy, Hepatology 14:963–968.

54. Haefely, W., Kyburz, E., Gerecke, M., and Mohler, M., 1985, Recent advances in the molecular pharmacology of benzodiazepine receptors and in the structure–activity relationships of their agonists and antagonists, Adv. Drug. Res. 14:165–322.

55. Gardner, C.R., 1988, Pharmacological profiles in vivo of benzodiazepine receptor ligands, Drug. Devel. Res. 12:1–28, 1988.

56. Jones, E.A., 1991, Benzodiazepine receptor ligands and hepatic encephalopathy: Further unfolding of the GABA story, Hepatology 14:1286–1290.

57. Grimm, G., Ferenci, P., Katzenschlager, R., Madl, C., Schneeweiss, B., Laggner, A.N., Lenz, K., and Gangl, A., 1988, Improvement in hepatic encephalopathy treated with flumazenil, Lancet ii:1392–1394.

58. Bansky, G., Meier, P.J., Riederer, E., Walser, H., Ziegler, W.H., and Schmid, M., 1989, Effects of the benzodiazepine receptor antagonist flumazenil in hepatic encephalopathy in humans, Gastroenterology 97:744–750.

59. Basile, A.S., Jones, E.A., and Skolnick, P., 1991, The pathogenesis and treatment of hepatic encephalopathy: evidence for the involvement of benzodiazepine receptor ligands, Pharm. Rev. 43:27–71.

60. Ferenci, P., Grimm, G., Meryn, S., and Gangl, A., 1989, Successful long–term treatment of portal–systemic encephalopathy by the benzodiazepine antagonist flumazenil, Gastroenterology 96:240–243.

61. Baker, B.L., Morrow, A.L., Vergalla, J., Paul, S.M., and Jones, E.A., 1990, Gamma–aminobutyric acid (GABA$_A$) receptor–function in a rat model of hepatic encephalopathy, Metabolic Brain Dis. 5:1285–1293.

62. Rossle, M., Deckert, J., and Jones, E.A., 1989, Autoradiographic analysis of GABA–benzodiazepine receptors in an animal model of acute hepatic encephalopathy, Hepatology 10:143–147.

63. Basile, A.S., 1991, The contribution of endogenous benzodiazepine receptor ligands to the pathogenesis of hepatic encephalopathy, Synapse 7:141–150.

64. Albrecht, J., Hilgier, W., and Rafalowska, U., 1990, Activation of arginine metabolism to glutamate in rat brain synaptosomes in thioacetamide–induced hepatic encephalopathy: an adaptive response? J. Neuroscience Res. 25:125–130.

65. Wysmyk, U., Oja, S.S., Saransaari, P., and Albrecht, J., 1992, Enhanced GABA release in cerebral cortical slices from rats with thioacetamide–induced hepatic encephalopathy, Neurochem. Res. 17:1187–1190.

66. Oja, S.S., Saransaari, P., Wysmyk, U., and Albrecht, J., 1993, Loss of GABA$_B$ binding sites in the cerebral cortex of rats with acute hepatic encephalopathy, Brain Res. 629:355–357.

67. Anderson, B., 1984, A proposed theory for the encephalopathies of Reye's syndrome and hepatic encephalopathy, Med. Hypotheses 15:415–420.

68. Bansky, G., Meier, P.J., Ziegler, W.H., Walser, H., Schmid, M., and Huber, M., 1985, Reversal of hepatic coma by benzodiazepine antagonist (Ro 15–1788), Lancet i:1324–1325.

69. Baraldi, M., Zeneroli, M.L., Ventura, E., Penne, A., Pinelli, G., Ricci, P., and Santi, M., 1984, Supersensitivity of benzodiazepine receptors in hepatic encephalopathy due to fulminant hepatic failure in the rat: reversal by a benzodiazepine antagonist, Clin. Sci. 67:167–175.

70. Bassett, M.L., Mullen, K.D., Skolnick, P., and Jones, E.A., 1985, GABA and benzodiazepine receptor antagonists ameliorate hepatic encephalopathy in a rabbit model of fulminant hepatic failure, Hepatology 5:1032.

71. Scollo–Lavizzari, G., and Steinmann, E., 1985, Reversal of hepatic coma by benzodiazepine antagonist (Ro 15–1788), Lancet i:1324.

72. van der Rijt, C.C.D., de Knegt, R.J., Schalm, S.W., Terpstra, O.T., and Mechelse, K., 1990, Flumazenil does not improve hepatic encephalopathy associated with acute ischemic liver failure in the rabbit. Metabolic Brain Dis. 5:131–141, 1990.

73. Mullen, K.D., Martin, J.V., Mendelson, W.B., Kaminsky–Russ, K., and Jones, E.A., 1989, Evidence for the presence of a benzodiazepine receptor binding substance in cerebrospinal fluid of a rabbit model of hepatic encephalopathy, Metabolic Brain Dis. 4:253–260.

74. Olasmaa, M., Rothstein, J.D., Guidotti, A., Weber, R.J., Paul, S.M., Spector, S., Zeneroli, M.L., Baraldi, M., and Costa, E., 1990, Endogenous benzodiazepine receptor ligands in human and animal hepatic encephalopathy, J. Neurochem. 55:2015–2023.

75. Basile, A.S., Pannell, L., Jaouni, T., Gammal, S.H., Fales, H.M., Jones, E.A., and Skolnick, P., 1990, Brain concentrations of benzodiazepines are elevated in an animal model of hepatic encephalopathy, Proc Natl Acad Sci (USA) 87:5263–5267.

76. Mullen, K.D., Szauter, K.M., and Kaminsky-Russ, K., 1990, "Endogenous" benzodiazepine activity in body fluids of patients with hepatic encephalopathy, Lancet 336:81–83.

77. Basile, A.S., Hughes, R.D., Harrison, P.M., Murata, Y., Pannell, L., Jones, E.A., Williams, R., and Skolnick, P., 1991, Elevated brain concentrations of 1,4–benzodiazepines in fulminant hepatic failure, N. Engl. J. Med. 325:473–478.

78. Yurdaydin, C., Gu, Z–Q., Nowak, G., Fromm, C., Holt, A.G., and Basile, A.S., 1993, Benzodiazepine receptor ligands are elevated in an animal model of hepatic encephalopathy: relationship between brain concentration and severity of encephalopathy, J. Pharm. Exp. Ther. 265:565–571.

79. Basile, A.S., Hughes, R.D., Harrison, P.M., Gu, Z–Q., Pannell, L., McKinnon, A., Jones, E.A., and Williams, R., 1994, Correlation between plasma benzodiazepine receptor ligand concentrations and the severity of hepatic encephalopathy in patients with fulminant hepatic failure, Hepatology 19:112–121.

80. Mullen, K.D., Martin, J.V., Mendelson, W.B., Bassett, M.L., and Jones, E.A., 1988, Could an endogenous benzodiazepine ligand contribute to hepatic encephalopathy? Lancet i:457–459.

81. Jones, E.A., Skolnick, P., Gammal, S.H., Basile, A.S., and Mullen, K.D., 1989, The gamma–aminobutyric acid A (GABA$_A$) receptor complex and hepatic encephalopathy. Some recent advances, Ann. Intern. Med. 110:532–546.

Neuropharmacologic Modulation of Hepatic Encephalopathy: Experimental and Clinical Data

Peter Ferenci, Andreas Herneth, Andreas Püspök and Petra Steindl

1. Introduction

Various neurochemical studies in hepatic encephalopathy (HE) (for review: 1) indicate that alterations of several neurotransmitter systems including the $GABA_A$–benzodiazepine-ergic, glutamatergic, dopaminergic, serotoninergic, noradrenergic and opiatergic neurotransmitter systems may contribute to the pathogenesis of this syndrome, but the precise role of each of these changes remains controversial. Using specific agonists and antagonists of these neurotransmitters the importance of altered neurotransmission in HE can be examined in vivo. Such experiments may improve our understanding of the pathophysiology of HE and can ultimately help to develop better treatments. In this paper the current status of neurobehavioural studies in experimental and in human HE will be reviewed.

2. Neurobehavioural Studies in Experimental Hepatic Encephalopathy

2.1. Animal Model and Neurobehavioural Testing

Several animal models of HE are currently used. They are reviewed elsewere in this book (Mullen, K). The parameters to assess drug effects include measurement of motor activity, clinical evaluation (behavioural score, neurological examination) and electrophysiologic methods (EEG, evoked responses).

In our laboratory drug effects were assessed in control rats, in rats 60 hrs after the first dose of thioacetamide (TAA) (HE I) and in rats with overt hepatic encephalopathy (HE III). This model has been characterized by clinical, light microscopic and electron microscopic investigations previously (2). Briefly, acute liver failure was induced in male Sprague Dawley rats by TAA (300 mg/kg BW given by gavage) on two consecutive days. Hypoglycaemia and renal failure were prevented by a supportive therapy. To evaluate progression of HE rats were tested clinically and the neurologic status was quantitated by a score based on 14 different reflexes, every 4 hours. At 60 hrs none of the rats has clinical overt HE but motor activity is decreased. HE develops usually after 67 hrs and is marked by a progressive neurologic deterioration (loss of reflexes).

Department of Internal Medicine IV, Gastroenterology and Hepatology, University of Vienna, Währinger Gürtel 18–20, A–1090 Wien, Austria

Hepatic Encephalopathy, Hyperammonemia, and Ammonia Toxicity
Edited by V. Felipo and S. Grisolia, Plenum Press, New York, 1994

103

For measurement of motor activity rats were put separately in an Animex Activity Meter (Farad Electronics), which counts every movement of the animal by means of magnetic induction. Rats were tested for ten minutes, thereafter coded drug was injected intraperitoneally and testing was repeated. During each test period the behavioural status was evaluated by a semiquantitative behavioural score (3), grading alertness, interest, walking, body–tension and nose poking from absent 0 points to apparently normal 3 points .

In untreated normal rats motor activity decreased in the first 30 minutes and remained stable thereafter (see Fig. 2). Rats 60 hrs after TAA have a lower initial motor activity but after 30 minutes in the cage their activity is not different from control rats. In stage HE III motor activity is significantly decreased (9.7±2.3) and does not change over an observation period of upto one hour. The behavioural score in control rats and rats 60 hrs after TAA is 15, and decreases in untreated rats with HE III to 2.5±0.4.

2.2. Benzodiazepine Receptor Ligands

Various observations in experimental liver failure like the similarities of changes of visual evoked potentials in rabbits and rats with HE and those induced in normal animals by drugs acting through the $GABA_A$–benzodiazepine receptor complex (4), the transient clinical improvement of HE associated with a normalization of abnormal visual evoked potentials (5,6) by specific antagonists, and the increased resistance to the convulsive action of bicuculline (6) can be readily explained by the presence of increased GABA–ergic tone. The mechanisms causing the activation of the $GABA_A$–ergic neurotransmission are unknown. Schafer and Jones (7) suggested that gut derived GABA with "supersensitive" postsynaptic GABA–receptors. Baraldi and Zeneroli (8) attributed the supersensitivity of postsynaptic $GABA_A$–receptors to a degeneration of presynaptic GABA–ergic terminals mediated by some toxines, excess glutamate, or zinc deficiency (9). None of these hypothesis could be confirmed sofar. More recently it was assumed that in HE agonistic compounds of endogenous origin binding to the $GABA_A$–benzodiazepine receptor ("endogenous benzodiazepines") are present in the brain. These substances were isolated, characterized and positively identified by gas chromatography–mass spectroscopy as benzodiazepines (10,11,12) both in brains, sera and CSF of men and experimental animals with liver failure.

The role of "endogenous" benzodiazepines to induce HE may be adressed by neurobehavioural studies using benzodiazepine receptor ligands. They can be classified according on their effects on the chloride ionophore to three different classes. The first class are benzodiazepine agonists like diazepam. They increase the affinity of GABA to its receptor and/or the coupling of the $GABA_A$–receptor to the chloride ionophore. The second type are inverse agonists like b–carbolines. They decrease the affinity of GABA receptors and GABA–induced chloride fluxes. The third type of benzodiazepine ligands are antagonists. These drugs are believed to stabilize the benzodiazepine receptor in a neutral state and competitively antagonize the binding of other benzodiazepine ligands. Consequently antagonists tend to normalize changes in GABA–ergic tone induced by agonists or inverse agonists. However, most benzodiazepine receptor antagonists have intrinsic effects (partial inverse agonistic (CGS 8216, Ro 15–4513, sarmazenil [Ro 15–3505]) or partial agonistic (flumazenil [Ro 15–1788])).

In rats 60 hrs after TAA and in control rats the injection of the benzodiazepine agonist flunitrazepam resulted in a continous loss of reflexes as shown by the decrease of the neurological score in both groups (see fig.1). However, the response in both groups was different: although controls remained completely normal up to and including a dosage of 0.25 mg/kg, the neurological score of TAA rats was significantly reduced already at the dose of 0.1 mg/kg. The difference became even more pronounced with increasing doses of flunitrazepam up to the highest dosage used (5 mg/kg) (13). Flunitrazepam–induced coma was completely

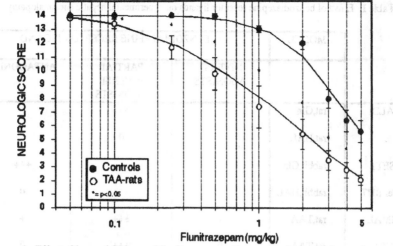

Figure 1. Effect of increasing doses of flunitrazepam on the neurologic status of control rats and rats 60 hrs after the first dose of thioacetamide (TAA). Taken from Püspök et al,1993 (13).

reversed by the pure benzodiazepine antagonist (Ro 14–7437) both in control and TAA rats. Flumazenil and "pure" antagonist (Ro 14–7437, ZK 93426) (at doses which completely reverse flunitrazepam induced coma) were ineffective to improve HE in our as well as in experiments by van der Rijt (14) and by Yurdaydin (15). In contrast, Bassett et al (6) and Bosman et al (16) reported an amelioration of HE. Thus the effect flumazenil on experimental HE remains controversial.

However, benzodiazepine antagonist with partial inverse agonistic properties (Ro 15–3505, Ro 15–513, Ro 19–4603, CGS–8216) unequivocally improve various neurobehavioural features of HE (3,5,13,15–18; see table 1). This improvement can be blocked by the concomitant administration of "pure" benzodiazepine antagonists (13). In contrast to HE coma due to renal failure in rats with bilateral ureteral ligation was not improved by these compounds (3). Inverse agonist (DMCM) were ineffective to improve HE.

Thus, the inverse agonistic effects and the displacement of an endogenous benzodiazepine–ligand from the receptor are equally important to achieve an amelioration of HE. Recently it was suggested that only benzodiazepine receptor ligands which interact with the "diazepam insensitive" subtype of the benzodiazepine receptor are effective to improve HE (15).

These observations do not support a direct role of "endogenous" benzodiazepines in the pathogenesis of HE. The fact that flumazenil may be effective in human HE (19,20) but not in experimental HE has been attributed to the higher concentrations of "endogenous" benzodiazepines in humans. Clearly further studies are needed to fully understand the role of "endogenous" benzodiazepines in the mediation of HE. The beneficial effects on HE of benzodiazepine antagonist with partial inverse agonistic properties do not necessarily imply an overactivity of the GABA$_A$–benzodiazepine neurotransmitter system. Another possible explanation would be an imbalance of excitatory and inhibitory neurotransmission.

2.3. Drugs acting on central serotonin receptors

In various animal models and in humans with HE elevated concentrations of serotonin and its metabolite 5–hydroxy–indol–acetic–acid were found in several brain areas (21,22), indicating and increased turnover–rate in HE (23). However, an increased turnover–rate does not necessarily imply an over–activity of this neurotransmitter system. Only serotonin

Table 1. Effect of benzodiazepine receptor ligands on experimental hepatic encephalopathy

	MODEL	BENZODIAZEPINE RECEPTOR LIGAND		
		INVERSE AGONISTS	PARTIAL INVERSE AGONISTS	ANTAGONISTS
BARALDI (5)	rat,Gln		+++	
ZIEVE (18)	rat,HAL		0	
BASSETT (6)	rabbit,Gln			+++
van der RIJT (14)	rabbit,HAL			0
GAMMAL (17)	rat,TAA	+	+++	+
STEINDL PÜSPÖK (3,13)	rat,TAA	0	+++	0
BOSMAN (16)	rat,HAL		+++	(+)
YURDAYDIN (15)	rat,TAA		+++	0

0= no effect; +++ = unequivokal effect; + = effect in some animals; (+) = unclear effect Gln= galactosamine, TAA= thioacetamide, HAL= hepatic artery ligation.

released from presynaptic vesicles into the synaptic gap can mediate the multiple biological effects of serotonin. Serotonin produced in larger quantities may not be taken up into presynaptic vesicle. This "free" serotonin is catabolised in the cytoplasm to 5–hydroxy–indol–acetic–acid. Furthermore, even if serotoninergic neurotransmission is activated, the various biological effects of serotonin may be unrelated to HE. The role of serotonin in the pathogenesis of HE in vivo can be investigated by neuro–behavioural studies. The serotonin neurotransmitter system is rather complex (24–26). According to binding studies there are at least 3 major receptor families, and in each receptor–family several subtypes can be distinguished. Each subtype modulates different biological effects (Table 2), of which many still are poorly characterised.

The $5-HT_{1A}$ agonist 8 OH–DPAT increases the motor activity dose dependently in all groups of rats tested. However, the motor response to his drug reflects not a normal

Table 2. Behavioural effects of serotonin agonists (+: increase, decrease, n.t.: not tested; ⁻: uncertain; 0: no-effect) according to E.Zifa and G.Fillion (24)

Receptor subtype	motor-activity	feeding	body-temperature	sexual behaviour
$5-HT_{1A}$	+	+	–	+
$5-HT_{1B}$	-	⁻	n.t.	–
$5-HT_{1D}$	-	-	-	-
$5-HT_2$	+	–	+	+
$5-HT_{1C}$	+	n.t.	n.t.	n.t.
$5-HT_3$	0	0	0	0

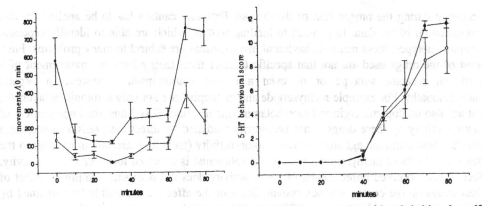

Fig.2. Effect of increasing doses of the 5–HT1A agonist 8–OH–DPAT on control rats (closed circle) and rats 60 hrs after TAA (open circle) n=4 in each group. From min 20 to min 70 rats were injected with increasing doses of 8–OH DPAT (0.001,0.01,0.05,0.1,0.5, and 1 mg/kg). Serotonin behavioural score according to Tricklebank (27).

behaviour but a specific syndrome induced by activation of postsynaptic $5 HT_{1A}$ receptors (serotonin behavioural syndrome). There was no difference in the sensitivity of control rats and of rats 60 hrs after TAA to 8–OH–DPAT (see fig. 2), indicating that the activity of this receptor system is not impaired in HE I. Even rats with HE III responded to 5 OH–DPAT by increased motor activity typical for the serotonin behavioural syndrome.

In control rats and in rats 60 hrs after TAA, except for spiroxantrine, none of the tested serotonin receptor antagonists had any effect on motor activity or the behavioural status.

However, impaired motor–activity and the behavioural status in rats with HE III was improved dose–dependently by methysergide. Metitepine showed similar effects, whereas metergoline further deteriorated the condition of the animals (see fig 3). The $5HT_{1A}$ antagonist NAN–190 increased motor–activity and the behavioural score dose–dependently, but another $5HT_{1A}$ antagonist, spiroxantrine, worsened the condition of the rats. The specific $5HT_2$ receptor antagonists ritanserin and seganserine, and the $5HT_3$ receptor antagonist odansetrone had no effect on measured parameters.

These findings suggest that changes of the serotoninergic neurotransmitter system are present in HE. Since not all antagonists tested were equally effective, apparently not all serotonin receptors are affected. However, this study cannot resolve whether changes in serotoninergic neurotransmission are direct consequences of liver failure or secondary events

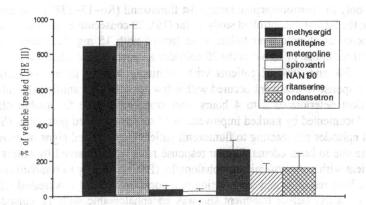

Figure 3. Effect of serotonin antagonists on motor activity of rats with HE III (each drug at the highest dose tested –1–10 mg/kg).

occurring during the progression of the disease. Extreme caution has to be applied for this interpretation of the data. In contrast to binding studies, which are able to identify especific receptor subtypes, these neuro–behavioural investigations are subject to many problems. First, most of the drugs used are not that specific to infer from their effects an involvement of a particular receptor subtype or of even a certain neurotransmitter system in hepatic encephalopathy. For example methysergide and metitepine are not only serotonin antagonists, but act also on dopaminergic and catecholaminergic neurones (28). Thus, the improvement of motor–activity by these drugs is not necessarily mediated by direct antagonism of serotonin effects. Most serotonin agonists increase motor–activity (table 2), therefore, in contrast to the observed effects of methysergide, a serotonin antagonist is expected to lower motor–activity. Second, the observed improvement of motor activity does not necessarily imply an effect of these drugs on the central nervous system. Some of the effects can possibly be explained by peripheral effects on blood pressure (29) or on the muscle tone. However, no changes in blood pressure by methysergide were observed in rats with liver failure (Herneth et al., unpublished observations). Also other peripheral effects of methysergide such as lowering body temperature (30) cannot explain the beneficial effects of the drug. Third, it is unknown how much of the applied drugs reach the brain. Thus, the lack of response to seganserine and odansetrone does not exclude with certainty a possible effect. Due to the experimental approach in this study rats could only be tested for 10 minutes. It is conceivable that some effects my occur lateron. Fourth, the observed effects occurred within a minute after application of methysergide which is in contrast to the pharmacokinetics of this drug in man where an effect is usually observed after a period of at least 20 minutes. The rapid onset of the action of methysergide may suggest that only minimal amounts of the drug are necessary to improve HE.

In spite of these problems inherent in such studies the marked effects on HE of certain serotonin antagonists are of potential importance in unravelling the pathogenesis of this syndrome and to develop better treatments.

2.4. Other drugs

Opiate receptor antagonist (31) may improve HE in rats with TAA induced liver failure. Preliminary data from our laboratory show also some effects of ß–blockers.

3. Flumazenil in Human Hepatic Encephalopathy

In humans only the benzodiazepine antagonist flumazenil (Ro–15–1788) was used for treatment of HE. In the largest uncontrolled study so far (19), 20 consecutive episodes of HE in 17 patients with acute or chronic liver failure were treated with 15 mg flumazenil infused intravenously over three hours. In 12 out of the 20 episodes an unequivokal amelioration of HE was observed (in 45% and 78% of patients with fulminant hepatic failure or cirrhosis, respectively). The response to treatment occured within few minutes after starting the infusion but 2/3 of the patient deteriorated 2 to 4 hours after stopping it. The favourable clinical response was also documented by marked improvement of sensory–evoked potencials (SEPs). In five of the eight episodes not reacting to flumazenil patients had marked signs of increased intracranial pressure due to brain edema. Similar response rates were observed by others (32). Furthermore, a patient with portosystemic encephalopathy (PSE) refractory to standard therapy following extensive liver resection and construction of a porto caval shunt was treated with 25 mg flumazenil twice daily. Before treatment she was encephalopathic with 12 episodes of coma within two years. On treatment with flumazenil all signs of HE abated in spite of unrestricted dietary protein intake (20).

These encouraging observations require controlled trials to document the effects of flumazenil in treatment of HE. HE is however a difficult syndrome to be studied by randomized controlled trials. The general difficulties were recognized in earlier trials on the effects of branched chain amino acids (33). With respect to flumazenil additional problems need to be adressed. The pharmakokinetics of flumazenil are altered in cirrhotics, changes being related to the severity of liver disease (34); this finding may account for possible individual differences in its duration of action. Furthermore, since flumazenil is effective to abolish the effects of benzodiazepine agonists, patients with i.e. diazepam induced encephalopathy have to be excluded. While this is logical, in practice it might be very difficult to identify patients with recent intake of a benzodiazepine. Methods include chart reviews and questionning of relatives as well as determination of benzodiazepines in urine or blood. None of these methods is entirely reliable. At present it is unknown how patients should be selected for treatment studies with benzodiazepine antagonist, since benzodiazepines may be present in blood of "drug-free" patients with liver failure (35). Less sensitive tests may miss some patients with benzodiazepine intake while HPLC or GCMS may detect benzodiazepine of presumable endogenous origin. Finally documentation of drug effects may require sophisticated methods, escpecially in patients with subclinical encephalopathy.

One controlled trial has been published as full paper so far (37), and the preliminary results of further four placebo controlled trials are available (see table 3).

All studies included only patients with cirrhosis. All five studies vary in design and exclusion criteria, and are therefore not directly comparable. Four studies are cross-over trials, only one a placebo-controlled double blind trial. Flumazenil was superior to placebo in three studies. (35-37). The largest study conducted so far was an international multicenter trial sponsored by Hoffmann-La Roche (35). An uncommon PSE score heavily based on neurologic signs (38) was used to document drug effects. 24 of 49 randomized patients had to be excluded from the final analysis, most of them because of inadequate benzodiazepine screening. Treatment included three bolus doses followed by each a one hour observation period and then a continous infusion over three hours. Flumazenil was superior to placebo whether the data were evaluated by standard analysis or an intent to treat analysis. The Canadian multicenter trial (36) had very strict exclusion criteria, which resulted in the rejection of 56 of 77 potential patients. The beneficial effect of flumazenil was not related to the presence of benzodiazepines in the blood. The positive results of this study in such a

Table 3. Randomized controlled trials (RCT) of flumazenil treatment of hepatic encephalopathy

AUTOR	Type of study	Dose	Efficacy parameter	Grade of HE	FLUMAZENIL		PLACEBO	
					Clinical	EEG	Clinical	EEG
					N improved/ N tested			
Gyr (Hoffman-La Roche) (36)	RCT Intent to treat	2mg + 1mg/h/ 3h	PSE-score	HE 2-4	5/14* (35%) 28%*		0/11 (0%) 0%	
Pomier-Layrarges (37)	crossover RCT	2mg	HE-grade EEG	HE 2-4	6/13* (46%)	4/12	0/15 (0%)	2/13
Cadranel (38)	crossover RCT	1mg	HE-grade EEG	HE 2-4	10/18* (56%)	10/18	2/12 (17%)	2/12
van der Rijt (40)	crossover RCT	1mg	HE-grade EEG	HE 0-4	6/17 (35%)	0/17	2/17 (12%)	0/17
Amodio (41)	crossover RCT	3mg /2h	NCT BAER	HE 0	0/9 (0%)	1/9	0/9 (0%)	0/9

*= p<0.05 NCT= number connection test, BAER= brainstem acoustic evoked responses.

highly selected group should be extrapolated with caution to cirrhotic patients as whole. In the third positive study (37) a not very sensitive test for benzodiazepines was used and not performed in all patients. Drug effects were evaluated on continous EEG recordings obtained before, during and 10 minutes after a bolus dose. Obviously a 10 minute observation is to short to obtain meaningful results. Two studies (39,40) were negative. Both studies included exclusively or predominantly patients with subclinical or mild HE. The study protocol of the Dutch trial (39) was changed during the study period. In this study there was a higher tendency for improval of HE by flumazenil than with placebo, but EEG remained unchanged in responding patients.

Thus, flumazenil may be a valuable new therapeutic approach in patients with acute or chronic HE. The publication of these trials as full papers is awaited. One other potentially useful indication for flumazenil may be differentiation of benzodiazepine induced coma from HE (20). No controlled trials were conducted sofar in patients with fulminant hepatic failure or in patients with chronic portosystemic encephalopathy.

References

1. Ferenci P., Püspök A., Steindl P: Current concepts in the pathophysiology of hepatic encephalopathy. Eur J Clin Invest 1992; 22:573–581.
2. Zimmermann C,Ferenci P,Pifl C,Yurdaydin C,Ebner J,Lassmann H,Roth E, et al. Hepatic encephalopathy in thioacetamide induced acute liver failure in rats: characterization of an improved model and study of amino acid–ergic neurotransmission. Hepatology 1989; 9:594–601.
3. Steindl P, Püspök A, Druml W, Ferenci P. Beneficial effect of pharmacological modulation of the GABA$_A$–benzodiazepine receptor on hepatic encephalopathy in the rat –comparison with uremic encephalopathy. Hepatology 1991; 14:963–968.
4. Schafer DF, Pappas SC, Brady LE, Jacobs R, Jones EA. Visual evoked potentials in a rabbit model of hepatic encephalopathy. I: Sequential changes and comparisons with drug induced comas. Gastroenterology 1984; 86:540–545.
5. Baraldi M, Zeneroli ML, Ventura E et al. Supersensitivity of benzodiazepine receptors in hepatic encephalopathy due to fulminant hepatic failure in the rat: Reversal by a benzodiazepine antagonist. Clin Science 1984; 67:167–175.
6. Bassett ML, Mullen KD, Skolnik P, Jones EA. Amelioration of hepatic encephalopathy by pharmacologic antagonists of the GABA$_A$–benzodiazepine receptor complex in a rabbit model of fulminant hepatic failure. Gastroenterology 1987; 93:1069–1077.
7. Schafer DF, Jones EA. Hepatic Encephalopathy and the γ–aminobutyric acid neurotransmitter system. Lancet 1982; ii:18–19.
8. Baraldi M, Zeneroli ML. Experimental hepatic encephalopathy –changes in gamma–amino–butyric acid. Science 1982; 216:427–431.
9. Baraldi M, Caselgrandi E, Borella P, Zeneroli ML. Decreased of brain zinc in experimental hepatic encephalopathy. Brain Res 1983; 258:170–172.
10. Basile AS, Pandl L, Jaouni T et al. Brain concentrations of benzodiazepines are elevated in an animal model of hepatic encephalopathy. Proc Natl Acad Sci USA 1990; 87:5263–5267.
11. Basile AS, Hughes RD, Harrison IM et al. Elevated brain concentrations of 1.4–benzodiazepines in fulminant hepatic failure. N Engl J Med 1991; 325:475–478.
12. Olasmaa M, Rothstein JD, Guidotti A et al. Endogenous benzodiazepine receptors ligands in human and animal hepatic encephalopathy. J Neurochem 1990; 55:2015–2023.
13. Püspök A., Herneth A., Steindl P., Ferenci P.: Hepatic encephalopathy in rats with thioacetamide induced acute liver failure is not mediated by endogenous benzodiazepines. Gastroenterology 1993; 105:851–857.
14. van der Rijt.CCD., de Knegt RJ., Schalm SW., Terpstra OT., Mechelse K. Flumazenil does not improve hepatic encephalopathy associated with acute ischemic liver failure in the rabbit. Metab Brain Dis 1990; 5:131–141.
15. Yurdaydin C., Wong G., Basile AS., Jones EA. Efficacy of benzodiazepine antagonists in

improving hepatic encephalopathy may be related to their affinity for diazepam insensitive receptors. Hepatology 1992; **16:**86A.

16. Bosman DK, Van den Buijs CACG, de Haan JG et al. Inverse benzodiazepine receptor agonists temporally restore hepatic encephalopathy in the rat. Gastroenterology 1991; **101:**772–781.

17. Gammal SH, Basile AS, Geller D, et al. Reversal of the behavioural and electrophysiological abnormalities of an animal model of hepatic encephalopathy by benzodiazepine receptor ligands. Hepatology 1990; **11:**371–378.

18. Zieve L.,Ferenci P.,Rzepczynski D.,Ebner J., Zimmermann Ch. Benzodiazepine antagonist does not alter course of hepatic encephalopathy nor neural GABA binding.Metabol Brain Dis 1987; **2:**201–205.

19. Grimm G, Ferenci P, Katzenschlager R et al. Improvement of hepatic encephalopathy treated with flumazenil. Lancet 1988; **ii:**1392–1394.

20. Ferenci P,Grimm G,Meryn S,Gangl A. Successful long–term treatment of portal systemic encephalopathy by the benzodiazepine antagonist flumazenil. Gastroenterology 1989; **96:**240–243.

21. Jellinger K, Riederer P, Kleinberger G, Wuketich ST, Kotbauer P. Brain monoamines in human hepatic encephalopathy. Acta Neuropathol (Berl) 1978; **43:**63–68.

22. Yurdaydin C, Hörtnagl H, Steindl P, Zimmermann C, Pifl C, Singer EA, Roth E, Ferenci P. Increased serotoninergic and noradrenergic activity in hepatic encephalopathy in rats with thioacetamide induced acute liver failure. Hepatology 1990; **12:**695–700.

23. Bugge M, Bengtsson F, Nobin A, Jeppsson B, Herlin P. The turnover of brain monoamines after total hepatectomy in rats infused with branched chain amino acids. World J Surg 1987; **11:**810–817.

24. Zifa E, Fillion G. 5–Hydroxytryptamine Receptors. Pharmacological Reviews 1992; **44,** 3:401–458.

25. Göthert M. Pharmacological, biochemical and molecular classification schemes of serotonin (5–HT) receptors with special reference to the $5-HT_2$ class. Progress in Pharmacology and Clinical Pharmacology,1990; **7,** 4:3–15.

26. Peroutka SJ. 5–Hydroxytryptamine Receptors. J Neurochem. 1993; **60,**2:408–416.

27. Tricklebank MD.: The motor properties and discriminative stimulus properties of 8 OH DPAT and their relationship to activation of the putative $5\ HT_{1A}$ receptor. in: Brain $5\ HT_{1A}$ Receptors. Dourish CT., Hutson PH and Ahlenius S (eds). Horwood Press, Chichester 1987; 140–151

28. Krulich L, McCann SM, Mayfield MA. On the mode of the prolactin release– inhibiting action of the serotonin blockers metergoline, methysergide and cyproheptadine. Endocrinology 1981. **108:** 1115–1124.

29. Saxena PR, Bolt GR, Dhasmana KM. Serotonin agonist and antagonists in experimental hypertension. J Cardiovasc Pharmacol. 1987; **10:** 12–18.

30. Myers RD. Hypothalamic control of thermoregulation: neurochemical mechanisms. In Handbook of the hypothalamus. Vol. 3, Morgane PJ, Pankseep J, eds., New York, Marcel Dekker 1980; 83–210

31. Lisker–Melman M, Moreno–Otero R, Fromm HC et al. Behavioural amelioration of hepatic encephalopathy by an opiate receptor antagonist in a rat model. Hepatology 1988; **8:**1247.

32. Bansky G, Meier PE, Riederer E et al. Effects of the benzodiazepine receptor antagonist flumazenil in hepatic encephalopathy in humans. Gastroenterology 1989; **97:**744–753.

33. Ferenci P. Critical evaluation of the role of branched chain amino acids in liver disease. In Thomas JC, Jones EA (eds) Recent Advances in Hepatology 1986, Churchill Livingstone, Edinburgh London Melbourne and New York.pp 137–154.

34. Pomier–Layrargues JF., Giguère J., Lavoie S., et al.: Pharmakokinetics of benzodiazepine antagonist Ro 15–1788 in cirrhotic patients with moderate or severe liver dysfunction. Hepatology 1989; **10:**969–972.

35. Basile AS., Harrison PM., Hughes RD.,et al. Relationship between plasma benzodiazepine receptor ligand concentrations and severity of hepatic encephalopathy. Hepatology 1994; **19:**112–121.

35. Gyr N. et al.: Synopsis of research report B–154'321 (Protocol N–12725a), Hoffmann–La Roche,1993.

36. Pomier–Layrargues JF., Giguère J., Lavoie S., et al.: Flumazenil in cirrhotic patients in hepatic coma: A randomized double–bild placebo–controlled crossover trial. Hepatology 1994; **19:** 32–37.

37. Cadranel JF., El Younsi M., Pidoux B., et al.: Immediate improvement of hepatic encephalopathy incirrhotic patients by flumazenil. Results of a double-bild cross-over study. J Hepatol 1991;13 (Suppl 2):S104.

38. Jones EA., Gammal SA.: Hepatic encephalopathy. in:The liver: Biology and pathobiology. Arias I, Jakoby WB., Popper H. (eds). Raven Press, New York, 1988.

39. Van der Rijt CCD, Schalm SW, Meulstee J, Stijnen T. Flumazenil therapy for hepatic encephalopathy: a double blind cross-over study. Hepatology 1989; 10:590A.

40. Amodio P., Marchetti P., Comacchio F., et al.: Effects of flumazenil on subclinical hepatic encephalopathy: preliminary data. Ital J Gastroenterol 1993; 25:183.

S–Adenosyl–L–Methionine Synthetase and Methionine Metabolism Deficiencies in Cirrhosis

José M. Mato, Luis Alvarez, Pablo Ortiz, Jesús Mingorance, Cristina Durán, María A. Pajares

Methionine metabolism impairment in human liver disease has been related with an alteration in SAM–synthetase. This deficiency is produced by a post–translational event since human liver cirrhosis presents normal levels of SAM–synthetase mRNA in spite of a more than 50% diminution in its activity. A series of different experiments on the structure and activity of this enzyme have provided strong evidence that SAM–synthetase is regulated by reduced/oxidized glutathione ratio. Restoration of glutathione levels by the addition of S–adenosyl–methionine or glutathione esters in various experimental conditions (buthionine sulfoximine and carbon tetrachloride intoxication) resulted in a normalization of the SAM–synthetase diminution caused by the toxics and an attenuation of the morfological alteration produced in the liver, including fiber production. This findings might have pharmacological implications in the treatment of liver diseases, since the possible beneficial effect of long term administration of SAM could include a reduction of fiber production.

1. Introduction

S–adenosyl–l–methionine synthetase (SAM–synthetase) is the enzyme that catalyzes the reaction in which the adenosyl moeity of ATP is transferred to methionine. The product of this reaction, S–adenosyl–methionine (SAM), is the methyl donor in most transmethylation reactions, the process in which methyl groups are added to compounds. The product of transmethylations is S–adenosyl–L–homocysteine (SAH), a potent inhibitor of transmethylation, which is subsequently converted into homocysteine and adenosine. Both molecules are quickly removed to mantain the ratio of SAM/SAH in normal rat liver above five. Homocysteine is converted into cystathionine and its derivatives (cysteine, glutathione, taurine, and inorganic sulphate) via the transsulfuration pathway or can be used for the resynthesis of methionine.

A methionine load in normal subjects produces an increase in SAM synthesis that is used to methylate glycine to sarcosine. The excess of SAH formed in this process is metabolized to cysteine, glutathione (GSH) and sulphate since homocysteine remethylation is blocked by SAM concentration (see fig. 1). In liver cirrhosis the clearance of methionine is delayed and the hepatic glutathione concentration and urinary sulphate excretion are reduced suggesting a block in the metabolism of this aminoacid (1,2). This hypothesis was confirmed by measuring SAM–synthetase activity in liver biopsies from cirrhotic patients and

Instituto de Investigaciones Biomédicas, CSIC, Arturo Duperier 4, 28029-Madrid. Spain

Hepatic Encephalopathy, Hyperammonemia, and Ammonia Toxicity
Edited by V. Felipo and S. Grisolia, Plenum Press, New York, 1994

113

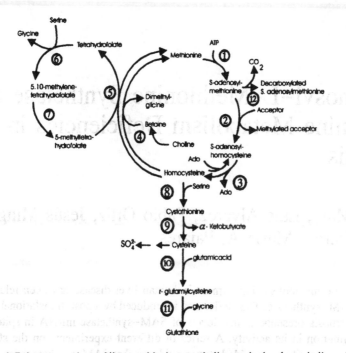

Figure 1. Relevant reactions of liver methionine metabolism and related metabolic pathways.

controls (3). Such alteration may have clinical consequences since a decreased conversion of methionine to cysteine may alter glutathione (GSH) availability and a diminution of the elimination of toxic substances. Furthermore, in total parenteral nutrition the transsulfuration pathway becomes essential and a failure to retain nitrogen can be observed unless exogenous cysteine and taurine are added to the diet (4). Recently, methionine metabolism has been studied by measuring the plasma clearance of exogenous methionine during steady–state conditions in cirrhotic patients. Methionine plasma clearance was reduced in approximately 20% and fasting plasma methionine increased 50% respect to normal controls. There was a significant correlation between fasting methionine and methionine clearance. Methionine utilization was also different in cirrhotics than in controls since infused methionine was not degraded to any significant extent to urea in patients, whereas a three fold increase of urinary urea nitrogen was observed in controls. Methionine clearance significantly correlated with hepatic impairment, as shown by the correlation with the Child–Pugh score or the galactose elimination test (5). The decreased formation of methionine end products as a result of an impairmet of methionine metabolism may play a major role in the liver cell function and could be the biochemical basis to explain the hypermethioninemia observed in severe hepatocellular failure. SAM–synthetase is the only site in the transmethylation/transsulfuration pathway that has been found to be altered in human cirrhosis (3). Thus it seems reasonable to assume that one or more of these metabolic abnormalities are responsible for some of the clinical complications of cirrhosis.

2. Structure of SAM–Synthetase

Human liver cytosol contains two different forms of SAM–synthetase, a high Mr and a low Mr. At physiological concentrations of methionine the high Mr form has a specific activity 15 times higher than the low Mr form (6). Kinetic behaviour of rat liver SAM–synthetase has been studied by several laboratories and results differ depending on the purification procedures and probably because the enzyme changes its kinetics properties according to the oxidation/reduction state of the preparation. Both forms are formed by the same polypeptide chain, which has a molecular mass of 43.7 kDa as determined both by SDS-PAGE and from the deduced amino-acid sequence of the cloned enzyme (7).

The gene for human liver SAM-synthetase appears to be present as a single copy and is expressed only in the liver. The cDNA of Human SAM-synthetase presents a high homology (89% in the coding region) with the rat liver cDNA SAM-synthetase but did not hybridize with mRNA from human kidney, spleen, ganglion, and gallbladder (8).

These results indicate the existence of at least two genes for SAM-synthetase in humans, one expressed in liver and the other expressed in non hepatic tissues. Two SAM-synthetases have also been identified in plants and yeasts (9-11) with an extensive similarity among all of them, indicating that the primary structure of this enzyme has been well preserved during evolution.

3. SAM-Synthetase and Glutathione

The presence of two sulfhydryl groups are essential for the activity of both oligomeric forms of SAM-synthetase. One of this sulfhydryl group, localized at cysteine 150, after oxidation with N-ethylmaleimide is responsible for a lost of 80% of the enzyme activity. Both forms of the enzyme are inhibited by oxidized glutathione (GSSG) and GSH is able to protect from the inhibitory effect of GSSG showing a possible regulatory role of the GSH/GSSG ratio in the activity of SAM-synthetase (12).

In vivo experiments using buthionine sulfoximine (BSO) to block GSH synthesis, have shown a 30% reduction of GSH in parallel with a 40% diminution of SAM levels and up to 60% reduction in SAM-synthetase activity. These biochemical alterations were accompanied with histological modifications such as mitochondrial swelling and vacuolization of smooth endoplasmic reticulum. All these changes were nearly completely prevented by increasing GSH concentration after administration of a monoethylester of GSH (10). A number of different compounds that reduced liver glutathione such as ethanol, galactosamine, or CCl4 are associated with lower SAM-synthetase activity and this effect was attenuated by the administation of drugs (e.g.,SAM, glutathione esters) that restore normal glutathione levels (13, 14, 15).

It is proposed that under normal condition, the cysteine groups of SAM-synthetase might be protected from oxidation by normal concentration of intracellular glutathione. However, when a reduction in liver GSH or the levels of GSSG increase occur, by a toxin or a disease, a vicious cycle might start. Depletion of GSH could lead to the inactivation of SAM-synthetase with a further decrease in GSH levels and thus worsen the deficiency in SAM-synthetase.

4. SAM-Synthetase and Glutathione Levels in Experimental Fibrosis: Effect of SAM Treatment

Liver fibrosis is common in most chronic liver diseases regardless of their ethiology. There is no established therapy for this process (16). There is an established rat model to study this process that induces liver fibrosis by a chronic intoxication (9 weeks) with sub-acute dosis of carbon tetrachloride. The CCl4 administration in the rat produced a 45% depletion of liver GSH and a 60% reduction in SAM-synthetase activity. Both alterations were prevented by SAM administration (15).

Moreover, this treatment was associated with a decreased number of rats that developed cirrhosis and an attenuation of hepatic collagen and prolylhydroxylase activity increase observerved in the intoxicated animals (15).

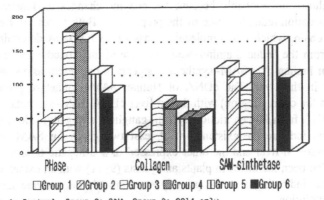

Group 1: Control. Group 2: SAM. Group 3: CCl4 only.
Group 4: CCl4+SAM 3 weeks (from week 6). Group 5: CCl4+SAM 6 weeks (from week 3).
Group 6: CCl4+SAM 9 weeks (from week 0).

Figure 2. Results after SAM administration (3–10 mg/kg i.m. daily) in an experimental model of fibrosis.

A second series of experiments in which SAM treatment started not at the beginning but 3 or 6 weeks after fibrosis induction showed again a normalization of hepatic SAM–synthetase and gluthation levels, together with a significant reduction of liver fibrosis parameters(Figure 2). This effect was particularly evident in the group that received SAM treatment from the 3rd to the 9th (6 weeks of treatment) suggesting a more pronounced effect of SAM in case of early treatment.

Despite the marked reduction of SAM–synthetase activity in the CCl4–treated rats the level of SAM–synthetase mRNA was not different from that in the control or the SAM–treated groups. These results suggest that the reduction observed in SAM–synthetase activity may be due to an inactivation of the enzyme rather than to a deficiency of its expression. The factors that regulate collagen accumulation in vivo are not very well understood. These results suggest that a reduction of SAM–synthetase together with a glutathione depletion are important concomitants of liver fibrosis in vivo.

In conclusion SAM administration may act as a precursor of GSH synthesis with the advantage, compared with methionine, of bypassing the deficit in SAM–synthetase activity mentioned above. It is now well stablished that exogenously administered SAM prevents GSH depletion in many different experimental conditions such as primates with alcoholic liver injury (13), rats treated with CCl_4 (15), the administration of GSH–depleting drugs (heroin, methadone, paracetamol and ethanol) to human hepatocytes (17) and in patients with liver disease (18). This could explain the beneficial effects of SAM administration in the treatment of liver disorders (19). Moreover, according with this hypothesis, GSH replenishment by other GSH precursors or by permeable derivatives of GSH should have similar or complementary beneficial effects on liver injury.

Acknowledgements: Work at the author's laboratory was supported by grants from Fondo de Investigaciones Sanitarias and Europharma, S.A.

References

1. Horowitz, J.H.; Rypins, E.B.; Henderson, J.M.; Heymsfield, S.B.; Moffitt, S.D.; Hain, R.P.; Chaela, R.K. et al.: Evidence for impairment of transsulfuration pathway in cirrhosis. Gastroenterology 1981; **81**:668–675.

2. Kinsell, L.W.; Harper, H.A.; Maton, H.C.; Michael G.D.; Weiss, H.A.: Rate of dissappearance from plasma of intravenously administered methionine in patients with liver damage. Science 1947; **106:**589–590.

3. Martin Duce, A.; Ortiz, P.; Cabrero, C.; Mato, J.M.: S–Adenosyl–L–Methionine synthetase and phospholipid methyltransferase are inhibited in human cirrhosis. Hepatology 1988; **8 (1):**65–68.

4. Rudman, D.; Kutner, M.; Ausley, J.; Jansen, R.; Chipponi, J. et al.: Hypotyrosinemia, hypocistinemia and failute to retain nitrogen during total parenteral nutrition of cirrhotic patients. Gastroenterology 1981, **81:**1025–1035.

5. Marchesini, G.; Bugianesi, E.; Bianchi, G.; Fabbri, A.; Marchi, E.; Zoli, M.; Pisi, E.: Impaired methionine elimination from plasma of patients with liver cirrhosis. Hepatology 1992, **16:**149–155.

6. Cabrero, C.; Alemany, S.: Conversion of rat liver S–adenosyl–methionine synthetase from high Mr to low–Mr from by LiBr. Biochem. Biophys. Acta 1988; **952:**277–281.

7. Alvarez, L; Asuncion, M; Corrales, F; Pajares, M.A; Mato, J.M. Analysis of the 5' non–coding region of rat liver SAM–synthetase mRNA and comparison of the Mr deduced from the cDNA sequence and the purified enzyme. FEBS Lett 1991; **290:**142–146.

8. Alvarez, L; Asuncion, M; Martin–Duce, A; Mato,J.M. Characterization of a full–length cDNA encoding human liver SAM–synthetase: tissue specific gene expression and mRNA levels in hepatopathies. Biochem Journal 1993; **293:**481–486.

9. Pajares, M.A; Corrales,F; Ochoa,P; Mato,J.M. The role of cysteine 150 in the structure and activity of rat liver SAM–synthetase.Biochem.J 1991; **274:**225–229.

10. Markham,G.D.; De Parasis J. Gatmaitan,J. The sequence of met K. the structural gene for S–adenosylmethionine synthetases in Sacchromyces cerevisae. J.Biol Chem. 1984; **259:**14504–14507.

11. Thomas,D.Surdin–Kerjan y.SAM I,the structural gene for one of the S–adenosylmethionine synthetases in Saccharomyces cerevisae. J.Biol:Chem.1987; **262:**16704–16709.

12. Thomas D.Rothstein R.Rosenberg N.Surdin–Kerjan Y.SAM 2 encodes the second methionine S–adenosyl transferase in Saccharomyces cerevisae. Mol Cell Biol 1988; **8:**5132–5139.

13. Pajares, M.A.; Corrales, F.; Durán, C.; Mato, J.M.; Alvarez, L.: How is rat liver S–adenosylmethionine synthetase regulated?. FEBS Letters 1992; **309:**1–4.

14. Lieber, C.; De Carlo, I.M.; Lowe, N.; Saraki, R.; Leo, M.A.: S–Adenosyl–L–Methionine attenuares alcohol–induced liver injury in the baboon. Hepatology 1990, **11:**165–172.4.

15. Stramentinoli, G; Gualano, M; Ideo, G. Protective role of SAM on liver injury induced by D–galactosamine in rats. Biochem Pharmacol 1978; **27:**1431–1433.

16. Corrales, F.; Giménez, A.; Alvarez, L.; Caballería, J.; Pajares, M.A.; Andreu, H.; Parés, A.; Mato, J.M.; Rodés, J.: S–adenosylmethionine treatment prevents carbon tetrachloride–induced S–adenosylmethionine synthetase inactivation and attenuates liver injury. Hepatology (1992), **16:**1022–1027.

17. Brenner, D. A; Alcorn JM. Therapy for Hepatic fibrosis.Semin.Liver. Disease 1990; **10:**74–83.

18. Ponsoda, X.; Jover, R.; Gómez–Lechón, M.J.; Fabra, R.; Trullenque, R.; Castell, J.V.: Intracellular glutathione in human hepatocytes incubated with SAMe and GSH–depleting drugs. Toxicology 1991, **70:**293–302.

19. Vendemiale, G.; Altomare, E.; Trizio, T.; Le Grazie, C.; Di Padova, C. et al.: S–adenosylmethionine on hepatic glutathione in patients with liver disease. Scand. J. Gastroenterol. 1989, **24:**407–415.

20. Frezza,M.Surrenti,C.Manzillo G. Fiaccadori F.Bartolini M.Di Padova C. Oral S–adenosylmethionine in the symptomatic treatment of intrahepatic cholestasis: a double–blind, placebo controlled study. Gastroenterology 1990; **99:**211–215.

Diagnosis and Therapy of Hepatic Encephalopathy

Antoni Mas, Joan Manuel Salmerón, Joan Rodés

1. Diagnosis

The diagnosis of Hepatic Encephalopathy (HE) is basically clinical, and consists in the detection of various degrees of mental impairment along with neuromuscular abnormalities. Three components of mental state may be impaired in HE: the level of consciousness, personality (behavior), and the upper intellectual functions (1). The most common neuromuscular abnormality is the so-called asterixis or flapping tremor, however other signs or symptoms such as impaired handwriting are usually present in the lower degrees of HE, with this being impossible to explore in cases of coma flapping tremor; in this situation muscular rigidity and hyperreflexia are common. In Table 1 the most common classification of HE is described. This classification is clearly useful in cases of acute HE, but in cases of chronic HE the four different stages of HE are less clear. It is important to know the existence of subclinical HE in some patients with chronic liver disease with apparent normal mental status, and this may only be documented by certain psychometric tests (2). These patients may have problems when performing activities requiring a correct degree of mental and neuromuscular status, such as driving cars (3).

To more accurately assess the severity of HE , usually for investigational purposes, in addition to the above mentioned classification of HE, based only on clinical data, a numerical "index" (Porto–Systemic Encephalopathy Index, or PSE Index) described by Conn (4) may be used. The PSE index scores the mental status (with a 3 x factor), the intensity of flapping tremor, the level of arterial ammonia, the Electroencephalogram, and the time wasted in completing a number–connection test (Table 2). The index is calculated by dividing the number of points obtained by the patient by 28 (the maximum score possible).

Other diagnostic procedures in HE, apart from those used in the calculation of the PSE index, are visual–evoked or somatosensory–evoked potentials, determination of glutamine in blood or cerebrospinal fluid, and others (5).

Differential diagnosis of HE is usually easy: a patient with a known (and usually advanced) liver disease develops changes in the mental status, has behavioral disturbances, or impairment in intellectual functions, along with an apparent asterixis, usually after a predisposal factor (gastrointestinal hemorrhage, hydroelectrolytic or renal complications, severe infection, use of sedatives, etc). However, the presence of such changes in a patient with liver disease can not always be atributed to HE, since similar symptoms may appear due to other causes of neurologic dysfunction, such as infections (meningoencephalitis), direct neurotoxins (alcohol abuse), metabolic changes (hypoglycemia), or cerebrovascular (hemorrhagic or thrombotic) accidents. Differential diagnosis should include accurate anamnesis, detection of specific signs on physical examination, and the adequate

Liver Unit, Hospital Clinic i Provincial, Universitat de Barcelona, Catalonia, Spain

Hepatic Encephalopathy, Hyperammonemia, and Ammonia Toxicity
Edited by V. Felipo and S. Grisolia, Plenum Press, New York, 1994

Table 1. Grades of Hepatic Encephalopathy.

Grade	Level of Consciousness	Behavior	Intellectual Function	Neuromuscular Abnormalities
1	Changes in sleep pattern	Euphoria Depression Irritability	Subtle changes Shortened Attention	Mild Asterixis Impaired handwriting
2	Slow responses Lethargy	Anxiety Inappropriate behavior	Loss of Time Amnesia	Asterixis Slurred speech Ataxia
3	Disorientation Somnolence Confusion	Bizarre behavior Paranoia	Disorientation Inability to compute	Asterixis Rigidity
4	Stupor Coma	None	None	Hyperreflexia Opisthotonus

complementary diagnostic procedure(s) in case of doubt (TC scan, cerebrospinal fluid examination, search of toxins in blood or urine, etc). Furthermore, HE may although rarely be the first clinical manifestation of liver disease. This may occur in a case of fulminant hepatic failure before jaundice is apparent, or in patients with unknown, previously well compensated chronic liver disease in whom HE appears after a precipitating cause (i.e. acute systemic infection).

Table 2. Porto-Systemic Encephalopathy Index (PSE Index).

Electroencephalogram (Cycles/sec)		Number Connection Test (sec.)	
Normal	0 points	< 30	0 points
8.5 – 12	1 point	31 – 50	1 point
7 – 8	2 points	51 – 80	2 points
3 – 5	3 points	81 – 120	3 points
< 3	4 points		
Flapping Tremor		**Arterial Ammonia (g/dl)**	
Absent	0 points	< 150	0 points
Isolated	1 point	150 – 200	1 point
Irregular	2 points	201 – 250	2 points
Frequent	3 points	251 – 300	3 points
Continous	4 points	> 300	4 points
Mental Status (according to the degrees of encephalopathy, see Table 1)			
	Grade 0	3 x 0 = 0 points	
	Grade 1	3 x 1 = 3 points	
	Grade 2	3 x 2 = 6 points	
	Grade 3	3 x 3 = 9 points	
	Grade 4	3 x 4 = 12 points	
INDEX = Points Obtained / 28 (maxim theoretic points)			

2. Therapy

The therapeutic approach of HE differs in some points depending upon whether the patient has an acute episode or carries a chronic HE status.

2.1. Management of Acute HE

Except for the case of fulminant hepatic failure, in which HE is a sign of "pure" hepatic dysfunction, tha vast majority of acute episodes of HE occur in cirrhotic patients who have a precipitating factor (the most common being gastrointestinal bleeding, renal and electrolyte abnormalities, use of sedatives, excess of dietary protein, infections, and constipation) (1). The prompt correction of such factors are crucial in the management of acute HE (1,5).

Measures directed to reduce the possible toxins (ammonia and many others) of intestinal origin are the most useful therapy, along with the above mentioned treatment of the precipitating cause. These measures include protein restriction and cleansing enemas, administration of non–absorbable antibiotics (neomycin, paromomycin, metronidazol or others) orally or via a nasogastric tube, and/or lactulose or related carbohydrates (lactitol) (1,5,6–8). The most common approach is to began with single therapy (lactulose or lactitol), and use combined therapy (non– absorbable antibiotics plus lactulose/lactitol) in cases of partial response to the first treatment. Lactulose or lactitol may also be administered with the cleansing enemas. Reduction of fecal flora producing ammonia and other toxins by antibiotics, and the laxative effect and acidification of colonic contents due to lactulose and related carbohydrates seems to be the mechanisms of action of these drugs (4,8).

Due to the evidence of aminoacid imbalance in advanced liver diseases and its possible relationship with HE, administration of branched amino acids have been employed as a "wake–up" therapy in this situation. Although there are some evidence of its effectiveness in clinical trials (total recovery of the episode of HE occurs more rapidly than other therapies), the real benefit of this approach in the treatment of HE seems to be poor (9).

The GABA–benzodiazepine theory of HE prompted some investigators to analyze the possible therapeutic use of flumazenil, a benzodiazepine antagonist, in this situation. Although there are good evidence of its efficacy (10), some authors have doubts concerning the possibility of recovery from HE with this drug being due to previous, and in some cases, subreptitious use of benzodiazepines rather than a direct effect (8). In our experience, benzodiacepine antagonists should be given to all cases of acute HE of unknown cause to exclude the above mentioned possibility. This is especially important in cases in which the presence and degree of HE is used in deciding very aggressive therapies, such as liver transplantation in fulminant hepatic failure (9).

2.2. Management of Chronic HE

The chronic use of non–absorbable antibiotics is dangerous, because of the possibility of oto or nephrotoxic effect by very low but continuous absortion. The therapeutic approach to chronic HE is based on two points: dietary protein restriction and the use of non–absorbable disaccharides (lactulose, lactitol, lactose in lactase deficient patients) (1,5,12–14).

Long–term reduction of protein intake may result in severe negative nitrogen balance. To obviate this problem, some different approaches have been proposed: reduction of meat ingestion and a lactovegetarian or strictly vegetarian diet, or supplementation of a highly protein–restricted diet with oral mixtures of branched chain amino acids (5,15,16).

Lactulose or lactitol should be given in a dose to achieve two soft bowel movements per day. Titration of fecal pH could be helpful in monitoring the efficacy of these drugs (fecal pH should be around 5). Lactose would achieve the same efficacy in cases of lactase deficiency. The secondary effects of these drugs are usually minor: flatulence, nausea and vomiting, aversion to lactulose due to its sweet taste (lactitol may therefore be preferable). Watery diarrhea and its possible consequences in hydroelectrolytic balance may be avoided by careful dose titration (1,8).

Oral flumazenil administration has been used exceptionally in the management of chronic HE, with apparent good results (17). However, the real efficacy of this therapy remains to be proved.

Other therapies have been postulated in the management of HE: zinc supplementation, L–dopa or bromocriptine, occlusion (with a balloon or surgically) of large porto–caval anastomosis (with the subsequent risk of bleeding for portal hypertension), use of keto–analogs of branched chain aminoacids, and others. The efficacy of some of these are doubtful, and others are applicable only in very selected cases (5).

Finally, the presence of HE may be a clear indication of liver transplantation, since this procedure eliminates the two basic causes of HE (hepatic insufficiency and porto–collateral circulation). In fulminant hepatic failure HE is a diagnostic criteria; after transplantation, patients usually recover a normal mental status very rapidly (within a few hours). In a cirrhotic patient with chronic HE (or frequent episodes of acute HE) liver transplantation should also be considered. Recovery is usually slower, but a frank improvement in mental status may be seen even in patients with advanced chronic HE and signs of organic brain damage (18).

References

1. Conn HO, Bircher J. Hepatic Encephalopathy: Management with Lactulose and Related Carbohydrates. Medi–Ed Press, East Lansing, Michigan, 1988.
2. Rikkers L, Jenko P, Rudman D, Freides D. Subclinical Hepatic Encephalopathy: detection, prevalence and relationship to Nitrogen Metabolism. Gastroenterology 1978; 75:462–469.
3. Schomerus H, Hamster W, Blunck H et al. Latent portsystemic encephalopathy. I. Nature of cerebral function deffects and their effect on fitness to drive. Dig Dis Sci 1981; 26:622–630.
4. Conn HO, Lieberthal MH. The Hepatic Coma Syndromes and Lactulose. Baltimore: Williams & Wilkins, 1979.
5. Ferenci P. Hepatic Encephalopathy. In Oxford Textbook of Clinical Hepatology. McIntyre N, Benhamou JP, Bircher J, Rizzetto M, Rodés J Eds. Oxford Univerty Press, Oxford 1991:473–483.
6. Morgan MY, Hawley KE. Lactitol vs. Lactulose in the treatment of acute hepatic encephalopathy: a double blind, randomized trial. Hepatology 1987; 7:1278–1284.
7. Heredia D, Caballería, Arroyo V, Ravelli G, Rodés J. Lactitol vs lactulose in the treatment of acute portal–systemic encephalopathy (PSE). A controlled trial. J Hepatol 1987; 4:293–298.
8. Bircher J, Sommer W. Portal–Systemic Encephalopathy. In Hepatobiliary Diseases. Prieto J, Rodés J, Shafritz DA eds. Springer–Verlag, Berlin, 1992:417–428.
9. Morgan MY. Branched chain amino acids in the management of chronic liver diseases. Facts and fantasies. J Hepatol 1990; 11:133–141.
10. Banski G, Meier PJ, Riederer E, Walser H, Ziegler WH, Schmid M. Effects of the benzodiacepine receptor antagonist flumazenil in hepatic encephalopathy in humans. Gastroenterology 1989; 97:744–750.
11. Castells A, Navasa M, Mas A, Rodés J. Flumacenil en la valoración del grado de encefalopatía hepática. Med Clin (Barc) 1991; 96:118.
12. Uribe M, Márquez MA, García–Ramos G et al. Treatment of chronic portal–systemic encephalopathy with lactose in lactase defficient patients. Dig Dis Sci 1980; 25:924–928.
13. Morgan MY, Hawley KE, Stambuck D. Lactitol versus lactulose in the treatment of chronic hepatic encephalopathy: a double–blind, randomized, cross–over study. J Hepatol 1987; 4:236–245.

14. Heredia D, Terés J, Orteu N et al. Lactitol vs. Lactulose in the treatment of chronic recurrent portal–systemic encephalopathy. J Hepatol 1988; **7**:106–110.

15. Horst D, Grace ND, Conn HO et al. Comparison of dietary protein with an oral, branched–chain enriched amino acid supplement in chronic portal–systemic encephalopathy: a randomized controlled trial. Hepatology 1984; **4**:279–287.

16. Marchesini G, Dioguardi FS, Bianchi GP et al. Long–term oral branched–chain amino acid treatment in chronic hepatic encephalopathy. A randomized double–blind casein–controlled trial. J Hepatol 1990; **11**:92–101.

17. Ferenci P, Grimm G, Meryn S, Gangl A. Successful long–term treatment of portal systemic encephalopathy by the benzodiacepine antagonist flumazenil. Gastroenterology 1989; **96**:240–243.

18. Lake JR. Changing indications for liver transplantation. In Advances in Liver Transplantation. Gastroenterology Clinics of North America. 1993; **22**:213–229.

Neomycin Reduces the Intestinal Production of Ammonia from Glutamine

Richard A. Hawkins, John Jessy, Anke M. Mans, Antonio
Chedid[†], Mary R. DeJoseph

The mechanism by which neomycin treatment reduces circulating ammonia concentrations was studied in normal and portacaval shunted rats. Rats were given neomycin for 3 days and then fasted for 24 hours to eliminate feces. Neomycin decreased arteriovenous differences of ammonia across the intestine even when the intestines were empty. Neomycin treatment lowered the activity of glutaminase in the intestinal mucosa and the rate of ammonia production from glutamine by isolated intestinal segments. The intestines from portacaval shunted rats had higher glutaminase activity (by 57%), and produced ammonia from glutamine at a greater rate (by 31%), than intestines from controls. Neomycin treatment lowered glutaminase activity and ammonia production in shunted rats, but glutaminase activity still remained higher than in controls (by 23%). The data indicate that the mechanism by which neomycin lowers plasma ammonia is owing, at least in part, to a direct effect on the intestines. Specifically, neomycin causes a reduction in mucosal glutaminase activity and thereby decreases the ability of the mucosa to consume glutamine and produce ammonia.

1. Introduction

Hepatocellular dysfunction or shunting of blood past the liver leads to a disturbance in nitrogen metabolism manifest by elevated concentrations of circulating ammonia [1, 2]. This occurs because the concentration of ammonia in the hepatic portal system is much higher than in the systemic circulation; a fact that was demonstrated almost 100 years ago by Nencki and Pavlov and their associates [3, 4] and confirmed by others. The first idea was that the amino acids resulting from protein digestion were deaminated in the intestinal wall, creating a high concentration of ammonia in the portal vein, which was delivered directly to the liver and converted into urea [3–6]. Subsequently, Folin and Denis took the position that the high concentration of ammonia in the portal vein was more likely to arise from bacterial degradation of "albuminous" material in the lumen of the colon [7]. The bacterial origin of portal ammonia gained popularity and remains the prevailing view today [8].

More recent investigations indicate that the intestinal metabolism of glutamine is an important, or perhaps the principal source of hepatic portal ammonia. One of the functions of glutamine is to transport ammonia [9]. Glutamine is released by peripheral tissues, especially muscle, as the end–product of amino acid metabolism [10]. In contrast, the intestinal mucosa preferentially consume glutamine as a source of energy for metabolism and thereby release large quantities of ammonia into the portal vein [11, 12]. While central venous

Department of Physiology and Biophysics and [†] Department of Pathology. Finch University of Health Sciences/ The Chicago Medical School. 3333 Green Bay Road, North Chicago, IL 60064

Hepatic Encephalopathy, Hyperammonemia, and Ammonia Toxicity
Edited by V. Felipo and S. Grisolia, Plenum Press, New York, 1994

125

ammonia concentrations are in the range of 20–35 μM [13], the ammonia concentration in the hepatic portal vein is about ten times as high [11, 12]; the high portal concentration is much more favorable for the synthesis of urea in the liver [14].

The major role that intestinal metabolism plays in ammonia production has been clearly illustrated in studies of germ–free animals. Warren and Newton showed that the ratio of portal–to–peripheral ammonia concentrations was about 5 to 1 in germ–free guinea pigs on a protein diet [15]. Nance and Kline demonstrated that after creating a portacaval shunt both ordinary and germ–free dogs developed high plasma ammonia concentrations and a comparable degree of encephalopathy [16]. Furthermore both ordinary and germ–free dogs with portacaval shunts showed the same rate of rise in plasma ammonia following the consumption of a blood meal [16]. Shalm and van der Mey found that the circulating level of ammonia and the time to onset of hyperammonemic coma following hepatectomy in germ–free and normal rats were indistinguishable [17]. These and other studies demonstrated definitively that pathological levels of ammonia can be produced without the participation of bacteria [18, 19].

Silen et al. conducted a comparative study of three antibiotics and found that neomycin was the most effective in reducing the ammonia content of portal venous blood [20]. Since that time neomycin has been used to treat patients on the assumption that it acted on bacteria [8]. The fact that neomycin treatment is often effective in ameliorating encephalopathy has further reinforced the idea that ammonia is produced primarily by bacteria.

Still, in view of the more recent information on the manner in which intestines produce large quantities of ammonia from glutamine, the question arises whether there is another mechanism by which neomycin acts in addition to that of killing bacteria. We addressed this issue in experiments on fasted rats and portacaval shunted rats. Our results confirmed that neomycin does lower portal and peripheral plasma ammonia levels, but that it acts on the intestinal mucosal cells. Specifically neomycin reduces the activity of glutaminase and thereby lowers the ability of the intestine to consume glutamine and produce ammonia.

2. Materials and Methods

2.1. Materials

Neomycin and glutaminase were obtained from Sigma Chemical Co., St. Louis, MO. The other enzymes and cofactors were bought from Boehringer Mannheim, GmbH Biochemica, Mannheim, West Germany. All other reagents used were of the best available grade.

2.2. Rats

Adult male Long–Evans rats were bought from Charles River Laboratories, Inc. Wilmington, MA, U.S.A. All rats were acquired, cared for and handled in conformance with the Public Health Service's "Guide for the Care and Use of Laboratory Animals.", (NIH Publication No. 86–23, revised 1985) and the "Guiding Principles for Research Involving Animals and Humans" (recommendations from the declaration of Helsinki) approved by the Council of the American Physiological Society. The rats were maintained on a 12 h–light–12 h–dark cycle under controlled conditions of temperature (20–22° C) and humidity. They were fed a commercial laboratory diet containing 22% protein, 4% fat, 5% fiber, 8% ash and 3% minerals (Purina Rat Chow, Purina Mills, Inc. St. Louis, MO) and tap water *ad libitum*. Unless otherwise stated rats were starved for 24 hours before measurements were made, at which time they weighed between 300 and 400 g.

2.3. Time Course of Response to Neomycin

Fed rats were given neomycin by gavage (500 mg/kg body weight in 0.15 M NaCl) every 24 hours. On day 1 (no treatment, 4 rats), day 2 (1 dose, 3 rats), day 3 (2 doses, 3 rats) or day 5 (4 doses, 3 rats) the rats were anesthetized with halothane (induction 4% in air), and anesthesia was maintained with 1.5–2.0% halothane in $N_2O:O_2$ (70:30) throughout all subsequent procedures. A catheter was placed in the femoral artery. The abdomen was opened and the hepatic portal vein was gently exposed. Blood samples were withdrawn simultaneously from the femoral artery and hepatic portal vein. The plasma was separated immediately and frozen at −70° C.

2.4. Arteriovenous Differences in Normal Rats

Fed rats (15 rats) were given neomycin by gavage (500 mg/kg body weight in 0.15 M NaCl) every day for 4 days, while control rats (15 rats) were given only 0.15 M NaCl. Food was withheld on day 4. On day 5 plasma samples were obtained from the femoral artery and hepatic portal vein as described above. The rats were anesthetized and decapitated. The brain was removed immediately and frozen at −70° C.

2.5. Arteriovenous Diferences in Portacaval Shunted Rats

Twenty portacaval shunted rats were prepared as described previously [21]. The operated rats were maintained in the animal quarters under normal conditions for 4 weeks. They were then divided into two groups of ten and treated as described in the preceding paragraph.

2.6. Tissue Preparation and Assays

Plasma and brain tissue were extracted with 0.5 M and 1.2 M $HClO_4$ respectively. The extracts were neutralized with 20% KOH in 0.1 M K_2HPO_4. Ammonia and glutamine were assayed enzymatically [22] and tryptophan fluorometrically [23].

2.7. Intestinal Ammonia Production and Glutaminase Activity *in vitro*

The intestines were removed from 10 normal and 12 portacaval shunted rats within 5 min of death. They were washed with ice cold 0.15M NaCl. Segments of intestine, about 2 mm wide, were cut from the jejunum. The segments, which formed rings with the villi protruding outwards, were suspended in 2 ml of cold Krebs–Henseleit buffer (40–60 mg fresh weight) and gassed with $O_2:CO_2$, 95%:5%. The segments were incubated at 37°C for 60 minutes with 20 mM glutamine. Metabolism was stopped with 200 μl of 10 M $HClO_4$. Ammonia was measured enzymatically in the neutralized supernatant. Controls had $HClO_4$ added before the incubation began.

The remainder of the intestine including jejunum and ileum was split open, laid out on a glass sheet on ice, and the mucosa scraped from the underlying muscle using a microscope slide. The mucosal scrapings were weighed and homogenized in 5 volumes of an extraction medium containing 150 mM K_2HPO_4, 50 mM Tris, 1 mM EDTA at pH 8.6 [24]. Glutaminase was assayed by incubating an aliquot of the homogenate from each group with 10 mM glutamine for 30 minutes at 37°C. The reaction was stopped with 100 μl of $HClO_4$

and the accumulation of glutamate was measured [25]. Controls were treated identically but without glutamine as substrate.

2.8. Pathology

Samples of the jejunum from four rats in each group were saved for histological examination by light microscopy. The examiners were unaware of the state of the rats while examining the slides. Staining was by hemotoxylin and eosin and by periodic acid Shiff.

2.9. Statistical Analysis

The data were analyzed by analysis of variance and tests of comparison (Least Significant Difference Test) using SAS procedures (Statistical Analysis System, SAS Institute, Cary, NC). Differences were considered to be significant at p < 0.05.

3. Results

3.1. Time Course

The time course of the response to neomycin was determined in a group of fed rats treated over 5 days (Figure 1). By day 3 the concentration of ammonia was clearly reduced in the portal vein and by day 5 there was a reduction in the arterial ammonia concentration as well. It was decided to treat all rats used in subsequent experiments for a period of 4 days and then starve them for 24 hours before making measurements. This was a sufficient period of time to eliminate all fecal material from the small and large intestines as was confirmed by direct inspection.

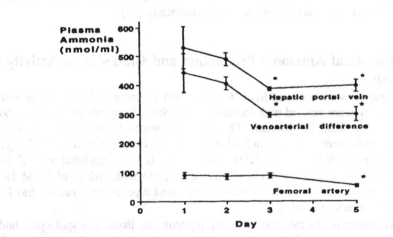

Figure 1. Neomycin decreases hepatic portal ammonia concentrations. Fed rats were given 500 mg of neomycin/kg body weight daily. Ammonia was measured in the femoral artery and hepatic portal vein before treatment (day 1) and one, two, and four days after treatment began. Points are the means of 3 – 4 rats with the S.E.M. indicated by the bars. * indicates statistical significance compared with the untreated control group.

Table 1. Neomycin treatment lowers ammonia production in normal and shunted rats

Variable	Normal Rats		Shunted Rats	
	Control(15)	Neomycin(15)	Control(10)	Neomycin(10)
Plasma:				
Ammonia				
Femoral artery	81±7	74±4	201±21^c	143±23^{c,sc}
Hepatic portal vein	380±18	252±14^c	550±82^c	398±80^{sc}
Arteriovenous	−300±19	−178±15^c	−350±68	−255±58
Glutamine				
Femoral artery	945±58	798±55	1,080±158	791±133
Hepatic portal vein	675±53	613±40	703±107	457±89^{sc}
Arteriovenous Difference	270±29	185±56	379±76	334±59
Brain:				
Glutamine	5,630±214	4,740±451	10,900±1,070^c	8,090±894^{c,sc}
Tryptophan	17.9±1.8	17.0±2.1	34.1±3.0^c	29.0±2.1^c

All values are means, ± SE, expressed in nmol/ml or g, with the number of rats in parentheses. Rats were given 500 mg of neomycin/kg body weight daily for 4 days. They were fasted overnight and plasma and tissue samples were taken for measurement on the fifth day after the treatment began. Four comparisons were of interest: normal control with all other groups (significant differences at the $p<0.05$ level indicated by c), and shunted control rats with shunted rats treated with neomycin (significant differences at the $p<0.05$ level indicated by sc).

3.2. Arteriovenous Differences of Ammonia and Glutamine

There were substantial arteriovenous differences of ammonia and glutamine in all groups (Table 1). The consumption of glutamine was sufficient to account for all the ammonia production, even if only the amide group of glutamine gave rise to ammonia. Treatment of normal rats with neomycin caused a significant reduction in the ammonia concentration of portal blood (by 34%) as well as in the arteriovenous difference (by 41%). There was no detectable decrease in the arterial ammonia concentration. The brain content of glutamine is related to the circulating ammonia concentration [26]. Although the brain glutamine content in treated rats appeared to be about 16% lower than that in control rats, the difference was not statistically significant (p = 0.09).

Portacaval shunted rats, as expected, had plasma ammonia concentrations that were significantly greater than in control rats (by 148%). The elevated plasma ammonia levels were also reflected by increased brain glutamine (by 94%). Brain tryptophan content, which is often closely correlated with hyperammonemia and brain glutamine content, was increased by 91%. Neomycin treatment reduced the arterial plasma ammonia (by 29%) and the brain glutamine content was also reduced by about the same fraction (26%). There was no detectable change in brain tryptophan content.

Ammonia, as mentioned, can be produced by the intestine from glutamine and the possibility was considered that neomycin reduced the use of glutamine by the mucosa [11, 12, 27]. The results on arteriovenous differences of glutamine were compatible with the

Table 2. Neomycin reduces glutaminase activity and ammonia production in the intestine

	Normal Rats		Shunted Rats	
	Control(5)	Neomycin(5)	Control(6)	(Neomycin(6)
Intact intestinal segments				
Ammonia production (μmol of ammonia.min.$^{-1}$g^{-1})	3.25±0.12	1.87±0.29^c	4.26±0.41^c	3.33±0.27^{9c}
Homogenate of intestinal mucosa				
Glutaminase (μmol of glutamate.min.$^{-1}$g^{-1})	4.08±0.23	3.42±0.06^c	6.40±0.12^c	5.03±0.21^{c,9c}

Values are means ± SE, with the number of observations in parenthesis. Intestines were removed from the rats described in Table 1. Glutaminase was measured as the rate of glutamate formation from glutamine (per minute per g fresh weight). Ammonia production was measured as net production from added glutamine (per minute per g fresh weight). Four comparisons were of interest: normal control with all other groups (significant differences indicated by ^{c}), and shunted control rats with shunted rats treated with neomycin (significant differences indicated by ^{9c}).

interpretation that neomycin interfered with the ability of intestine to consume glutamine, but they did not provide conclusive evidence. If neomycin reduced the ability of the intestine to metabolize glutamine, the arteriovenous differences of glutamine should have been reduced by 61 μmol/ml and 48 μmol/ml in the normal and shunted groups respectively (on the basis of the effect of neomycin on the arteriovenous differences of ammonia shown in Table 1). The actual decreases in the arteriovenous differences were 85 μmol glutamine/ml and 45 μmol glutamine/ml for normal and portacaval rats respectively, but these changes were not statistically significant (Table 1). Moreover, because of the relatively large standard deviation of glutamine determinations it was calculated that it would have been necessary to make measurements in more than 600 rats to detect differences of the order of 50 μmol/ml (at p < 0.05) with a power of 90%. For these reasons the following experiments on isolated intestine were done.

3.3. *In vitro* Studies

The experiments on isolated intestinal segments incubated *in vitro* showed that treatment of normal rats with neomycin lowered the rate of ammonia production from glutamine by 42% (Table 2).

Portacaval shunted rats had a 31% greater ability to produce ammonia compared with untreated controls. Treatment of portacaval shunted rats with neomycin reduced ammonia production (by 22%) to a level similar to that in untreated normal rats.

Glutaminase activity in the intestinal mucosa was greater in shunted rats compared with controls by 57%, and glutaminase activity was reduced in both groups by neomycin. Nevertheless after shunted rats were treated with neomycin, which reduced glutaminase activity by 21%, the final enzyme activity was still 23% greater than that found in normal untreated rats.

Examination of the jejunum of the various groups did not reveal any remarkable changes in morphology at the light microscopic level.

4. Discussion

The results confirmed that plasma ammonia levels are reduced by neomycin [18, 20, 28], that glutamine is consumed by the intestine in large quantities, and that this consumption of glutamine is sufficient to account for all the ammonia produced [11, 12, 27]. The novel findings were that portacaval shunted rats had a greater capacity to produce ammonia from glutamine, that neomycin reduced the activity of glutaminase in normal and portacaval shunted rats, and that neomycin decreased the ability of the intestine to produce ammonia from glutamine.

There are three potential sources of ammonia in the portal circulation: bacterial degradation of nitrogenous materials in the intestinal lumen (e.g., protein), urea that has leaked from the circulation and entered the intestinal lumen, and glutamine, produced by various tissues in the body, and used as a source of energy by the intestinal mucosa. In the present experiments the rats were fasted overnight to eliminate feces as a significant source of nitrogen.

If urea passed across the intestinal mucosa and was hydrolyzed it could contribute to the portal ammonia concentrations. Early studies of humans provided evidence for urea recycling [29, 30]. On the other hand, more recent studies have shown that the intestines are impermeable to urea, casting doubt on urea as a significant source of nitrogen [30–32]. Furthermore, as mentioned, ammonia can be produced in considerable quantities in germ–free animals in which the bacterial degradation of urea or other substances was ruled out.

In the present experiments the most likely source of the high concentrations of ammonia nitrogen was glutamine; the arteriovenous differences of glutamine were more than sufficient -- with an excess of 40 to 50% -- to account for the production of ammonia in both normal and portacaval shunted rats (Table 1). The additional nitrogen potentially available from glutamine, which was unaccounted for in our experiments, could have been contained by amino acids that are produced by the intestine such as citrulline, proline and alanine [11, 12, 27].

Neomycin has been assumed to be effective through its ability to reduce the intestinal bacterial population, but there has been skepticism regarding this theory because neomycin does not eliminate the intestinal flora and there is no correlation between bacterial flora and the clinical efficacy of neomycin (see [18] for a review). Neomycin does have other effects in the intestine. It has been reported to cause morphological changes in intestinal cells [33–35] (although we found no evidence of this) as well as changes in absorptive function [36–38]. Several biochemical changes were shown to be caused by neomycin in both normal and germ–free rats by van Leeuwen who concluded that explanations for the beneficial effects of neomycin on hyperammonemia should take into account not only the bactericidal action of neomycin, but also its effect on the metabolic functions of the mucosal cells [35]. On the basis of our data we suggest that one of the primary effects of neomycin is on mucosal cell function; specifically the ability of neomycin to reduce glutaminase activity in mucosal cells and consequently the ability of enterocytes to make use of glutamine and produce ammonia as a by–product.

One of the more intriguing observations was that the intestines from portacaval shunted rats have a greater ability to produce ammonia from glutamine. This may be related to the existence of a futile cycle in shunted animals in which it is necessary for the intestine to metabolize more glutamine than normal in order to provide ammonia for urea synthesis.

Urea synthesis does not take place at the concentrations of ammonia that ordinarily exist in the systemic circulation. The first enzyme of urea synthesis, carbamyl phosphate synthetase, has a relatively low affinity for ammonia and urea synthesis is nil when the ammonia concentration drops below 50 μM [14]. Yet, if the concentrations in the circulation were to rise significantly above 50 μM, cerebral dysfunction would occur [13, 26]. This physiological dilemma is solved by keeping the high ammonia concentrations necessary for urea synthesis restricted to the hepatic portal system [27]. Glutamine serves as an ammonia scavenger in the body, keeping the ammonia concentrations in general circulation low [9]. The consumption of glutamine by the intestinal mucosa raises the portal ammonia to about ten times the arterial concentration thereby providing the periportal hepatocytes with the ammonia concentration necessary for urea synthesis [12, 14]. Ammonia that escapes the periportal cells is synthesized to glutamine by perivenous liver cells [14].

With complete shunting the high concentration of ammonia in the portal blood is delivered directly to the general circulation. Because under these circumstances liver receives blood only from the hepatic artery, the ammonia concentration in the systemic circulation must rise considerably above normal levels before the liver will be capable of synthesizing urea. But, when the circulating concentrations of ammonia rise some of the ammonia will be re–incorporated into glutamine by non–hepatic tissues. Portacaval shunting creates an inefficient situation where some futile recycling of glutamine occurs. The degree to which a futile cycle operates is indicated by data recently published by Coy et al. who measured blood flow and ammonia concentrations in normal and portacaval shunted rats [39]. Their data show that intestines of control rats produced ammonia at a rate of 22 μmoles·min^{-1}·kg^{-1} while the comparable group of portacaval shunted rats produced 31 μmoles·min^{-1}·kg^{-1}. It appears that portacaval shunted rats must hydrolyze about 40% more glutamine than normal to maintain circulating ammonia concentrations high enough for urea synthesis. Our observation that portacaval shunted rats have more glutaminase and a 31% greater capacity for ammonia production from glutamine fits well with the data.

Neomycin treatment of portacaval shunted rats reduced mucosal glutaminase activity, the rate of ammonia production from glutamine and most importantly the arterial ammonia concentration (by 29%). It has been shown that the cerebral dysfunction caused by portacaval shunting is more closely correlated with brain glutamine than it is with plasma ammonia [26, 40, 41]. It is when ammonia is metabolized to glutamine that abnormal signs appear. In this regard it is significant that neomycin treatment of portacaval shunted rats resulted in a distinct reduction in brain glutamine (by 26%).

The idea that hyperammonemia can be reduced by the action of a drug on the intestinal mucosa could be important in treating patients with liver disease or portacaval shunting. The success of neomycin probably rests on two factors: first its ability to inhibit glutaminase in mucosal cells, and second the relative impermeability of the intestine to neomycin. Because of the second factor, neomycin is in a situation to be effective on the intestinal mucosal cells only and cannot disturb the other phosphate–dependent glutaminases of the body. The net effect of neomycin in the present experiments was to reduce the portal ammonia concentration thereby causing the liver to use glutamine and perhaps other amino acids as a source of ammonia for urea synthesis [9]. It is our hope that an appreciation of the biochemical mechanism by which neomycin is effective in diminishing hyperammonemia will stimulate the development of other more effective therapies.

Acknowledgement: This work was supported by a grant from the National Institutes of Neurological Disorders and Stroke NS 16389.

References

1. McDermott Jr. WV, Adams RD. Episodic stupor associated with an Eck fistula in the human with particular reference to the metabolism of ammonia. J Clin Invest 1954;33:1–9.
2. Sherlock S, Summerskill WHJ, White LP, Phear EA. Portal–systemic encephalopathy. Neurological complications of liver disease. Lancet 1954;2:453–457.
3. Nencki M, Pawlow JP, Zaleski J. Ueber den Ammoniakgehalt des Blutes und der Organe und die Harnstoffbildung bei den Säugethieren. Arch Exp Path Pharm 1896;37:26–51.
4. Hahn M, Massen O, Nencki M, Pawlow J. Die Eck'sche Fistel zwischen der unteren Hohlvene und der Pfortader und ihre Folgen für den Organismus. Arch Exp Path Pharm 1896;32:161–210.
5. Horodynski W, Salaskin S, Zaleski J. Ueber die Vertheilung des Ammoniaks im Blute und den Organen normaler und hungernder Hunde. Zeitschr Physiol Chem 1902;35:246–263.
6. Salaskin S. Ueber das Ammoniak in physiologischer und pathologischer Hinsicht und die Rolle der Leber im Stoffwechsel stickstoffhaltiger Substanzen. Zeitschr Physiol Chem 1898;25:449–491.

7. Folin O, Denis W. Protein metabolism from the standpoint of blood and tissue analysis. J Biol Chem 1912;**11**:161–167.

8. Sherlock S. Chronic portal systemic encephalopathy: update 1987. Gut 1987;**28**:1043–1048.

9. Smith RJ. Glutamine metabolism and its physiologic importance. J Parenter Enteral Nutr 1990;**14**:40s–44s.

10. Felig P, Wahren J, Karl I, Cerasi E, Luft R, Kipnis DM. Glutamine and glutamate metabolism in normal and diabetic subjects. Diabetes 1973;**22**:573–576.

11. Hanson PJ, Parsons DS. Transport and metabolism of glutamine and glutamate in small intestine. In: Kvamme E, eds. Glutamine and Glutamate in Mammals, I. Boca Raton: CRC Press, Inc., **1988**:235–253.

12. Windmueller HG. Metabolism of vascular and luminal glutamine by intestinal mucosa in vivo. In: Gayssubgerm D, Sies H, eds. Glutamine Metabolism in Mammalian Tissues, Berlin: Springer–Verlag, **1984**:61–77.

13. Cooper AJ, Plum F. Biochemistry and physiology of brain ammonia. Physiol Rev 1987;**67**:440–519.

14. Sies H, Haüssinger D. Hepatic glutamine and ammonia metabolism. Nitrogen redox balance and the intracellular glutamine cycle. In: Haüssinger D, Sies H, eds. Glutamine Metabolism in Mammalian Tissues, New York: Springer–Verlag, **1984**:78–97.

15. Warren KS, Newton WL. Portal and peripheral blood ammonia concentrations in germ–free and conventional guinea pigs. Am J Physiol 1959;**197**:717–720.

16. Nance FC, Kline DG. Eck's fistula encephalopathy in germfree dogs. Ann Surg 1971;**174**:856–861.

17. Schalm SW, Van Der Mey T. Hyperammonemic coma after hepatectomy in germ–free rats. Gastroenterology 1979;**77**:231–234.

18. van Leeuwen PAM. Ammonia generation in the gut and the influence of lactulose and neomycin. 1985, University of Maastricht (Thesis)

19. Weber FLJ, Veach GL. The importance of the small intestine in gut ammonium production in the fasting dog. Gastroenterology 1979;**77**:235–240.

20. Silen W, Harper HA, Mawdsley DL, Weirich WL. Effect of antibacterial agents on ammonia production within the intestine. Proc Soc Exp Biol Med 1955;**88**:138–140.

21. DeJoseph MR, Hawkins RA. Glucose consumption decreases throughout the brain only hours after portacaval shunting. Am J Physiol 1991;**260**:E613–E619.

22. Bergmeyer HU, ed. Methods of Enzymatic Analysis. 2nd ed. Vol. I–IV. 1974, Academic Press: New York. 2299.

23. Eccleston EG. A method for the estimation of free and total acid soluble plasma tryptophan using an ultrafiltration technique. Clin Chim Acta 1973;**48**:269–272.

24. Ardawi MSM, Newsholme EA. Maximum activities of some enzymes of glycolysis, the tricarboxylic acid cycle and ketone–body and glutamine utilization pathways in lymphocytes of the rat. Biochem J 1982;**208**:743–748.

25. Curthoys NP, Lowry OH. The distribution of glutaminase isoenzymes in the various structures of the nephron in normal, acidotic, and alkalotic rat kidney. J Biol Chem 1973;**248**:162–168.

26. Jessy J, Mans AM, DeJoseph MR, Hawkins RA. Hyperammonemia causes many of the changes found after portacaval shunting. Biochem J 1990;**272**:311–317.

27. Souba WW. Glutamine: A key substrate for the splanchnic bed. Annu Rev Nutr 1991;**11**:285–308.

28. Fisher CJ, Faloon WW. Blood ammonia levels in hepatic cirrhosis. Their control by the oral administration of neomycin. N Engl J Med 1957;**256**:1030–1035.

29. Walser M, Bodenloos LJ. Urea metabolism in man. J Clin Invest 1959;**38**:1617–1626.

30. Wolpert E, Phillips SF, Summerskill WHJ. Transport of urea and ammonia production in the human colon. Lancet 1971;**2**:1387–1390.

31. Vince A, Down PF, Murison J, Twigg FJ, Wrong OM. Generation of ammonia from non–urea sources in a faecal incubation system. Clin Sci Mol Med 1976;**51**:313–322.

32. Bown RL, Gibson JA, Fenton JCB, Snedden W, Clark ML, Sladen GE. Ammonia and urea transport by the excluded human colon. Clin Sci Mol Med 1975;**48**:279–287.

33. Dobbins WO, Herrero BA, Mansbach CM. Morphologic alterations associated with neomycin induced malabsorption. Am J Med Sci 1968;**255**:63–77.

34. Jacobson ED, Prior JT, Faloon WW. Malabsorptive syndrome induced by neomycin: morphologic alterations in the jejunal mucosa. J Lab Clin Med 1960;**56**:245–250.

35. van Leeuwen PA, Drukker J, van der Kleyn NM, van den Boogaard AE, Soeters PB. Morphological effects of high dose neomycin sulphate on the small and large intestine. Acta Morphol Neerl Scand 1986;24:223–234.

36. Faloon WW, Paes IC, Woolfolk D, Nankin H, Wallace K, Haro EN. Effect of neomycin and kanamycin upon intestinal absorption. Ann N Y Acad Sci 1966;132:879–887.

37. Hayman H, Fisher CJ, Duggan KC, Rubert MW, Faloon WW. Effect of fat–poor diet upon neomycin induced malabsorption. Gastroenterology 1964;47:161–165.

38. Jacobson ED, Chodos RB, Faloon WW. An experimental malabsorption syndrome induced by neomycin. Am J Med 1960;28:524–533.

39. Coy DL, Srivastava A, Gottstein J, Butterworth RF, Blei AT. Postoperative course after portacaval anastomosis in rats is determined by the portacaval pressure gradient. Am J Physiol 1991;261:G1072–G1078.

40. Vergara F, Plum F, Duffy TE. a–Ketoglutaramate: Increased concentrations in the cerebrospinal fluid of patients in hepatic coma. Science 1974;183:81–83.

41. Hawkins RA, Jessy J. Hyperammonemia does not impair brain function in the absence of net glutamine synthesis. Biochem J 1991;277:697–703.

N–Acetylglutamate Synthetase (NAGS) Deficiency

J. P. Colombo

1. Introduction

N–Acetylglutamate synthetase (NAGS) deficiency is a genetic disorder of ammonia detoxication. These disorders result in acute and chronic hyperammonemia, becoming evident in early infancy. They are associated with a high mortality and morbidity.

Hyperammonemia ensues when there is an imbalance between ammonia production and its removal. In congenital disorders of urea cycle enzymes and certain organic acidurias, a disturbed removal is the main reason for the accumulation of ammonia in extracellular fluids and tissues. Hyperammonemia is found in many congenital syndromes (Table 1).

Ammonia at elevated levels is particularly toxic to the nervous system and an important factor in the pathogenesis of hepatic encephalopathy, particularly in young children, where we might speculate that the developing brain is more sensitive to this toxic effect.

In contrast to liver failure with hyperammonemia in adults most frequently due to acquired different types of cirrhosis, in congenital hyperammonemia metabolic processes in the liver function normally and there is no liver bypass or portocaval shunt (PCS). Substances generated in the GI–tract such as methanthiol and dimethylsulfide can not act as hepatic encephalopathy (HE) promotors. We therefore believe that in urea cycle disorders ammonia is the major component causing the acute disturbances of the central nervous system, leading to lethargy and coma. Furthermore the accumulation of the amino acid not metabolized by the deficient enzyme as well as the deficiency of amino acids after the enzyme block, may play an additional fundamental role causing long term psychomotor retardation as may be observed in argininemia (1).

The clinical course of these disorders in the neonatal period may be lethal. The symptoms include poor sucking, vomitting, lethargy (somnolence to coma), muscular hypo- and hypertonicity, seizures, hyperpyrexia and hyperreflexia. Some of these patients show an acute clinical course leading without appropriate treatment to psychomotor retardation.

These symptoms are precipitated by increased protein intake and catabolism (infections, recurrent illness). The severity varies greatly, depending on the genetic variant of the enzyme defect.

An evaluation of the neurologic outcome at 12 months of age in patients with urea cycle disorders showed an inverse correlation of the IQ and a direct correlation of CT–abnormalities with the duration of neonatal hyperammonemic coma (stage III and IV) (2). In blood normal ammonia concentrations are between 50 and 80 $\mu mol/l$, in hyperammonemia concentrations up to 2000 $\mu mol/l$ can be found. Newborns have higher concentrations than adult people (3). When the venous blood ammonia is over 100 $\mu mol/l$ measured by an enzymatic method, we talk about hyperammonemia.

Dept. of Clinical Chemistry. Inselspital. University of Berne. 3010 Berne. Switzerland

Hepatic Encephalopathy, Hyperammonemia, and Ammonia Toxicity
Edited by V. Felipo and S. Grisolia, Plenum Press, New York, 1994

135

Table 1. Disorders leading to hyperammonemia in infancy and chidhood

---

A. DECREASED DETOXICTION OF AMMONIA

1. Congenital Defects of Urea Cycle Enzymes
- carbamoylphosphate synthetase deficiency
- ornithine carbamoiltransferase deficiency
- argininosuccinate synthetase deficiency (citrullinemia)
- argininosuccinase deficiency (argininosuccinic aciduria)
- arginase deficiency (argininemia)
- N–acetylglutamate synthetase deficiency

2. Disorders Affecting the Transport of Intermediary Metabolites of the Urea Cycle
- lysinuric protein intolerance
- hyperammonemia hyperornithinemia homocitrullinuria syndrome

3. Organic Acidemias/–urias
- isovaleric acidemia
- 3–methylcrotonylglycinuria
- 3–methylglutaconic aciduria
- 3–hydroxy–3–methylglutaric aciduria
- 2–methylacetoacetic aciduria
- propionic acidemia
- methylmalonic acidemias (including defects of cobalamine metabolism)
- pyroglutamic aciduria
- glutaric aciduria type II
- systemic carnitine deficiency
- multiple acylCoA dehydrogenase defect
- pyruvate carboxylase deficiency
- multiple carboxylase deficiency:
  - biotinidase defect
  - holocarboxylase synthetase defect
- valproate therapy

4. Insufficient Arginine Supply: diet, parenteral nutrition

5. Liver Bypass
- transient hyperammonemia of the premature (?)
- cirrhosis

6. Liver Insufficiency (infection, infestation)

B. INCREASED PRODUCTION OF AMMONIA

1. Augmented Muscular Activity:
- seizures
- respiratory (IRDS, Crying)

2. Bacterial Production:
- dermatitis
- cystitis (urease positive bacterias)

Since ammonia is toxic, powerful mechanisms are at disposal for its detoxication. Bolus injections of $N13-NH_4^+$ in the portal vein of rats have shown that during a single pass 93% is already extracted by the liver (4).

Two detoxication mechanisms of ammonia are of importance: The synthesis of urea and the synthesis of glutamine.

2. Urea Synthesis

To have a constant flux through the urea cycle, bicarbonate, NH_4^+ and aspartate must be available in stoichiometric amounts in the presence of ornithine. (Fig. 1). Carbamylphosphate is formed in the mitochondria from ammonia, ATP and bicarbonate. It condenses then with ornithine to citrulline, which leaves the mitochondrion and in a further reaction is metabolized via argininosuccinic acid to arginine. Arginase splits urea from this amino acid, leading again to ornithine, which is then recycled within the mitochondrion. As a consequence the overall pathway of urea formation involves enzyme reactions in both the cytosol and the mitochondria, which are controlled by the concentration of substrates, activators and inhibitors. In addition, compartmentation of the urea cycle enzymes necessitates transport of the intermediates across the mitochondrial membrane. Hence, many factors contribute to the regulaton of urea synthesis under different metabolic conditions.

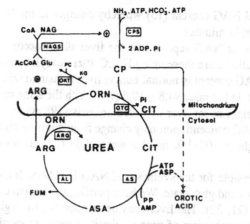

Figure 1. Urea cycle. OTC = ornithinetranscarbamylase; AS = argininosuccinate synthetase; AL = argininosuccinate lyase; Arg = arginase; OKT = ornithineketoacid transaminase; NAGS = N-acetylglutamate synthetase; CPS = carbamylphosphate synthetase; CP = carbamylphosphate; ORN = ornithine; CIT = citrulline; ASA = argininosuccinic acid; ARG = arginine; AcCoA = acetyl coenzyme A; Glu = glutamate; NAG = N-acetylglutamate; PC = pyrrolinecarboxylic acid; KG = α-ketoglutarate; ASP = asparate; FUM = fumarate; PP = pyrophosphate; Pi = phosphate.

Congenital defects of the urea cycle involve the following enzymes (Fig. 1): Carbamyl phosphate synthetase (CPS), ornithine carbamyl transferase (OCT), argininosuccinic acid synthetase (AS), argininosuccinate lyase (AL), arginase (ARG) and N-acetylglutamine synthetase (NAGS). The latter enzyme is not directly a part of the cycle, but is essential for its function. Our laboratory was involved in the first report of NAGS and arginase deficiency (argininemia) (5, 6). OCT deficiency is the most frequent inborn error of urea cycle and best studied on the molecular level, and most apt for prenatal diagnosis. Today, at least 35 single base mutations and several larger deletions associated with impaired enzyme functions are known. We have recently described four new mutations on Exon 2 and three on Exon 5, using the PCR-reaction (7, 8).

The rate limiting enzymatic step in the urea cycle is the enzyme argininosuccinate synthetase (AS), when it is fully saturated with subtrates such as ornithine, ammonia and aspartate.

Men on a normal protein diet produce about 14 mg urea/kg BW/h or 235 μmol/kg/h (Newborns: 210 μmol/kg/h) (9). With an average BW of 70 kg and a liver weight of 1'500 g, an adult produces 395 mmol/d. AS-activity averages 90 ± 12 μmol/h/g liver w.w. (10), which corresponds to an urea synthetizing capacity of 3'240 mmol/d, that is 8 times more than the daily urea production. According to this calculation the overcapacity of the urea cycle is not very large. However, in vivo the relationship between urea cycle flux and the concentration of the cycle intermediates indicates, that under physiological conditions urea cycle enzymes are far from being saturated by their substrates.

In vivo the rate through the urea cycle flux is mainly regulated by CPS. CPS constitutes about 24% of the total matrix protein of liver mitochondria. Recent experiments have shown that a CPS-OCT complex exists at the mitochondrial inner membrane, allowing a rapid channelling of substrates (11). CPS has an absolute requirement for N-acetylglutamate (NAG) (12). One mol of NAG binds to one mol of the enzyme subunit leading to conformational changes with allosteric activation of the enzyme CPS (13). In the presence of ATP, Mg^{2+}, K+ and NAG, CPS forms a high affinity complex (enzyme-ATP-ATP-carboxylphosphate – NAG), whereby NAG is tightly bound to the enzyme. The enzyme complex reacts very rapidly with ammonia to yield carbamylphosphate and Pi (14). The capacity of rat liver mitochondria to synthetize citrulline from ammonia, ornithine and HCO_3^- is a direct function of the intramitochondrial NAG content (15) whereby changes in the NAG concentration are rapid and may occur within minutes.

The concentrations of NAG reported in the liver differ according to the measuring techniques used. Most reliable are those using HPLC after deacylation of the compound (16) or GC–MS (17). The NAG content in normal human liver measured with GC–MS was 19,3 – 67,1 nmol/g wet weight, in fed mice 94,8 ±19,8 (18). With the same technique we measured 27 to 32 nmol/g wet weight in rat liver of fasted animals (19), which corresponds with the biological assay (17). NAG concentration may change from a low to high protein intake from 10–20 nmol/g wet weight to 100–150 nmol g wet weight (15), as does the enzyme NAGS (20).

The enzyme responsible for the synthesis of NAG is NAGS. It catalyzes the synthesis of NAG from acetyl–CoA and glutamate. We have purified the human enzyme and developed a method to measure it (21, 22). The liver enzyme is activated by arginine (23), disclosing thus a positive feedback mechanism of urea synthesis. Kinetic properties in the absence of arginine are compatible with a rapid equilibrium random bibi menchanism. The K_m of the forward reaction of the human amino acyl transferase for glutamate and acetyl CoA are 8,1 and 4,4 mmol/l respectively. Arginine increases the V_{max} of the enzyme and has no effect on the K_m values for the substrates. At a concentration of 0,7 mmol/l of acetyl CoA, corresponding to the level present in the mitochondrion (0,6–0,8 mmol/l), the K_m for glutamate was 0,8 mmol, similar to the concentration found in rat liver mitochondria (3–15 mmol/l) (15). With a highly purified rat liver enzyme Sonoda and Tatibana found a K_m for acetyl CoA of 0,7 mmol/l (24). Small changes in the concentration of the two substrates might therefore markedly affect the initial velocity of NAGS.

The regulation of the mitochondrial NAG concentration depends on the rate of its intramitochondrial synthesis and its efflux out of the mitochondrion. Since NAG is mainly degraded by amino acylase in the cytosol it must cross the mitochondrial membrane. The rate of efflux is about 0,05 nmol $\cdot$ min^{-1} $\cdot$ mg^{-1} mitochondrial protein in energized mitonchondria (25).The activity of NAGS in human liver according to our reference values amounts from 0,4–0,9 nmol $\cdot$ min^{-1} .mg^{-1} mitochondrial protein (22).

NAG synthesis has also been found in rat and human intestinal mucosa (26), but not in rat kidney and brain, two organs that do not synthetize citrulline because of lack of CPS (27). In brain however, NAG is found in the cytosol and is probably synthetized by L–aspartate–N–acetyl transferase and may be a modulator compound for neurotransmission (27).

3. Diagnosis and Course of NAGS–Deficiency

The diagnosis of NAGS–deficiency can be assumed when, in the presence of hyperammonemia, the amino acid pattern in plasma shows no specific increase of urea cycle intermediates, there is a normal orotic acid excretion, and organic aciduria is excluded. Up to now we have examined ca 75 liver specimen for NAGS activity. We have been involved in the diagnosis by enzyme analysis of 7 cases out of 10 presented in table 2.

There is some heterogeneity as to the outcome of the clinical course. The late onset form had an as rapid a lethal course as normally the neonatal forms, whereas some neonatal onset forms appeared to do well. Despite of severe symptoms, 5 patients had a residual enzyme activity between 15–40% of the lower normal range. In four of them, NAGS could not be stimulated by arginine in vitro. This may be due to enzyme variants. However it has also been shown, that in the fasted state, rat liver NAGS is not stimulated by arginine, whereas the activity increases significantly in fed animals. Since patients with hyperammonemia crisis often are in a catabolic state, stimulation by arginine might not occur. A conclusive interpretation of the lack of NAGS stimulation is not possible at the present time.

Table 2. Patients with NAGS–deficiency

	patients	sex	age at onset	age at death	late neurological symptoms	NAGS % of normal	references
1.	F.Ph.	M	birth	9 y	psychomotor retardation	o	5, 28
2.	P.C.	M	6 d	8 d	seizures, coma	o	29
3.	D.R.	F	13 mo	13½ mo	coma, apnoe	33 % (arg–)	30
[4.	D.	F	11 mo	13 mo	coma	n.m.]	
5.		M	5 w	---	18 mo, normal growth and	o	31
[6.		M	2 w	---	6 mo, retarded growth,	n.m.]	
7.	B.L.	M	1 d	---	1 mo, retarded growth,	15 % (arg–)	
8.	D.B.	M	3 w	---	4 mo, normal growth	10 % (arg–)	
9.	E.	M	1 d	3 d	coma	34 % (arg+)	
10.	S.E.	F	2 mo	---	2 y, psychomotor retardation	40 % (arg–)	32

Patients with initials: NAGS determinded in our laboratory.
[ ]: Siblings of proven NAG patients with the similar clinical picture.
o: NAGS activity could not be distinguished from zero.
n.m.: NAGS was not measured.
arg–/+: activation by arginine.

The first case we described has been observed during 8 years, when he suddenly died (28). The growth development was on the 50% percentile (Fig. 2), whereas the psychomotor development was greatly retarded (Fig. 3) (33). The child presented the following evelopmental milestones: because of extreme muscular hypotonicity sat with one year, walked with three years. Apraxia of the hand movements, recognized colors at 4 years, at 5 years he

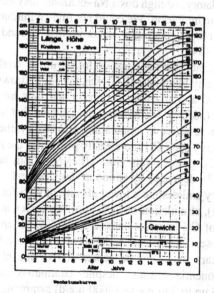

Figure 2. Growth curve of patient F.Ph. with NAGS–defociency (28).

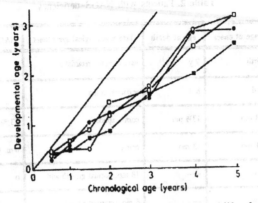

Figure 3. Psychomotor evaluation during the first 5 years of life of patient F.Ph. with NAGS–deficiency (Denver Developmental Screening Test). O, Language; ●, personal–social; □, fine motor–adaptive; ■, gross motor (28).

was not able to design, with 3 years he spoke a few words which never exceeded three–word–sentences up to the age of 8 years. He presented an anxious basic mood. He was able to attend a special school for retarded children where he felt good. He was always difficult to feed. At the age of 4 1/2 years the nasal tube feeding could be replaced by normal oral feeding.

4. Treatment

The uniqueness of NAGS deficiency lies in the possibility of therapy by oral supply of a carbamyl phosphate synthetase activator such as N–carbamylglutamate and a balanced diet (low protein, arginine resp. citrulline supplementation) (28).During hyperammonemic crisis Na–benzoate may be mandatory. At high dosis Na–benzoate may exert toxic symptoms which were attributed to urea cycle inhibition. We could not find an inhibition of mitochondrial urea cycle enzymes in the rat at benzoate concentrations found in plasma of treated hyperammonemic patients (34).

It has been shown in rats that the capacity for citrulline synthesis in the mitochondria increased, when a N–carbamylglutamate (CG) was fed (35). Brown et al. as well as Kim et al. advocated the use of CG and ariginine to prevent and treat hyperammonemia in clinical conditions of liver disease (36, 37). Mejier et al. have shown that in mitochondria of rats fed a standard diet, CG was more active in stimulating citrulline synthesis than NAG itself (25). In a low mitochondrial energy state CG more easily penetrates the mitonchondrial membrane than NAG. Furthermore CG protects rats more efficiently from ammonia intoxication than NAG, since it is less rapidly degraded by amino acylase, present in the cytosol (37). On the basis of the facilitated entry and despite a lower affinity of CPS for CG (K_a = 4 mmol/l) than for NAG (0,1–0,2 mmol/l), stimulation of CPS must take place at high doses of CG (25).

The administration of CG lowers ammonia in NAGS–patients. However it is difficult to elaborate the correct dose. Table 3 shows the standard treatment of our patient at the age of 13 months and 4 years and may be representative for other cases. When CG is discontinued, hyperammonemia ensues, despite continuous arginine supplementation. Increasing the dose of CG up to 750 mg/kg (3600 mg/d) symptoms of intoxication occurred, evoking a Chinese–Restaurant Syndrome with tachycardia, profuse sweating, increased bonchial secretion, increased temperature and permanent screaming. Initially in untreated

Table 3. Nutrition in NAGS-deficiency (daily requirements). According to the experience in the case F.Ph. (28)

		13 mo (10 kg BW)	4 1/4 y (17,5 kg BW)
FEEDING		gastric tube	oral
	carbohydrates, g	144	155
	fat, g	24	35
	protein, g	15	25
	total calories, kcal	914	1035
MEDICATION	N–carbamylglutamate	1800 mg = 9,5 mmol (3 x 600 mg)	2400 mg = 12,6 mmol (9–6–9 x 10^2 mg)
	Arginin–hydrochloride	7 g = 40 mmol	
	L–Citrulline		7,3 g = 42 mmol

carbamylphosphate production which even continues shortly after CG is withdrawn. This is probably due to the longer biological half life of CG, compared to NAG. Arginine supplementation additionally stimulates NAGS. But it may also provide ornithine due to the splitting by arginase located near the external mitochondrial surface.

A balanced treatment, using CG, arginine resp. citrulline, a moderate protein supply and enough calories can contribute to the wellbeing of these children. However, hyperammonemic crisis must be treated very rapidly to avoid or minimize psychomotor retardation. We still have to await the outcome in further cases to evaluate the efficiency of these therapeutic trials.

References

1. Colombo, J.P. Argininaemia: clinical and biochemical aspects. Guanidino compounds in Biology and Medicine, eds. by De Deyn PP, Marescau V, Stalon V, Qureshi I.A. John Libbey and Company Ltd. 1992; 343–8.
2. Msall M, Batshaw ML, Suss R, Brusilow SW, Mellits ED. Neurologic outcome in children with inborn errors of urea synthesis. Outcome of Urea–Cycle Enzymopathies. N Eng J Med. 1984, **310**:1500–5.
3. Colombo JP, Peheim E, Kretschmer R, Dauwalder H, Sidiropoulos D. Plasma ammonia concentrations in newborns and children. Clin Chim Acta. 1984; **138**:283–91.
4. Cooper AJL, Nieves E, Coleman AE, Filc–De Ricco S, Gelbard AS. Short–term metabolic fate of [13N] ammonia in rat liver. J Biol Chem. 1987; **262**:1073–80.
5. Bachmann C, Krähenbühl S, Colombo JP. N–Acetylglutamate synthetase deficiency: A disorder of ammonia detoxication. N Eng J Med. 1981, **304**:543.
6. Terheggen HG, Schwenk A, Lowenthal A, Van Sande M, Colombo JP. Argininemia with arginase deficiency. Lancet ii. 1969, 748

7. Oppliger E, Liechti–Gallati S, Colombo JP, Wermuth B. Ornithine transcarbamylase deficiency: Identification of four new mutations in exon 2. Abstract, XV International Congress of Clinical Chemistry, Melbourne, Australia, 1993.

8. Oppliger E, Wermuth B, Colombo JP, Liechti–Gallati S. Ornithine transcarbamylase deficiency: Identification of three new mutations in exon 5. Abstract, XV International Congress of Clinical Chemistry, Melbourne, Australia, 1993.

9. Kalhan SC. Rates of Urea Synthesis in the Human Newborn: Effect of Maternal Diabetes and Small Size for Gestational Age. Ped Res. 1993, **34**:801–4.

10. Nuzum CT, Snodgrass PJ. Multiple Assays of the Five Urea–Cycle Enzymes in Human Liver Homogenates. The Urea Cycle, eds. by Grisolia S, Báguena R, Mayor F. John Wiley & Sons, Inc., New York, 1976.

11. Meijer AJ, Lamers WH, Chamuleau R. Nitrogen Metabolism and ornithine cycle function. Physiol Reviews. 1990; **70**:701–48.

12. Grisolia S, Cohen PP. Catalytic role of glutamate derivatives in citrulline biosynthesis. J Biol Chem. 1953, **204**:753–7.

13. Guadalajara AM, Rubio V, Grisolia S. Inactivation of carbamoyl phosphate synthetase (ammonia) by elastase as a probe to investigate binding of the substrates. Biochem Biophys. Res. Comm. 1983, **117**:238–44.

14. Britton HG, Rubio V. Carbamoyl–phosphate synthetase I. Kinetics of binding and dissociation of acetylglutamate and of activation and deactivation. Eur J Biochem. 1988, **171**:615–22.

15. Meijer AJ, Hensgens H. Ureogenesis, in Metabolic compartmentation. Sies H, Ed. Academic Press, London 1982.

16. Alonso E, Rubio V. Determination of N–Acetyl–L–glutamate Using High–Performance Liquid Chromatography. Anal Biochem. 1985, **146**:252–9.

17. Tuchmann M, Holzknecht RA. Human hepatic N–acetylglutamate content and N–acetylglutamate synthase activity. Biochem J. 1990, **271**:325–9.

18. Tuchmann M, Holzknecht RA. N–Acetylglutamate Content in Liver and Gut of Normal and Fasted Mice, Normal Human Livers, and Livers of Individuals with Carbamyl Phosphate Synthetase or Ornithine Transcarbamylase Deficiency. Ped Res. 1990, **27**:408–12.

19. Bühlmann R. Personal communication.

20. Colombo JP, Pfister U, Cervantes H. The regulation of N–Acetylglutamate synthetase in rat liver by protein intake. Biochem Biophys Res Comm. 1990, **172**:1239–1245.

21. Bachmann C, Krähenbühl S, Colombo JP. Purification and properties of acetyl–CoA: L–glutamate N–acetyltransferase from human liver. Biochem J. 1982, **205**:123–7.

22. Colombo JP, Krähenbühl S, Bachmann C. N–Acetylglutamate Synthetase: Enzyme Assay in Human Liver. J Clin Chem Clin Biochem. 1982, **20**:325–9.

23. Freedland RA, Crozier GL, Hicks BL, Meijer AJ. Arginine uptake by isolated rat liver mitochondria. Biochim Biophys Acta. 1984, **802**:407–12.

24. Sonoda T, Tatibana M. Purification of N–Acetyl–L–glutamate Synthetase from Rat Liver Mitochondria and Substrate and Activator Specificity of the Enzyme. J Biol Chem. 1983, **258**:9839–44.

25. Meijer AJ, Van Woerkom GM, Wanders RJA, Lof C. Transport of N–Acetylglutamate in Rat–Liver Mitochondria. Eur J Biochem. 1982, **124**:325–30.

26. Wakabayashi Y, Iwashima A, Yamada E, Yamada R. Enzymological Evidence for the Indispensability of Small Intestine in the Synthesis of Arginine from Glutamate. Arch Biochem Biophys. 1991, **291**:9–14.

27. Alonso E, García–Pérez MA, Bueso J, Rubio V. N–Acetyl–L–Glutamate in Brain: Assay, Levels, and Regional and Subcellular Distribution. Neurochem Res. 1991, **16**:787–94.

28. Schubiger G, Bachmann C, Barben P, Colombo JP, Tönz O, Schüpbach D. N–Acetylglutamate synthetase deficiency: diagnosis, management and follow–up of a rare disorder of ammonia detoxication. Eur J Pediatr. 1991, **150**:353–6.

29. Bachmann C, Brandis M, Weissenbarth–Riedel E, Burghard R, Colombo JP. N–Acetylglutamate Synthetase Deficiency, A Second Patient. J Inher Metab Dis. 1988, **11**:191–3.

30. Elpeleg ON, Colombo JP, Amir N, Bachmann C, Hurvitz H. Late–onset form of partial N–acetylglutamate synthetase deficiency. Eur J Pediatr. 1990, **149**:634–6.

31. Pandya AL, Koch R, Hommes FA, Williams JC. N–Acetylglutamate Synthetase Deficiency: Clinical and Laboratory Observations. J Inher Metab Dis. 1991, **14**:685–90.

32. Burlina AB, Bachmann C, Wermuth B, Bordugo A, Ferrari V, Colombo JP, Zacchello F. Partial N-Acetylglutamate synthetase deficiency: A new case with uncontrollable movement Disorders. J Inher Metab Dis. 1992, **15**:395-8.
33. Barben P. N-Acetyl-Glutamat-Synthetase-Mangel. Dissertation Bern, 1989.
34. Colombo JP, Bachmann C, Pfister U, Gradwohl M. Mitochondrial urea cycle enzymes in rats treated with sodium benzoate. Biochem Biophys Res Comm. 1988, **151**:872-7.
35. Koritz SB, Cohen PP. The effect of diet on citrulline synthesis in vitro. J Biol Chem. 1953, **200**:551-7.
36. Brown R, Manning R, Delp M, Grisolia S. Treatment of hepatocerebral intoxication. Lancet i. 1958, 591-2.
37. Kim S, Paik WK, Cohen PP. Ammonia Intoxication in Rats: Protection by N-Carbamoyl-L-Glutamate Plus L-Arginine. Proc Nat Acad Sci. 1972, **69**:3530-3.

Ornithine Transcarbamylase Deficiency: A Model for Gene Therapy

Manal A. Morsy and C. Thomas Caskey

1. Introduction

Ornithine transcarbamylase (EC 2.1.3.3.) deficiency (OTCD) is the most common and severe defect of the urea cycle disorders. It is an X–linked disorder with a high new mutation rate and variable phenotypic consequences. The enzyme catalyses the condensation of carbamyl phosphate and ornithine to citrulline in the second step of the urea cycle. It is expressed mainly in the liver and intestine (approximately 30% of liver levels), and is targeted to the mitochondria in which it assumes its homotrimeric active form.

Despite progress in dietary and pharmacological therapy the prognosis for OTCD patients remains poor. In the neonatal period, affected males develop hyperammonemia, acidosis, orotic aciduria and coma. The consequences include death if untreated, and mental retardation or cerebral palsy in the surviving treated newborns (1, 2). Less severe forms of OTCD may present during infancy, childhood or adulthood and are a consequence of mutation heterogeneity. These mutations can be responsible for life–threatening hyperammonemic comas in late onset males (3) and carrier females (4). As in the case of treated neonates it is reported that most of the late–onset OTCD patients who have had one or more episodes of hyperammonemic encephalopathy suffer some degree of brain damage or death (4–6).

It is therefore essential to develop alternative therapeutic approaches for treatment and control of OTCD. Transient or permanent correction can be beneficial in relieving the metabolic consequences of a catabolic crisis and may be life–saving during hyperammonemic episodes. Rapid transient correction may be followed by conventional therapy or liver transplantation.

2. Methods of Gene Delivery

There are several possible strategies for the delivery of nucleic acid sequences to accomplish somatic gene therapy. In the context of OTC, for *in vivo* delivery these include viral vectors such as adenovirus (Ad) and adeno–associated viral (AAV) vectors. Retroviruses can be used but in an *ex–vivo* approach is necessary because of their inefficiency of infecting quiescent cells (such as liver cells). *Ex–vivo* delivery involves isolation of hepatocytes from the patients' liver, infection with the vector of interest *in vitro*, followed by autologus infusion. This is a complex and invasive approach. Alternative liver–targeted gene delivery methods employ chemically modified DNA. Conjugates of asialo–orosomucoid and poly–L–

Department of Molecular and Human Genetics, Baylor College of Medicine, Houston, TX 77030. Telephone (713) 798–4774. Fax (713) 798–7383

Hepatic Encephalopathy, Hyperammonemia, and Ammonia Toxicity
Edited by V. Felipo and S. Grisolia, Plenum Press, New York, 1994

lysine achieve DNA delivery by binding to the hepatic asialoglycoprotein receptor. Each delivery system has individual merits and limitations (7).

Typically, viral vectors such as Ad are rendered defective (e.g. in replication) by various deletions in their genome, into which genes of interest along with desired regulatory elements are then inserted. The recombinant vectors must then be propagated and produced in packaging (helper) cell lines, which complement the missing functions of the defective vector. Such defective viral vectors unable to replicate in non–helper cells, thus the undesirable effect of the virus in the target tissue is lost and therapeutic gene expression achieved.

As the liver plays a central role in the pathogenesis of many human disorders, it has been a target for gene therapy in experimental animals. The liver has been targeted for treatment of disorders such as OTCD, citrullinemia, hypercholesterolemia, α1–antitrypsin deficiency, hemophilia and others. Ponder and colleagues evaluated the *ex vivo* method of gene transfer to hepatocytes (8). They utilized two transgenic mice, one expressing β–galactosidase and the other expressing human α1–antitrypsin (hAAT). Hepatocytes isolated from the two transgenic models were transplanted into the livers of non–transgenic mice of the same strain. A large fraction of these cells was identified at 2 months following transplantation and serum hAAT was detected for more than 6 months. Treatment of Watanabe rabbits defective in the LDL receptor has been successfully achieved by Chowdhury and colleges (9). Following a 30% partial hepatectomy and intrasplenic injection of autologous, retroviraly–transduced hepatocytes expressing the human LDL receptor, a 30–50% reduction in total serum cholesterol lasting 4 months was demonstrated. Although the *ex vivo* delivery approach is technically challenging, and the therapeutic expression is transient, two clinical protocols have been approved for *ex vivo* liver gene transfer. One protocol by Ledley and associates will genetically mark hepatic cells in order to study the utility of hepatocellular transplantation in acute hepatic failure patients (10). A second protocol by Wilson and colleges is directed at treatment for familial hypercholesterolemia (11).

Gene delivery to hepatocytes using conjugated DNA complexes was examined by Cristiano *et al.* (12). This group used asialoorosomucoid–poly(L–lysine) conjugated to DNA molecules coding for canine factor IX and very low concentrations of adenoviral particles. Following infection of primary mouse hepatocytes, significant concentrations of the factor were expressed in the culture medium, indicating efficiency of delivery and expression of the exogenous gene. However, although non–viral mediated gene transfer approaches are relatively safer than viral approaches, in general they are transient in mediating expression and of limited *in vivo* efficiency. These methods therefore await further modifications.

3. The Adenoviral Vector and Gene Therapy

Over the past few years, the adenovirus has been one of the most extensively studied gene delivery systems. Adenoviral vectors efficiently deliver recombinant genes to multiple targets tissues *in vitro* and *in vivo*, including liver, lung, muscle, blood vessels, and brain and have proven to be very powerful as gene transduction agents. To date there are at least five human gene therapy clinical trials approved for the use of recombinant Ad vectors as the gene delivery vehicle (13).

Adenoviruses are large (38 kb) DNA viruses that are very stable and infect both dividing and non–dividing cells. These are extremely favorable traits for drug development, especially in comparison to retroviruses which infect only dividing cells. Adenoviruses which have been extensively studied at the molecular levels and have been used safely for vaccine preparations. The Ad genome has late (transcribed after DNA replication) and early expressed genes which are required for DNA replication and viral propagation. The early genes include an immediate early gene subset (E1A), a multifunctional regulator of genes which themselves regulate other genes required for adenovirus replication. In the adenovirus life cycle the virus binds to cell surface receptors and enters the cell by lysing its endosome prior to lysosomal degradation. If E1A is active, transcription of early genes induces DNA replication, late gene expression, virus particle assembly, and cell lysis. This is undesirable for gene therapy. Recombinant replication–defective vectors are constructed by the replacement of the E1A region of the adenovirus with the therapeutic gene. Defective adenoviruses can be produced at very high titers (10^{11} viable particles per ml) from helper cells (293) which themselves express E1A. These defective vectors have the capacity to incorporate up to 7 kb of the therapeutic gene. Current adenovirus vectors, however, do not integrate into nuclear DNA of the recipient cell, and thus their therapeutic genes are expressed transietly. The duration of expression depends on cell type (14, 15).

Recombinant adenoviral vectors containing reporter genes such as β–galactosidase or luciferase were used by many groups to study the efficacy and longevity of adenoviral–mediated gene expression. Injected mouse muscles expressed β–gal 75 days post Ad–mediated transfection (16), and intravenous injection into mice resulted in expression of the reporter gene up to 12 months after recombinant Ad–β–gal delivery (17). Ragot *et al.* used a human dystrophin minigene to show efficient Ad–mediated delivery and expression in mouse skeletal muscles for up to 98 days post injection (18).

Successful Ad–mediated LacZ expression was also achieved in respiratory epithelium. Bout *et al.* showed Ad–mediated β–gal expression in the lung epithelium of Rhesus monkeys, with no virus–mediated toxicity to lungs or any other organ tested (19). Ad–mediated delivery and expression of the cystic fibrosis transmembrane conductance regulator (CFTR) gene was extensively evaluated by several groups. Efficient expression was achieved *in vitro* (20) and *in vivo* in lungs of cotton rats (21). Such studies lead to the development of clinical trials using recombinant Ad vectors for treatment of cystic fibrosis (13).

In targeting the liver, a recombinant Ad vector carrying the rat OTC cDNA was shown to mediate gene expression in newborn OTCD mice (22). *In vitro*, Kozorsky *et al.*, achieved highly efficient Ad–mediated expression of LDL receptor protein in hepatocytes derived from patients suffering from familial hypercholestorolemia (23). *In vivo*, Ishibashi *et al.* reported restoration of functional LDL receptor protein expression in the liver of LDL receptor knockout mice. Ad–encoded receptors were capable of reversing the hypercholesterolemic effects of the LDL receptor deficiency (24). Kay *et al.*, demonstrated *in vivo* transient adeno–mediated correction of hemophilia B dogs (25).

These studies illustrate the potential usefulness of the adenovirus as gene therapy vectors. Taking into consideration the numerous advantages of the adenoviral system, we have recently concentrated our efforts on evaluating the efficacy of this system in mediating human OTC gene expression and have examined its potential utility in correcting the enzymatic and metabolic defect in the OTCD mouse model.

4. Progress Towards OTC Gene Therapy

Progress towards OTC gene therapy has been facilitated by the availability of two mouse models for OTCD, the sparse fur (*spf*), and the sparse fur–abnormal skin and hair (*spf/ash*) mutants. Both models are phenotypically small in size, display delayed development, and possess little or no fur together with wrinkled skin. The phenotype is most pronounced in the first 3 weeks of life. Survival rates of newborns are low, and biochemically both models are characterized by reduced enzymatic activity and pronounced orotic aciduria, one of the hallmarks of OTCD shared by mouse and man (26). The molecular defect in the *spf* model is a point mutation in exon 4 which alters the pH optimum for the enzyme activity. This results in only 20% wild type activity at physiological pH despite high levels of expressed protein (150% of wild–type) (27, 28). In contrast the *spf/ash* OTC gene carries a splice junction mutation, leading to expression of 5–15% wild–type levels of active enzyme

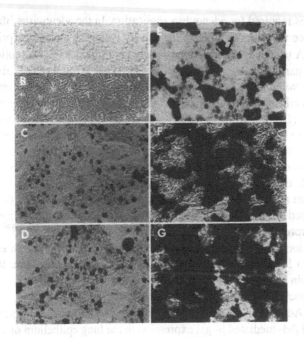

Figure 1. Human hepatocyte – Panels (C–G) show cultures infected with AdHCMVsp1LacZ at 10, 20, 50,100 and 200 multiplicities of infection (moi) respectively. Panel (A) shows cultures stained immunohistochemically after incubation with α1–antitrypsin antibodies. Panel (B) shows control hepatocytes infected with AdSRαhOTC at moi of 200.

(29). The abnormal precursors are properly imported into the mitochondria, but fail to form enzymatically active trimers (30). Both models are fundamental to designing approaches for human OTCD gene therapy and have been instrumental for our work.

There is good evidence that successful correction of OTCD can be achieved by gene transfer. Germline correction of OTCD homozygous mice was achieved in our laboratory by injecting a truncated segment of the mouse OTC promoter coupled to human OTC cDNA. These transgenic mice were corrected both phenotypically and metabolically despite exclusive enzyme expression in the small intestine, presumably due to the different tissue specificity

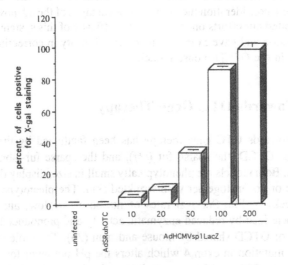

Figure 2. Primary human hepatocytes cultures (n=3) were evaluated for βgal activity 72 hours post–AdHCMVsp1LacZ infection by scoring the percentage of blue stained cells. Vertical error bars show standard deviations from the mean.

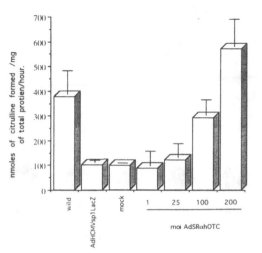

Figure 3. Livers of two–month–old *spf* (OTC–deficient) and C3H/HENCRMTV mice (wild–type) (Jackson Laboratories ME) were used for the hepatocyte cultures. OTC–deficient hepatocytes were infected 48 hours post–plating with different mois of AdSRαhOTC, AdHCMVsp1LacZ or suspension media (mock) and evaluated for OTC enzyme activity one week post–infection (n=3). Vertical error bars show standard deviations from the mean.

conferred by the truncated promoter (31). Carvard *et al.* had succeeded in creating corrected transgenic mice by germline transfer of rat OTC cDNA coupled to the strong viral SV40 promoter (32). Somatic gene transfer to OTCD primary hepatocytes has been evaluated using retroviruses (33). However due to the limitations of retroviruses as mentioned above, *in vivo* retroviral–mediated liver infection would be inadequate.

Currently we are using an Ad construct driven by the SRα promoter which is a combination of the SV40 early region promoter linked to human T cell leukemia virus–1 enhancer sequences.(34) This promoter has proven utility in the correction of OTC deficiency both *in vitro* (35) and *in vivo*. Using this promoter in the context of an E1–deleted E3 mutant Ad5, we have achieved high levels of human OTC gene expression in hepatocyte cell culture. *In vivo*, phenotypic and metabolic correction in OTC–deficient mice was observed in greater than 50% of animals treated.

Initially we evaluated the efficiency of Ad–mediated gene expression, by determining the percentage of cells expressing a reporter gene at different multiplicities of infection. Using an Ad expressing the β–galactosidase gene, AdHCMVsp1LacZ, we achieved expression in 100% of primary hepatocytes 72 hours post infection at multiplicities of 100–200 viral particles per cell (figures 1 and 2).

This led us to test the efficacy of AdSRαhOTC in mediating gene activity *in vitro*. Reconstitution of wild–type levels of enzyme activity was observed in primary mouse hepatocytes derived from OTC–deficient mice (figure 3). This level of activity was achieved when hepatocytes were infected at multiplicities of 100–200 viral particles per cell. In addition, we were able to reconstitute OTC gene expression (otherwise undetectable) in primary hepatocytes derived from an OTC–deficient patient undergoing liver transplantation (figure 4).

In vivo, using the reporter AdHCMVsp1LacZ virus, greater than 40% of hepatocytes expressed β–gal when adult mice (20–25 grams) were injected intraportally with 2×10^{10} viral particles per animal as detected by a colorometric β–gal assay (figures 5 and 6) (36). The viral dose – ranging from 4–8×10^8 particles per gram weight – was not associated with pathological findings in newborn (2–4 grams) or adult mice (20–25 grams). Subsequently, a large study was conducted in newborn *spf/ash* mice to evaluate the efficacy of AdSRαhOTC in mediating OTC gene expression *in vivo*, using titers between $\leq 0.1 \times 10^9$ – 3.0×10^9 viral particles per newborn. With this dose range there were no significant differences in the

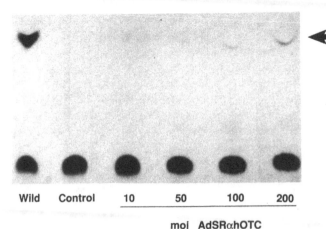

Wild   Control   10   50   100   200

moi AdSRαhOTC

Figure 4. This is an autoradiograph of a TLC plate used to separate the product citrulline (arrow) from the substrate ornithine of the OTC enzyme reaction assay. Human hepatocytes were isolated from both the donor (wild–type) and recipient (control and AdSRαhOTC–infected at different mois) liver. The recipient was a severely affected OTC–deficient male with an exon 3 *Taq* I site mutation. Hepatocytes were assayed 6 days post plating (4 days post Ad vector infection). The first lane (wild–type) represents wild type enzyme activity found in the hepatocyte cultures from the normal donor liver specimen. The second lane (control) represents the enzyme activity found in the patient's OTC–deficient liver specimen cultures uninfected with AdSRαhOTC. The remaining lanes represent OTC–deficient cultures infected with AdSRαhOTC at different mois.

survival rates of animals treated with the recombinant virus or those treated with suspension buffer alone (table 1).

We have recently succeeded in correcting the biochemical defect in newborn treated *spf/ash* mice using AdSRαhOTC. The extent of biochemical correction was assessed by measurement of two specific parameters: 1) orotic acid levels in urine, and 2) OTC enzyme levels in liver and intestine. Reduced utilization of carbamyl phosphate by the mutant enzyme results in the accumulation of orotic acid, which has a high urinary clearance rate. This underlines the basic biochemical similarity of these animals to their human counterpart. The increase in functional OTC levels with concomitant utilization of carbamyl phosphate are directly reflected by the urinary orotic acid excretion, providing a highly sensitive index of the biochemical phenotype (37).

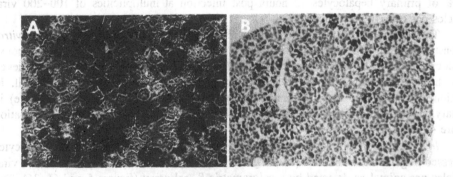

Figure 5. Livers were analyzed 72 hours post–*in vivo* infection for βgal expression. Panel (A), hepatocytes were cultured 72 hours post–infection and evaluated for βgal expression. Panel (B), liver frozen section evaluated 72 hours post–injection.

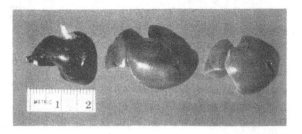

Figure 6. Whole liver was perfused *in situ* with PBS followed by 2.5% glutaraldehyde, PBS and stain. After dissection, livers were incubated for an additional 2 hours in X-gal stain. From left to right: *in vivo* intraportal transfer of 2 x 10¹⁰, 1 x 10¹⁰ pfu of AdHCMVsp1LacZ and 2 x 10¹⁰ pfu AdSRαhOTC followed 72 hours post-infection, by *in situ* fixing and X-gal staining of the liver.

A rapid response in reduction of orotic acid levels was observed within 24 hours after a single injection and lasted at least up to 15 weeks post-treatment (data not shown). These findings are critical in evaluating this therapeutic approach, especially during hyperammonemic crises when such a rapid response would be life-saving.

Increase in enzyme activity was observed in liver and intestine (data not shown) of treated animals and was associated with phenotypic correction (hair growth and weight gain relative to control litter mates) (figure 7).

5. Conclusion

Gene therapy is coming of age, and several viral systems and technologies are merging to generate the most efficient, safe and persistent gene delivery and expression vector. At the present time the adenovirus is proving to be one of the most powerful gene delivery systems. Our laboratory has long searched alternative therapeutic approaches for OTCD. Taking into account the strengths and weaknesses (possible short-term episomal persistence in target cells) of the Ad system we tested the efficacy of recombinant Ad viral vectors in mediating gene expression in hepatocytes *in vitro* and *in vivo*.

Table 1. Survival rates of mice treated with recombinant Ad-vectors and sham-treated.

	Survivors	Deaths	Total Viral pfu/animal	Total Number of animals
Treatment: AdSRαhOTC	70 (74%)*	24 (25%)+	0.1–3.0 x 10⁹	94
Control: AdCMVsp1LacZ	36 (75%)*	12 (25%)+	0.025–1.0 x 10⁸	48
Sham: Suspension Buffer	9 (64%)*	5 (36%)+	---------	14
*+ no significant difference among groups				

**Adenoviral - Mediated
In Vivo Phenotypic Correction of OTC
Deficiency in Mouse Model**

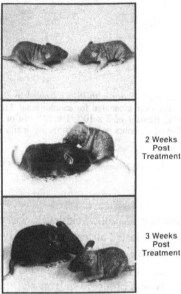

2 Weeks
Post
Treatment

3 Weeks
Post
Treatment

Figure 7. This photograph illustrates the phenotypic difference in two litter mates 2 and 3 weeks post-treatment.The mouse on the left (treated) and the one on the right (control) were injected with equivalent titers of AdSRαhOTC and AdHCMVsp1LacZ virus respectively.

We have shown highly efficient β–galacosidase and OTC gene expression in human and mouse primary hepatocytes in vitro. Gene expression was mediated by replication deficient Ad vectors. These vectors supported delivery and expression in the target organs *in vivo*. Single injections to OTCD newborn mice using the AdSRαhOTC vector resulted in correction of the phenotypic and metabolic defect. Metabolic correction was evaluated by measurements of orotic acid levels in urine and OTC enzyme activity in liver and intestine (data not shown). The reductions in orotic acid levels were dramatic (greater than 60% reduction) and rapid (within 24 hours). These observations are significant since such a rapid response may be essential in patients suffering from severe hyperammonimic crisis.

Our findings suggest that the Ad system may have clinical utility and that gene therapy can be used for correction or control of OTCD. It is important to stress that in such a devastating disorder, although long term correction is desirable, transient correction may be life saving in cases of catabolic crisis.

Acknowledgments: We thank Dr. BJF Rossiter for her review of the manuscript and Elsa Perez for preparation of the manuscript. CT Caskey is an Investigator with the Howard Hughes Medical Institute. This work was supported in part by a grant from the NIH.

References

1. Maestri N., Hauser E., Bartholomew D., Brusilow S.W., 1991, Prospective treatment of urea cycle disorder, J. Pediatr. **119:**923–928.

2. Brusilow, S. W. and Horwich, A. L. In: The metabolic basis of inherited disease, Vol 6 (Scriver CR, Beaudet AL, Sly WS and Valle D, Eds) New York: McGraw-Hill, pp 629-670. (1989)

3. Finkelstein J., Hauser E., Leonard C., Brusilow S., 1990, Late-onset ornithine transcarbamylase deficiency in male patients, J. Pediatr. 117(6):(6)897-902.

4. Batshaw M., Msall M., Beaudate A., Trojak J., 1986, Risk of serious illness in heterozygotes for Ornithin Transcarbamylase deffeciency, J. Pediatr. 108:236-241.

5. Rowe P., Newman S., Brusilow S.W., 1986, Natural history of symptomatic partial ornithine transcarbamylase deficiency, New Engl Med, 314:541-547.

6. Arn P.H., Hauser E.R., Thomas G.H., Herman G., Hess D., Brusilow S.W., 1990, Hyperammonemia in women with a mutation in the ornithine transcarbamylase locus: a cause of postpartum coma., New Engl J Med, 322:1652-1655.

7. Morsy M.A., Mitani K., Clemens P., Caskey C.T., 1993, Progress towards human gene therapy, JAMA, 270:2338-2345.

8. Ponder K.P., Gupta S., Leland F., Darlington G., Finegold M., DeMayo J., Ledley F.D., Chowdhury J.R., Woo S.L.C., 1991, Mouse hepatocytes migrate to liver parenchyma and function indefinitely after intrasplenic transplantation. Proc. Natl. Acad. Sci. USA, 88:1217-1221.

9. Chowdhury J.R., Grossman M., Gupta S., Chowdhury N.R., Baker J.R. Jr., Wilson J.M., 1991, Long-term improvement of hypercholesterolemia after ex vivo gene therapy in LDLR-deficient rabbits, Science, 254:1802-1805.

10. Ledley F.D., Woo S.L.C., Ferry G.D., Whisennand H.H., Brandt M.L., Darlington G.J., Demmler G.J., Finegold M.J., Pokorny W.J., Rosenblatt H., Schwart P., Anderson W.F., Moen R.C., 1991, Clinical protocol: hepatocellular transplantation in acute hepatic failure and targeting genetic markers to hepatic cells, Hum. Gene. Ther., 2:331-358.

11. Wilson J., Grossman M., Raper S., Baker J.J., Newton R., Thoene J., 1992, Ex vivo gene therapy of familial hypercholesterolemia, Hum. Gene. Ther., 3:179-222.

12. Cristiano R., Smith L., Kay M., Brinkley B., Woo S., 1993, Hepatic gene therapy: efficient gene delivery and expression in primary hepatocytes utilizing a conjugated adenovirus-DNA complex, Proc. Natl. Acad. Sci. USA, 90:11548-11552.

13. Human gene marker/therapy clinical protocols, 1994, Hum. Gene Ther., 5(2):271-280.

14. Graham, F. L. and Prevec, L. Manipulation of adenovirus vectors. In: Methods in Molecular Biology, edited by E.J.Clifton, NJ: The Humana Press Inc., 1991, p. 109-128.

15. Horwitz, M. S. Field's Virology (2nd), edited by B. N. Fields and D. M. Knipe, NY: Raven Press, 1990, p. 1679-1721.

16. Quantin, B., Perricaudet, L.D., Tajbakhsh, S., Mandel. J.L., 1992, Adenovirus as an expression vector in muscle cells in vivo, Proc. Natl. Acad. Sci. USA. 89:2581-2584.

17. Stratford-Perricaudet, L., Makeh, I., Perricaudet, M., Briand, P., 1992, Widespread long-term gene transfer to mouse skeletal muscles and heart, J. Clin. Invest., 90:626-630.

18. Ragot, T., Vincent, N., Chafey, P., Vigne, E., Gilgenk-Rantz, H., Couton, D., Cartaud, J., Briand, P., Kaplan, J.-C., Perricaudet, M., Kahn, A., 1993, Efficient adenovirus-mediated transfer of a human minidystrophin gene to skeletal muscle of mdx mice, Nature, 361:647-650.

19. Bout, A., Perricaudet, M., Baskin, G., Imler, J.-L., Scholte, B.J., Pavirani, A., Valerio, D, 1994, Lung gene therapy: in vivo adenovirus-mediated gene transfer to Rhesus monkey airway epithelium, Hum. Gene. Ther., 5(1):3-10.

20. Rich, D.P., Anderson, M.P., Gregory, S.H., Cheng, S.H., Paul, S., Jefferson, D.M., McCann, J.D., Klinger, K.W., Smith, A.E., Welsh, M.J., 1990, Expression of cystic fibrosis transmembrane conductance regulator corrects defective chloride channel regulator in cystic fibrosis airway epithelial cells. Nature, 347:358-363.

21. Rosenfeld, M.A., Yoshimura, K., Trapnell, B.C., Yoneyama, K., Rosenthal, W., Dalemans, W., Fukayama, M., Bargon, J., Stier, L.E., Stratford-Perricaudet, L., et al., 1992, In vivo transfer of the human cystic fibrosis transmembrane conductance regulator gene to the airway epitheluim. Cell, 68:143-155.

22. Stratford-Perricaudet, L.D., Levrero, M., Chasse, J.-F., Perricaudet, M., Briand, P., 1990, Evaluation of the Transfer and Expression in Mice of an Enzyme-Encoding Gene Using a Human Adenovirus Vector. Hum. Gene Ther., 1:241-256.

23. Kozarsky K., Grossman M., Wilson J.M., 1993, Adenovirus-mediated correction of the genetic defect in hepatocytes from pateints with familial hypercholesterolemia, Somat. Cell Mol. Genet., 19:449-458.

24. Ishibashi S., Brown M.S., Goldstein J.L., Gerard R.D., Hammer R.E., Herz J., 1993, Hypercholesterolemia in low density lipoprotein receptor knockout mice and its reversal by adenovirus–mediated gene delivery, J. Clin. Invest., **92**:883–893.

25. Kay M.A., Landen C.N., Rothenberg S.R., Taylor L.A., Leland F., Wiehle S., Fang B., Bellinger D., Finegold M., Thompson A.R., Read M., Brinkhous K.M., Woo S.L., 1994, *In vivo* hepetic gene therapy: complete albeit transeint correction of factor IX deficiency in hemophilia B dogs, Proc. Natl. Acad. Sci. USA, **91**:2353–2357.

26. Gushiken T., Yoshimura N., Saheki T., 1985, Transient hyperammonemia during ageing in ornithine transcarbamylase–deficient, sparse–fur mice, Biochem. Int., **11**:637–643.

27. DeMars R., LeVan S.L., Trend B.L., Russell L.B., 1976, Abnormal ornithine carbamoyltransferase in mice having the sparse–fur mutation, Proc. Natl. Acad. Sci. USA, **73**:1693–1697.

28. Briand P., Cathelineau L., Kamoun P., Gigot D., Penninckx M., 1981, Increase in ornithine transcarbamylase protein in sparse–fur mice with ornithine transcarbamylase deficiency, FEBS lett., **130**:65–68.

29. Hulbert, L., Cordy, C. & Doolittle, D., 1974, A new allele of the sparse fur gene in the mouse, J. Hered., **65**:194–195.

30. Hodges, P. E. & Rosenberg, L. E., 1989, The spf^{ash} mouse: A missence mutation in the ornithine transcarbamylase gene also causes aberrant mRNA splicing, Proc. Natl. Acad. Sci. USA, **86**:4142–4146.

31. Jones S.N., Grompe M., Munir M.I., Veres G., Craigen W.J., Caskey C.T., 1990, Ectopic correction of ornithine transcarbamylase deficiency in sparse fur mice, J. Biol. Chem., **265**:14684–14690.

32. Carvard C., Grimber G., Dubois N., Chasse J.F., Bennoun M., Minet T.M., Kamoun P., Briand P., 1988, Correction of mouse ornithine transcarbamylase deficiency by gene transfer into the germ line, Nucl. Acids. Res., **16**:2099–2110.

33. Grompe M., Jones S.N., Loulseged H., Caskey C.T., 1992, Retroviral–mediated gene transfer of human ornithine transcarbamylase into primary hepatocytes of spf and spf–ash mice, Hum. Gene Ther., **3**:35–44.

34. Takebe Y., Seiki M., J.–I. F., P. H., Yokota K., Arai K.–I., Yoshida M., Arai M., SRα promoter: an efficient and versatile mammalian cDNA expression system composed of the simian virus 40 early promoter and the R–US segment of human T–cell leukemia virus type–1 long terminal repeat, Mol. Cell. Biol., **8**:466–472.

35. Morsy M.A., Alford E.L., Bett A., Graham F.L., Caskey C.T., 1993, Efficient adenoviral–mediated OTC expression in deficient mouse and human hepatocytes, J. Clin. Invest., **92**:1580–1586.

36. MacGregor, G. R. and Caskey, C. T., 1989, Construction of plasmids that express E. coli β–galactosidase in mammalian cells, Nucl. Acids. Res., **17**:2365.

37. Quershi, I. A., Letarte, J., Ouellet, R., 1979, Ornithine transcarbamylase deficiency in mutant mice: Studies on the charecterization of enzyme defect and suitability as animal models of human disease, Pediatr. Res., **13**:807–811.

Retroviral Gene Transfer for LDL Receptor Deficiency into Primary Hepatocytes

Jean-Christophe Pages[‡], Marion Andreoletti[‡], Myriam Bennoun[‡], Dominique Franco[§], Pascale Briand[‡], and Anne Weber[‡]

Although the pharmacological approach has proven its efficacy for most diseases there are still situations where praticians remain helpless. Among these, genetic diseases are the more difficult to deal with as correction of the defect requires the precise targeting of a protein. As far as the liver is concerned, genetic lesions may affect two kinds of products, excreted proteins and cellular proteins. Whereas the latter need to be produced in the affected cell the former could be delivered by subcutaneous injection or produced by a nonphysiological organ easier to target (myoblast, fibroblast ..). Gene therapy is the most attractive therapy as it restores function in a stable manner by introducing alongsides the dysfunctional gene its wildtype counterpart (1). In recent years, systems have been developed for gene transfer. Of particular interest are recombinant viruses among which retroviruses and adenoviruses are the more widely used.

Retroviruses are diploid RNA viruses widespread in vertebrates. Studies on their cycle have permitted the definition of both structural and biological structures indispensable for their replication. Although of variable complexity their genomes share common features. (Fig. 1). The main characteristics of these particles are: a viral genome resembling eukaryotic mRNA; a reverse transcription step providing double stranded DNA; a stable and random integration of the viral DNA genome into the host chromosome which is thus transmitted as a regular locus during mitosis (2). In the 80's it appeared possible to use retroviruses as vectors for expression of foreign genes in infected cells (3). To avoid the spread of such recombinant vectors, viruses were rendered defective for replication. Thus production of recombinant particles implies a transcomplementation for viral functions. This was achieved by transfection of NIH 3T3 with viral structural genes leading to stable encapsidation cell lines. (Fig. 2). After transfection of this producing cell line with a recombinant provirus, a selection allows the isolation of a high titer-producing clone. The supernatant of this producer which contains the recombinant particles is used for cell infection. The tropism of these therapeutic viruses is directed by the envelope glycoprotein of the particle, the amphotropic envelope being used for human targeting. Since the first experiments performed, both encapsidation cell lines and backbone structure of the retrovirus vectors have evolved. The main modifications concern the production of helper free recombinant retrovirus with cell

[‡] ICGM, INSERM U380, 22 rue Méchain, 75014 Paris, FRANCE
[§] Hôpital A. Beclère, Service de Chirurgie, 157 rue de la Porte de Trivaux, 92141 Clamart, FRANCE

Hepatic Encephalopathy, Hyperammonemia, and Ammonia Toxicity
Edited by V. Felipo and S. Grisolia, Plenum Press, New York, 1994

155

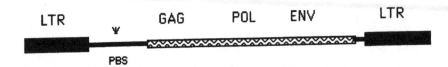

Structural genes

Figure 1. Normal structure of a wildtype simple retrovirus. Bold lines and black rectangles are cis–acting sequences indispensable for viral encapsidation and replication. These structures are: the LTR which contains the enhancer and promoter driving the transcription of the viral genomic RNA; the primer binding site (PBS) for the initiation of reverse transcription by the tRNA; the Y region which is necessary for encapsidation of the viral RNA. These sequences are conserved in vectors. Wavy lines rectangle contains genes for structural viral proteins: GAG: matrix, nucleocapsid and capsid; POL: reverse transcriptase and integrase; ENV: viral envelope. These functions can be provided in trans.

lines containing structural viral genes at different loci (4). This modification together with suppression of the encapsidation signal increases the number of recombination events necessary for the production of infectious retrovirus. Improvement of the viral titer has been obtained with vectors that harbor an extended and mutated GAG region to achieve high encapsidation rate. Another frequent modification is the enhancer deletion in the 3' LTR which leads to transcriptionally inactive LTRs in infected cells. This modification is useful for expression from an internal promoter and to avoid insertional activation after integration. Concerning safety of retroviral vectors the occurence of insertional mutation is statistically very low when compared with that potentially induced by endogenous mobile retroelements.

Adenoviruses are double stranded DNA viruses responsible for acute respiratory diseases. The cycle of these viruses exhibit two phases. Knowledge of the genomic structure and the pattern of expression have permitted the design of adenoviral vectors (5). In these vectors the gene of interest is inserted in a deletion of the E 1 region which codes for proteins

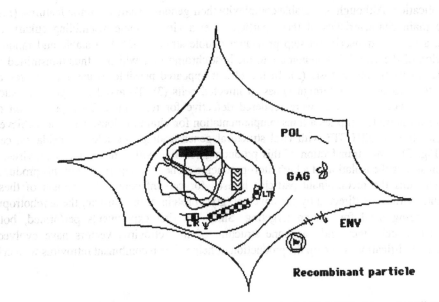

Figure 2. Encapsidation cell line. Black rectangle represents the GAG–POL cistron; wavy lines rectangle the Env gene; mosaic rectangle stands for recombinant viral genome.

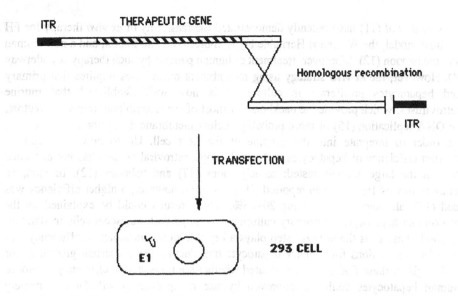

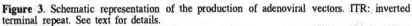

Figure 3. Schematic representation of the production of adenoviral vectors. ITR: inverted terminal repeat. See text for details.

responsible for the regulation of transcription of the viral genome. The production of the recombinant vector is obtained after cotransfection of linearised plasmids, the first containing the gene of interest and part of the adenovirus sequence, and the second composed of adenoviral overlapping DNA sequences with the rest of the viral genome in a permissive cell. *In vivo* homologous recombination between overlapping sequences results in the formation of stable viruses which are amplified in the 293 cells that constitutively produce E1 proteins (Fig. 3). Adenoviruses are of interest as they provide vectors at high titer with a wide range of infectivity. As they do not integrate into the genome of infected cells they are attractive for gene transfer into quiescent cells (neurons). *In vivo* injection of adenovirus vectors has proven its efficacy for liver gene transfer in different models: LDL receptor deficiency (6) and OTC deficiency (7) which is treated in a chapter of this issue.

To study the feasibility of retrovirus–mediated gene transfer into the liver we focused on a single gene defect, familial hypercholesterolemia (FH). Familial hypercholesterolemia (8) is an autosomal dominant disorder due to a defect in the cellular receptor that binds low density lipoprotein (LDL). Homozygous FH patients suffer from premature, life–threatening coronary heart disease. Hepatocytes are the appropriate target cells for gene therapy in FH, since they are responsible for the catabolism of LDL and are the only cells capable of excreting cholesterol and bile acids into the bile.

One strategy for such hepatic therapy is represented by the transplantation of autologous cells that have been genetically modified *in vitro*. This *ex vivo* strategy involves partial hepatectomy and isolation of hepatocytes from the patient with defective gene function, retroviral transduction of the normal gene and finally transplantation of the genetically modified cells. *In vivo* retroviral gene transfer for liver diseases has also been attempted with success. The major difficulty in the *in vivo* approach using retroviruses is the low number of transduced cells mainly as a result of low viral titer (9) This raises the question of the minimal level of expression needed for a clinical correction or attenuation of a disease. Kay et al. (10) have reported that the production of 0,1% of the normal amount of factor IX results in a diminution of 40% in the whole blood clotting time. Nevertheless higher transduction efficiency should give best results, providing an expression approaching the physiological level.

Wilson *et al* (11) have recently demonstrated the feasibility of *ex vivo* therapy for FH in an animal model, the Watanabe Heritable Hypercholesterolemic Rabbit, and a non–human primate, the baboon (12). Moreover, treatment of human patients by such therapy is underway (13,14). However, the *ex vivo* strategy using recombinant retroviruses requires that primary cultured hepatocytes proliferate in culture. It is now well established that murine oncoretroviruses, which provide the backbone for most of the recombinant retroviral vectors, require DNA replication (15) or more probably nuclear membrane disruption during mitosis (16) in order to integrate into the genome of the host cell. Up to now, the reported transduction efficiency of hepatocytes with amphotropic retroviral vectors has not exceeded 20–25% in the large animals tested; namely, dogs (17) and baboons (12). In man, an efficiency as low as 1% has been reported (18); recently, however, a higher efficiency was obtained (13), although not exceeding 20–25%. These results could be explained by the observation that hepatocytes in primary culture are, in large part, quiescent cells in standard culture conditions. Thus the *in vitro* step plays a key role in the transduction efficiency. All current culture conditions for primary hepatocyte transduction use epidermal growth factor (EGF). In light of these findings, we evaluated whether the transduction efficiency of mouse and human hepatocytes could be improved by use of specific growth factors, namely hepatocyte growth factor (HGF). We also ensured that culture conditions which would lead to an increase in the transduction efficiency of the isolated hepatocytes would not affect their differentiation status. For this purpose, we employed a β–galactosidase–expressing retroviral vector for the infection of primary hepatocytes. In order to achieve a high level of expression of the transferred gene, we have designed a new retroviral vector incorporating the human LDL receptor under the transcriptional control of the L–type pyruvate kinase promoter which is liver–specific. The choice of the internal promoter driving the therapeutic gene is very important as it has been shown that a promoter which is functional *in vitro* can lose its property *in vivo*; this feature is more particularly observed with viral promoters (19,20). Among the growth factors tested, hepatocyte growth factor (HGF) proved to be the most potent for efficient transduction. With this factor we obtained 80% and 40% of mouse and human primary hepatocytes infected, respectively. Furthermore, using these conditions with the LDL–R vector we obtained an elevated expression of the recombinant gene(results submitted for publication).

In the future the knowledge of mechanisms underlying the infectivity of lentiviruses in quiescent cells will help in the construction of new retroviral vectors. Another important goal is the design of tissue specific vectors which can be obtained by modifying the retroviral envelope.

Acknowledgement: We are grateful to Jennifer Richardson for critical review of the manuscript.

References

1. Mulligan, R. C. 1993. The basic science of gene therapy. *Science.* **260:**926–932.
2. Coffin J. M. Retroviridae and their replication. In: Fields B, Knipe D, Chanock R, eds. *Virology*, 2nd New York: Raven Press, 1990; 1437–500.
3. Cepko, L. C., Roberts, B. E. and Mulligan, R. C. 1984: construction and application of a highly transmissible murine retrovirus shuttle vector. *Cell* **37:**1053–1062.
4. Danos, O. and Mulligan, R. C. 1988. Safe and efficient generation of recombinant retrovirus with amphotropic and ecotropic host ranges. *Proc. Natl. Acad. Sci. USA.* **85:**6460–6464.
5. Berkner, K. L. 1988 Development of adenovirus vectors for the expression of heterologous genes. *Bio/Techniques* **6:**n°7; 616–629.

6. Ishibashi, S., Brown, M. S., Goldstein, J., Gerard, R. D. Hammer, R. and Herz, J. 1993. Hypercholesterolemia in low density lipoprotein receptor knock out mice and its reversal by adenovirus–mediated gene delivery. *J. Clin. Invest.* **92**:883–893.

7. Straford–Perricaudet, L. D., Levrero, M., Chasse, J. F., Perricaudet, M. and Briand, P. 1990; Evaluation of the transfer and expression in mice of an enzyme–encoding gene using a human adenovirus vector. *Hum. Gene Ther.* **1**:241–256.

8. Brown, M. S. and Goldstein, J. L. 1986. A receptor–mediated pathway for cholesterol homeostasis. *Science.* **232**:34–47.

9. Ferry, N., Duplessis, O., Houssin, D., Danos, O. and Heard, J. M. 1991. Retroviral–mediated gene transfer into hepatocytes in vivo. *Proc.   Natl. Acad. Sci. USA.* **88**:8377–8381.

10. Kay, M. A., Rothenberg, S., Landen, C. N. et *al*; 1993: *In vivo* gene therapy of hemophilia B: sustained partial correction in factor IX– deficient dogs. *Science* **262**:117–119.

11. Wilson, J. M., Johnston, D. E., Jefferson, D. M. and Mulligan, R. C. 1988. Correction of the genetic defect in hepatocytes from the watanabe heritable hyperlipidemic rabbit. *Proc. Natl. Acad. Sci. USA.* **85**:4421–4425.

12. Grossman, M., Raper, S. and Wilson, J. M. 1992. Transplantation of genetically modified autologous hepatocytes in nonhuman primates: feasability and short–term toxicity. *Hum. Gene Ther.* **3**:501–510.

13. Grossman, M., Raper, S. E. and Wilson, J. M. 1991. Towards liver–directed gene therapy: retrovirus–mediated gene transfer into human hepatocytes. *Som. Cell and Mol. Genet.* **17**:601–607.

14. Wilson, J. M. 1992. *Ex vivo* gene therapy of familial hypercholesterolemia. *Hum. Gene Ther.* **3**: 179–222.

15. Miller, D. G., Adam, M. A. and Miller, A. D. 1990. Gene transfer by retrovirus vectors occurs only in cells that are actively replicating at the time of infection. *Mol. Cell Biol.* **10**:4239–4242.

16. Roe, T. Y., Reynolds, T. C., Yu, G. and Brown, P. O. 1993. Integration of murine leukemia virus DNA depends on mitosis. *EMBO J.* **12**:2099–2108.

17. Kay, M. A., Baley, P., Rothenberg, S., Leland, F., Flemin, F., Ponder, K. P., Liu, T. J., Finegold, M., Darlington, G., Pokorny, W. and Woo, S. L. C. 1992. Expression of human alpha–1–antitrypsin in dogs after autologous transplantation of retroviral transduced hepatocytes. *Proc. Natl. Acad. Sci. USA.* **89**:89–92.

18. Adams, R. M., Soriano, H. E., Wang, M., Darlington, G., Steffen, D. and Ledley, F. D. 1992. Transduction of primary human hepatocytes with amphotropic and xenotropic retroviral vectors. *Proc. Natl.   Acad. Sci. USA.* **89**:8981–8985.

19. Dai, Y., Roman, M., Naviaux, R. K. and Verma, I. M. 1993. Gene therapy via primary myoblasts: long–term expression of factor IX protein following transplantation in vivo. *Proc. Natl. Acad. Sci. USA.* **89**:10892–10895.

20. Scharfmann, R., Axelrod, J. and Verma, I. M. 1991. Long–term *in vivo* expression of retrovirus–mediated gene transfer in mouse fibroblast implants. *Proc. Natl. Acad. Sci. USA.* **88**:4626–4630.

The "Carnitine System": Recent Aspects

Noris Siliprandi *, R. Venerando ** and V. Tassani *

Carnitine is one of the most widely occurring constituents of biological systems in living beings (1,2): "a vitamin for an insect, vital for men" (2). Carnitine is the factor necessary for the transport of fatty acids into the mitochondria where they are completely oxidized to CO_2 and H_2O with energy production. In all its functions carnitine operates in tandem with coenzyme A, so as creatine does with ATP: "CoA regulator". Indeed under a variety of conditions, e. g. in hypoxia, carnitine is necessary for the maintenance of the minimum requirement of free CoA.

1. Biosynthesis

ε-N-trimethyllysine (TML) is the common precursor of carnitine both in microorganisms and in mammals. However while microorganisms (e.g. *Neurospora crassa*) obtain TML by methylation of free lysine (catalyzed by methylase I), mammals derive TML destined for carnitine synthesis by methylation of proteic lysine (as catalyzed by methylase III) (3). After liberation by proteolytic digestion, TML is converted to carnitine in a process consisting of 4 reactions (Fig 1).

In mammals all tissues are capable of transforming TML into deoxycarnitine, the immediate precursor of carnitine, but only liver, brain and, in humans, kidneys are also capable of hydroxylating deoxycarnitine into carnitine (4).

It has been estimated that the amount of carnitine synthesized in 24 hours by a rat is around 20 µmoles/Kg (5) and from 3 to 28 µmoles/Kg by dogs (6). According to Rebouche (7) the TML released from methylated proteins is sufficient to support carnitine biosynthesis.

The largest amount of proteic TML is present in muscle (3). This lends weight to the idea that, although a part of TML is metabolized by muscles themselves, some is also taken up by kidneys and converted into carnitine. Evidence for this is that in man at least, kidneys have considerable β-hydroxylase activity, much higher than that found in other tissues and also a high capacity to take up TML from the blood (7). Which proteins are the source of TML is still ignored, but a possible candidate could be the adenylate translocase which contains one residue of TML. Due to its great abundance it could contribute to the TML level, hence to the control of carnitine formation. The mechanism(s) underlying the regulation of carnitine biosynthesis is poorly understood. Nevertheless two factors must regulate the disposition of TML released from proteic digestion either into the pathway of carnitine biosynthesis or the excretion by kidney (8). The first control is the entry of the amino acid into mitochondria where it is hydroxylated (9). Even if no study has been reported on TML transport in mitochondria, the entry of TML into these organelles may represent a significant rate limiting obstacle. The second control is represented by the affinity of the hydroxylase for

* Dept. Chimica Biologica, Università di Padova
** Sigma Tau Ind. Farm. Riun, Research and Developement, Pomezia, Roma

Hepatic Encephalopathy, Hyperammonemia, and Ammonia Toxicity
Edited by V. Felipo and S. Grisolia, Plenum Press, New York, 1994

161

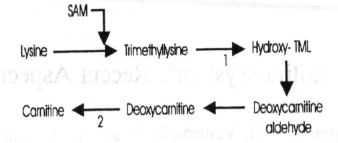

Figure 1. Schematic pathway of carnitine biosynthesis. 1 and 2 indicate the two hydroxylation steps requiring, in addition to the specific hydroxylases, α–ketoglutarate, ascorbate and Fe^{2+}. SAM = S–adenosylmethionine.

TML. According to Melegh et al (8), the enzyme is probably not saturated under most conditions and fluctuations in substrate concentration should be reflected in changes in the rate of β–hydroxy–ε–N–trimethyllysine formation. Availability of increased substrate, by oral administration of TML, significantly increased the rate of carnitine synthesis in both rats (10) and humans (11). This suggests that the capacity both to transport TML into mitochondria and to hydroxylate this substance is not fully used under normal conditions. This implies that only a severe deficiency of lysine, associated with a very poor carnitine introduction, as it occurs in conditions of malnutrition, may significantly affect carnitine biosynthesis. The reason why, unlike microorganisms, mammals can obtain TML only from protein lysine belongs to the field of teleology. It is tempting to speculate that the proteins in which lysine residues become susceptible of methylation by methylases III are aged proteins near to death, or in excess in respect to the cellular demand. It seems otherwise paradoxical that the synthesis of carnitine might imply the proteolytic breakdown of physiological active proteins.

2. Transport

The concentration of carnitine in tissues is generally related to their capacity to oxidize fatty acids (e.g. skeletal and cardiac muscles, 16). It appears paradoxical therefore that the tissues richest in carnitine are unable to synthesize it and must take it up from blood. Since the concentration in blood is considerably lower, active transport might be thought to occur. We have recently provided evidence that the transport of carnitine, its esters and analogues, across the sarcolemma may occur in an exchange–diffusion process in which the extracellular carnitine pool exchanges with the intracellular one (13). Most significant is the exchange between deoxycarnitine, synthesized by muscle, and carnitine. This exchange may occur bidirectionally in a ratio close to 1:1, but at a higher rate when deoxycarnitine is the internal partner, thus reflecting the physiological condition whereby muscles export deoxycarnitine and import carnitine. Such an exchange seems to be also occurring "in vivo" as shown by the observation that carnitine administration to rats induces a transient but significant depletion of deoxycarnitine in tissues, whereas administration of equivalent amounts of deoxycarnitine induces an analogous depletion in carnitine (13). This may be relevant to our understanding of the primary carnitine deficiencies and particularly the myopathic form. This latter syndrome could be due either to an alteration of the sarcolemma carrier responsible for the exchange or to an insufficient synthesis of deoxycarnitine in muscles.

3. Functions

The fundamental function of carnitine is the transport of long-chain and short-chain acyls (the activated forms of fatty acids) across the mitochondrial membrane. The transport of the former requires the preliminary activity of CPT (Carnitine Palmitoyl Transferase), that of the latter the activity of CAT (Carnitine Acetyl Transferase) (14). Both the transferases catalyze the reversible transfer of long- and respectively short-chain acyls from CoA to carnitine. The transport of the neoformed acyl carnitines is mediated by Carnitine Translocase (15) which catalyzes the exchange between intra- and extra- mitochondrial carnitines. Under physiological conditions the system CPT dependent transports the long-chain acyls into the mitochondria where they are oxidized in the β-oxidation process with energy production: energetic function. In the CAT dependent transport short-chain acyls are exported from mitochondria thus buffering the Acyl CoA/CoA ratio: buffer function. In humans the importance of the energic function of carnitine clearly emerges in the "primary carnitine deficiency" characterized by muscular weakness, caused by the inhibited transport of fatty acids to the intramitochondrial β-oxidation process, and muscular steatosis, consequent to the accumulation of fatty acids in the extramitochondrial compartment. Accumulation of long-chain acyl CoA has per se deleterious effects on the integrity of mitochondrial membrane; moreover when long-chain acyl CoA accumulation is associated with an increase of Ca^{2+} concentration the so-called "permeability transition" (16) does occur. This consists of the opening of pores through which solutes (ions and small proteins) pass outward and inward inducing a collapse of electrochemical gradients and a large amplitude swelling. The pores may be resealed by the action of either Mg^{2+} or the immunosuppressant cyclosporin A (17). Also free carnitine by converting acyl CoA into the undamaging acyl carnitines has analogous preventive and restorative action (17). The synergistic action of long-chain acyl CoA and Ca^{2+} may help to elucidate the mechanism of cellular damage induced by anoxia, during which both these substances increase in concentration (18).

The other important function of carnitine is the export of short-chain acyls from mitochondria. This process is seen in mitochondria of tissues endowed with short-chain CoA: carnitine acyl transferase (CAT) (19) and has the function of exporting acetyl-propionyl- and branched-chain acyls (20). When free carnitine is (largely) available, the preexisting short-chain acyl CoA's are transformed into the corresponding acyl carnitines and the free CoA concurently formed may further generate acyl carnitines readily diffusable in blood and urines. The export of branched-chain acyls from mitochondria in form of acyl-carnitines is not only relevant for the catabolism of leucine, isoleucine and valine in muscles but also for the preservation of normal mitochondrial metabolism (21).

The removal of short-chain acyls from mitochondria by the "carnitine-CAT" system has another relevant implication in conditions, e.g. maximal exercise, leading to lactate accumulation (22). Owing to the limited oxygen supply one of the end products of pyruvate dehydrogenase, acetyl CoA, accumulates in mitrochondria, progressively inhibiting the activity of this key enzyme. Free carnitine takes over the acetyl moiety by forming acetyl-carnitine, readily diffusable into the blood, thus maintaining the tissue level of free CoA compatible with a minimal degree of pyruvate dehydrogenase activity. This explains the concurrent decrease of lactate and increase of acetyl-carnitine in blood (22). In this regard it is important to stress that the wash-out of the acetyls by carnitine may occur independently of any increase of carnitine in the tissue. The point at issue is that carnitine transport across both mitochondrial membrane (15) and muscle sarcolemma (13) occurs, as mentioned above, chiefly (or exclusively) by a 1:1 exchange with a carnitine ester. A priori the rate of this process, implying an increase of esterified/free carnitine ratio could increase without any change in muscle total carnitine content. The exchange is instead expressed by the increase of acetyl-carnitine both in plasma and urine (22). Another pertinent observation is the finding that carnitine, given orally to patients with isovaleric aciduria, rapidly induced a large increase in plasma and urine isovaleryl-carnitine (23). We would also attribute this to an increased rate of exchange of external carnitine with endogenous isovaleryl–carnitine formed from the excess of isovaleryl CoA.

References

1. Frenkel, R.A. and McGarry, J.D., 1980, Carnitine biosynthesis, metabolism and functions, Academic Press Publ., New York, London.
2. Pande, S. and Murtny, M.S.R., 1989, Carnitine: vitamin for an insect, vital for man, Biochem Cell. Biol., 67:671–673.
3. Paik, W.K. and Kim, S., 1975, Protein methylation: chemical enzymological and biological significance, Adv. Enzymol., 42:227–228.
4. Rebouche, C.J. and Engel, A.G., 1980, Tissue distribution of carnitine biosynthetic enzyme in man, Biochim. Biophys. Acta 630:22–29.
5. Cederblad, G. and Lindstet, S., 1976, Metabolism of labeled carnitine in rat, Arch. Biochem. Biophys. 175:173–180.
6. Rebouche, C.J. and Engel, A.G., 1983, Kinetic compartmental analysis of carnitine metabolism in the dog, Arch. Biochem. Biophys. 220:60–70.
7. Rebouche, C.J., 1982, Sites of regulation of carnitine biosynthesis in mammals, Fed. Proc. 41:2848–2852.
8. Melegh, B., Pap, M., Bock, I., and Rebouche, C.J., 1993, Relationship of carnitine and carnitine precursors lysine, ε–trimethyllysine and γ–butyrobetaine in drug–induced carnitine depletion, Pediatric Research 34:460–464.
9. Hulse, J.D., Ellis, S.R., and Handerson, L.M., 1978, Carnitine biosynthesis, hydroxylation of trimethyllysine by an α–ketoglutarate dependent mitochondrial dioxygenase, J. Biol. Chem. 253:1654–1659.
10. Rebouche, C.J., Lehman, L.J., and Olson, A.L., 1986, ε–N–trimethyllysine availability regulates the rate of carnitine biosynthesis in the growing rats, J. Nutr. 116:751–759.
11. Rebouche, C.J., Bosch, E.P., Chenard, C.A., Schabold, K.J., and Nelson, S.E., 1989, utilization of dietary precursors for carnitine synthesis in human adults, J. Nutr. 19:1907–1913.
12. Bohmer, T. and Mølstad, P., 1980, Carnitine transport across the plasma membrane, in: "Carnitine biosynthesis, metabolism and function", Frenkel, R.A. and McGarry, J.D., Eds., Academic Press, New York, pp. 73–89.
13. Siliprandi, N., Sartorelli, L., Ciman, M., and Di Lisa, F., 1989, Carnitine: metabolism and clinical chemistry, Clinica Chimica Acta 183:3–12.
14. Bieber, L.L., 1988, Carnitine, Ann. Rev. Biochemistry 57:261–283.
15. Pande, S.V., Parvin, R., 1980, Carnitine–acylcarnitine translocase catalyzes an equilibrating unidirectional transport, J. Biol. Chem. 255:2994–3001.
16. Gunter, T.E. and Pfeiffer, D.R., 1990, Mechanism by which mitochondria transport calcium, Am. J. Physiol. 258:C755–C786.
17. Silliprandi, D., Biban, C., Testa, S., Toninello, A., and Siliprandi. N., 1992, Effects of Palmitoyl CoA and palmitoylcarnitine on the membrane potential and Mg^{2+} content of the rat heart mitochondria, Molec. and Cell. Biochem. 116:117–123.
18. Neely, J.R., Garber, D., McDonough, K., and Idell Wenger, J., 1979, Ischemic myocardial and antianginal drugs, Winburg and Abiskoy, Eds., Raven Press, New York, pp. 25–234.
19. Ferri, L., Valente, M., Ursini, F., Gregolin, C., and Siliprandi, N., 1981, Acetyl–carnitine formation and pyruvate oxidation in mitochondria from different rat tissues, Bull. Mol. Biol. Med. 6:16–23.
20. Lysiak, W., Toth, P.P., Svelter, C.H., and Bieber, L.L., 1986, Quantitation of the efflux of acylcarnitine from rat heart, brain and liver mitochondria, J. Biol. Chem. 261: 13698–13703.
21. Waiajtys–Rode and Williamson, J.R., 1980, Effects of branched chain α–ketoacids on the metabolism of isolated rat liver cells III. Interaction with pyruvate dehydrogenase. J. Biol. Chem. 255:413–418.
22. Siliprandi, N., Di Lisa, F., Pieralisi, G., Ripari, P., Maccari, F., Menabò, R., Giamberardino, M.A., Vecchiet, L., 1990, Metabolic changes induced by maximal exercise in human subjects following L–carnitine administration, Biochim. Biophys. Acta 1034:17–21.
23. De Sousa, C., Chalmers, R.A., Stacey, T.E., Tracey, B.N., Weaver, C.H., and Bradley, D., 1986, The response to L–carnitine and glycine therapy in isovaleric acidemia, Eur. J. Pediatr. 144:451–465.

Use of Hepatocyte Cultures for Liver Support Bioreactors

Jörg C. Gerlach

Chirurgische Klinik, Universitätsklinikum Rudolf Virchow, Freie Universität Berlin.

Summary

Hybrid artificial liver systems are being developed as extracorporeal temporary liver support therapy. Here, an overview is given with emphasis on hepatocyte culture models for bioreactors, in vitro studies, animal studies and the clinical application of hybrid liver support systems. In vitro studies show long term external metabolic functions of primary isolated hepatocytes in bioreactors. These systems are capable of supporting essential liver functions. Animal experiments show the possibility of upscaling the bioreactors for clinical treatment. Since there is no reliable animal model for investigations on the treatment of acute liver failure, the promising results of these studies have limited relevance. The small number of clinical studies are not sufficient to give statements about a clinical improvement of therapy of acute liver failure. Although important progress has been made in the development of the systems, multiple different hepatocyte culture models and bioreactor constructions are discussed in the literature, indicating competition in this field of medical research.

Keywords: Hepatocyte Culture Models, Bioreactors, Cell Perfusion Systems, Hybrid Liver Support Systems

1. Introduction

Despite improvements in intensive care therapy, the mortality of acute fulminant liver failure (1) still remains around 80% (2,3,4). Therefore, liver transplantation is the primarily chosen therapy. In addition to transplantation, three fields of therapy were investigated in the past. Extracorporeal methods as the hemoperfusion were investigated for an artificial suport. As a biological aid, auxiliary perfusion with animal livers were investigated. So called hybrid systems are currently in development.

The aim of the present article is to give an overview of the development of hybrid liver support bioreactors for a temporary extracorporeal liver assistance.

Hybrid systems combine biologically active cell cultures with artificial devices. In hybrid liver support systems (LSS) hepatocytes are cultivated in bioreactors. These reactors enable an extracorporeal use of detoxification, metabolism, synthesis and regulation of these cell performances.

Chirurgische Klinik, Universitätsklinikum Rudolf Virchow, Freie Universität Berlin. Address: Dr. med. J. Gerlach, Forschungshaus Experimentelle Chirurgie, Chirurgische Klinik, Universitätsklinikum Rudolf Virchow, Spandauer Damm 130, D–14050 Berlin 19

Hepatic Encephalopathy, Hyperammonemia, and Ammonia Toxicity
Edited by V. Felipo and S. Grisolia, Plenum Press, New York, 1994

The main interest for extracorporeal liver assistance would be liver transplantation, where such systems might act as a bridge for temporary extracorporeal support. Since fulminant liver failure is potentially reversible (5), extracorporeal bridging of liver function would also be beneficial until the patient's own liver resumes functional activity.

2. Isolation of Primary Hepatocytes

In principle, the use of hepatoma cells (6,7) would be of interest. However, since problems of dedifferenciation and possible metastasis are not yet solved, we focus, in the following text, on primary isolated hepatocytes from a donor liver.

Isolation of hepatocytes from the parenchyma of the liver started half a century ago with mechanical methods but failed with respect to viability of the isolated cells. The methods of enzymatic collagenase perfusion introduced by Howard & Pesch et al.(8), sophisticated by Berry & Friend (9,10) and Seglen (11,12), are today the standard method of choice. However, chemical methods using citrate, EDTA or EGTA which are more economical, are still in discussion.

To enable a mass hepatocyte culture, we investigated the cell isolation from larger organs (13), in order to develop a method for pig livers (14) and for human livers (15). Since the co-cultivation of hepatocytes with endothelial cells appears beneficial, we developed a combined cell isolation method which provides also sinusoidal endothelial cells from the organ (16).

3. Hepatocyte Culture

Freshly isolated parenchymal liver cells, the hepatocytes, retain many of the metabolic characteristics of the tissue in vivo. As isolated cells, they are generally in a catabolic stage and therefore care is essential in fully maintaining their activity.

Basic investigations on improvement of the external in-vitro functions of hepatocytes mainly dealt with cell adhesion substrates (17, 18,19,20,21), co-culture (22,23), culture media formulations (24) and growth factors (25), whereas the standard culture technique on flat culture substrates was mostly retained.

A limiting problem in the development of LSS systems is that hepatocytes cultivated in-vitro lose their external functions with time. As a consequence, different culture models were introduced. The use of appropriate cell adhesion techniques, using artificial substrates as membranes, microcarriers (26) or biological matrix as connective tissue preparations (27,28,29) have been studied.

Bioreactors enable an upscaling of culture models to a larger scale. Knazek (30,31) introduced in 1972 a first construction for cell culture which utilizes capillary membranes. Using the discussed culture models, different bioreactors were constructed. They are based on microcarrier beads (32), membranes (33), gel sandwiches (34,35) or utilize spheroids (36).

If a culture model could enable a free three-dimensional cell rearrangement of the microenvironment of hepatocytes by hepatocyte self aggregation (37), the reconstruction of junctional complexes, re-localisation of the cytoskeleton and the re-orientation of the cell organelles in-vitro (38) may be more beneficial to the cells. In the development of culture models for hepatocyte culture, various aspects of the physiological macroenvironment of the hepatocytes must be taken into account. In the majority of bioreactors developed, metabolite exchange is performed by diffusion with large gradients of gas, nutrients, toxins and cell products, while the hepatocytes in-vivo function under perfusion conditions. The local organisation and orientation of hepatocytes, as found in the three dimensional liver lobulus, are impossible in standard culture techniques; and vectorial metabolite transfer is therefore disturbed.

4. Animal Experiments

The use of bioreactors in hybrid LSS was investigated in different animal models, i.e acetaminophen (39) –or galactosamin– intoxification (40) or surgical models. These experiments were performed on pigs (41), dogs (42), or rats (43,44). The studies showed that hybrid systems can be scaled up for a clinical use. Typical biochemical performances of the liver were demonstrated in all models and acute immunological reactions were not described. In our own studies, TNF–alpha liberation was found to be moderate (45).

Since there is no reliable animal model available, animal studies have limited relevance for giving information about the treatment of hepatic encephalopathy.

5. Hybrid Liver Support in Human Application

The first application of bioreactors in hybrid LSS was demonstrated by Matsumura et al.(46) in 1987. Metabolic encephalopathy due to a bile duct occlusion was improved. In a controlled clinical study (47,48) survival rate of hepatic failure was improved by using hepatocytes in a cell suspension technique. Further successful application of LSS was demonstrated recently by Demetriou et. al (49) and Sussmann et al. (50). It seems to be too early to give statements about clinical applications of LSS, because the small number of applications allow no safe statistical presentation or, as with Margulis, the technique has been already discharged.

6. Own Bioreactor Construction

We have introduced a bioreactor concept (fig. 1) which can integrate known techniques of hepatocyte culture in vitro, including the use of hepatocyte adhesion supporting capillaries (51), extracellular basement membrane matrix (52), hepatocyte aggregation (53) and the use of nonparenchymal liver cells in co–culture. In addition, direct membrane contact oxygenation (54), a three dimensional orientation of cells, perfusion around the cells and low metabolite gradients were achieved. The culture model has the following characteristics:

–   Perfusion of the cells between independent capillary membrane systems.
–   Identical units for few hepatocytes in parallel, analog to the liver lobuli.
–   Decentral metabolite in– and outflow with low gradients.
–   Decentral oxygen supply and carbon dioxide removal with low gradients.
–   Cell adhesion on hepatocyte compatible membranes, coated with biomatrix and aggregation between the capillaries.
–   Co–culture compartment for sinusoidal endothelial cells.
–   Possibility for upscaling the construction to a large cell mass bioreactor for therapeutic liver support.
–   Possibility of further capillary functions, such as dialysis and heat–exchange for DMSO–freezing of the reactor with the cells.

In summary, the results of studies with a cell mass of 2.5 x10^9 hepatocytes in each reactor indicate that the culture model will enable the external metabolism to be maintained for up to five weeks. The specified construction allows long–term, sterile handling and enables scale–up to a large cell mass bioreactor for therapeutic use.

This culture model results in prolonged and enhanced activity of hepatocytes in comparison to the standard culture technique (55). This may be explained by the closer approximation to the in vivo situation of hepatocytes in our bioreactor: The capillary systems create a three dimensional artificial framework as a macroenvironment, in which the cells can

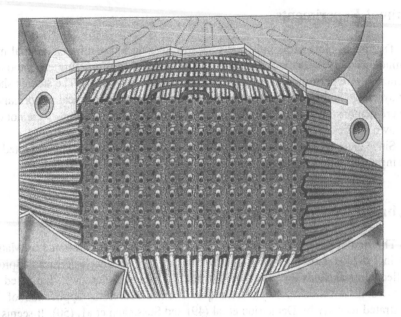

Figure 1. Culture model for hepatocytes. Capillary systems create a three dimensional artificial framework in which the cells can aggregate and reorganize tissue structures. The capillaries leave the reactor in differently arranged bundles, so that they can independently serve different functions: independent plasma inflow–outflow as well as independent oxygen supply/ carbon dioxide removal. Many identical small units are perfused with low gradients simultaneously and in parallel. Using an additional capillary system, a co–culture with sinusoidal endothelial cells is possible.

aggregate and reorganize tissue structures. Capillaries and potting material (56) were shown to be cell compatible. Additional coating by basement membrane matrix improves the microenvironment of each cell. The capillaries leave the reactor in differently arranged bundles, so that they can independently serve different functions. Therefore, the cells can be perfused and independent plasma inflow–outflow as well as independent oxygen supply/ carbon dioxide removal are thus possible. Identical units supply few hepatocytes. Analog to the liver lobuli, many identical small units are perfused with low gradients simultaneously and in parallel. Using an additional capillary system, a co–culture with sinusoidal endothelial cells is possible, thus preventing the negative side effect of the hepatocytes being overgrown.

The specific bioreactor construction allows the introduction of a further three-dimensionally woven capillary system. Therefore, further functions can be integrated e.g. decentral dialysis with low gradients or decentral heat exchange capillaries for deep freezing of the reactors with cultured cells.

Acknowledgements: I cordially thank Mrs. E. Heber, Mr. J. Encke, Mr. J. Lehnert and Ing. Mr. F. Zartnack for their technical support. In addition, I would like to thank Akzo AG, Wuppertal, FRG, for supplying membrane materials, the scientific support of Dr. J. Vienken is especially appreciated.

References

1. Trey C, Davidson LS.,1970, In: Popper H, Schaffner F (eds): Progress in liver diseases. Grune and Stratton, New York: p. 282.

2. European association for the study of the liver, 1987, Randomized trial of steroid therapy in acute liver failure. Gut **20**:20–23.

3. O'Grady JG, Gimson AES, O'Brien CJ et al., 1988, Controlled trials of charcoal hemoperfusion and prognostic factors in fulminant hepatic failure. Gastroenterology **94**:1186–1192.

4. Ring–Larsen H, Palazzo V., 1985, Renal failure in fulminant hepatic failure and terminal cirrhosis. Gut **22**:585–591.

5. Jones EA, Schaefer DF. Fulminant hepatic failure. In: Zakim D, Boyer TD, eds. Hepatology. Philadelphia: Saunders, **1990**:460–475.

6. Wolf CFW, Munkelt BE., 1975, Bilirubin conjugation by an artificial liver composed of cultured cells and synthetic capillaries. ASAIO Transactions **21**:16–27.

7. Sussman NL, Chong MG, Koussayer T, He DE, Shang TA, Hartwell H, Whisennhalld, Kelly JH, 1992, Reversal of fulminant hepatic failure using an extracorporeal liver assist device, Hepatology **16**:60–65.

8. Howard RB, Christensen AK, Gibbs FA und Pesch LA., 1967, The Enzymatic Preparation of Isolated Intact Parenchymal Cells from Rat Liver. The Journal of Cell Biology **35**:675–684.

9. Berry MN und Friend DS, 1969, High–Yield Preparation of Isolated Rat Liver Parenchymal Cells. J.Cell Biol. **43**:506–520.

10. Berry MN, 1974, High–Yield Preparation of Morphologically Intact Isolated Parenchymal Cells from Rat Liver. In "Methods in Enzymology" (S.Fleischer and L.Packer,eds.), Volume 32, pp.625–632, Academic Press, New York, 625–632.

11. Seglen PO., 1972, Preparation of Rat Liver Cells: I. Effect of calcium on enzymatic dispersion in perfused liver. Experimental Cell Research **74**:450–454.

12. Seglen PO., 1973, Preparation of Rat Liver Cells: III. Enzymatic requirements for tissue dispersion, Experimental Cell Research **82**:391–398.

13. Gerlach J, Brombacher J, Courtney JM, Neuhaus P., 1993, Nonenzymatic versus enzymatic hepatocyte isolation from pig livers for larger scale investigation of liver cell perfusion systems, Int. J. Artificial Organs. **16**:677–681.

14. Gerlach J, Klöppel K, Schön MR, Brombacher J, Courtney JM, Unger J, Neuhaus P., 1993, Comparison of pig hepatocyte isolation using intraoperative perfusion without warm iscemia and isolation of cells from abattoir organs after warm iscemia, Artificial Organs. **17**:950–953.

15. Gerlach J, Brombacher J, Klöppel K, Schnoy N, Neuhaus P., 1994, Comparison of four methods for mass hepatocyte isolation from pig and human livers, Transplantation. **57**:1318–1322.

16. Gerlach J, Grehn S, Neuhaus P., 1993, Endothelial cell kinetics after anoxia and hypothermia in preservation solutions as indicator for endothelial repair. Transpl. Proc. **25/11**:1593–1594.

17. Gjessing R, Seglen PO, 1980, Adsorption, simple binding and complex binding of rat hepatocytes to various in vitro substrata, Exp. Cell Res. **129**:239–240.

18. Rubin K, Golderg A, Höök M, Öbrink B., 1978, Adhesion of rat hepatocytes to collagen, Exp. Cell Res. **117**:127–135.

19. Roijkind M, Gatmaitan Z, Mackensen S, Giambrone MA, Ponce P, Reid LM., 1980, Connective tissue Biomatrix: Its isolation and utilisation for long term cultures of normal rat hepatocytes, J Cell Biol **87**:225–263.

20. Enat R, Jefferson DM, Ruiz–Opazo N, Gatmaitan Z, Leinwand LA, Reid L., 1984, Hepatocyte proliferation in vitro: its dependence on the use of hormonally defined medium and substrata of extracellular matrix, Proc Natl Acad Sci USA, **81**:1411–1415.

21. Bissel DM, Arenson DM, Maher JJ , Roll FJ., 1987, Support of cultured hepatocytes by a laminin-rich gel. Evidence for a functionally significant subendothelial matrix in normal rat liver, J Clin Invest **79**:801–812.

22. Guguen–Guillouzo C, Clement B, Baffet G, Beaumont C, Morel–Chaney E, Glaise D, Guillouzo A., 1983, Maintenance and reversibility of active albumin secretion by adult rat hepatocytes co-cultured with another liver specific cell type, Exp Cell Res. **143**:47–54.

23. Clement B, Gugen–Guillouzo C, Campion JP., 1984, Long term co–cultures of adult human hepatocytes with rat liver epithelial cells: Modulation of albumin secretion and accumulation of extracellular meterial, Hepatology **4**:373–380.

24. Leffert HL. Koch KS., 1982, Hepatocyte growth regulation by hormones in chemically defined media: A two signal hypothesis. In: Sato GH, Sirbasku AA, eds. Growth of cells in hormonally defined media. Cold Spring Harbour NY, Cold Spring Laboratory: 597–613.

25. Koch KS, Lu X, Brenner DA., 1990, Mitogens and hepatocyte growth control in vivo and in vitro. In Vitro Cell Dev Biol **26:**1011–1022.

26. Shnyra A, Bocharow A, Bochkova N, Spirov V., 1991, Bioartificial liver using hepatocytes on biosilon microcarriers: treatment of chemically induced acute hepatic failure in rats, Artif. Org. **15:**189–197.

27. Yanagi K, Ookawa K, Mizuno S, Ohshima N., 1989, Performance of a new hybrid artificial liver support system using hepatocytes entrapped within a hydrogel. ASAIO Transactions **35:**570–572.

28. Dunn JCY, Yarmush ML, Koebe HG, Tompkins RG., 1989, Hepatocyte function and extracellular matrix geometry: long–term culture in a sandwich configuration. FASEB **3:**174–177.

29. Nyberg SL, Shatford RA, Peshwa MV, White JG, Cerra FB, Hu WS.,1993, Evaluation of a hepatocyte entrapment hollow fiber bioreactor: a potential artificial liver. Biot. Bioeng. **4:**194–203.

30. Knazek, RA, PM. Gullino, PO. Kohler, RL. Dedrick, 1972, Science **178:**65–67.

31. Knazek, R. A., P. O. Kohler, P. M. Gullino., 1979, Exp. Cell Res. **84:**251–254.

32. Rozga J, Williams F, Ro MS, Neuzil DF, Giorgio TD, Backfisch G, Moscioni AD, Hakim R, Demetriou AA., 1993, Development of a bioartificial liver: Properties and function of a hollow–fiber module inoculated with liver cells, Hepatology **17:**258–265

33. Jauregiou HO, Naik S, Solomon BA, Duffy RL, Lipski M, Galetti PM., 1983, Attachment of adult rat hepatocytes to modified Amicon XM–50 membranes. ASAIO Transactions **19:**698–702.

34. Shatford RA, Nyberg SL, Payne WD, Hu WS, Cerra FB.,1991, A hepatocyte bioreactor as a potential bioartificial liver: Demonstration of prolonged tissue–specific functions. In: Gere MA: Surgical Forum XLII, Chicago:54–56.

35. Yanagi K, Ookawa K, Mizuno S, Ohshima N., 1989, Performance of a new hybrid artificial liver support system using hepatocytes entrapped within a hydrogel. ASAIO Transactions **35/3:**570–572.

36. Takabatake H, Koide N, Tsuji T., 1991, Encapsulated multicellular speroids of rat hepatocytes produce albumin and urea in a spouted bed circulating culture system, Artif. Org. **15:**474–480.

37. Koide N, Sakagucci K, Koide Y., 1990, Formation of multicellular spheroids composed of adult rat hepatocytes in dishes with positive charged surfaces and under other nonadherent environments. Exp. Cell Res. **186:**227–235.

38. Berry MN, Edwards AM, Banit GJ., 1991, Isolated hepatocytes preparation, properties and applications. In: Burdon RH, van Knippenberg PH eds. Laboratory techniques in biochemistry and molecular biology. Amsterdam: Elsevier.

39. Kelly JH, Koussayer T, He DE, Chong MG, Shang TA, Hartwell H, Whisennand, Sussman NL., 1992, An improved model of acetaminophen–induced fulminant hepatic failure in dogs. Hepatology **15:**329–335.

40. Jauregui HO., 1991, Treatment of hepatic insufficiency based on cellular therapies. Artif. Org. **14:**321–326.

41. Filipponi F, Fabbri LP, Marsili M, Falcini F. Benassai C. Nucera M, Romagnoli P., 1991, A new surgical model of acute liver failure in the pig: Experimental procedure and analysis of liver injury. Eur. Surg. Res. **23:**58–64.

42. Uchino J, Tsuburaya T, Kumagai F, Hase T, Hamada T, Komai T, Funatsu A, Hashimura E, Nakamura K, Kon T., 1988, "A hybrid bioartificial liver composed of multiplated hepatocyte monolayers", ASAIO Transactions **34:**972–977.

43. Arnaout WS, Moscioni AD, Barbour RL, Demetriou AA., 1990, Development of bioartificial liver: Bilirubin conjugation in gunn rats. Journal of Surgical Research **48/4:**379–382.

44. Demetriou A. et al., 1986, New method of hepatocyte transplantation and extracorporal liver support. Annals of Surgery, Vol. **204:**259–271.

45. Gerlach J, Jörres A, Vienken J, Gahl GM, and Neuhaus P., 1993, Side effects of hybrid liver support therapy: TNF liberation in pigs, connected with extracorporeal bioreactors. Int. J. Artif. Org. **16:**604–608.

46. Matsumura KN, Guevara GR, Huston H, Hamilton WL, Riliimaru M, Yamasaki G, Matsumura MS., 1987, "Hybrid bioartificial liver in hepatic failure: Preliminary clinical report" Surgery 101, **No.1:**99–103.

47. Margulis MS, Erukhimov EA, Andreiman LA, Kuznetsov KA, Viksna LM, Kuznetsov AI, Devyatov VV., 1990, Hemoperfusion through suspension of cryopreserved hepatocytes in a treatment of patients with acute liver failure. Research in Surgery 2:99–102.

48. Margulis MS, Erukhimov EA, Andreiman LA., 1989, Temporary organ substitution by hemoperfusion through suspension of active donor hepatocytes in a total complex of intensive therapy in patients with acute hepatic insufficiency. Resuscitation 18:85–94.

49. Neuzil D, Rozga J, Moscioni AD, Ro MS, Hakim R, Arnaout WS, Demetriou AA., 1993, Use of a novel bioartificial liver in a patient with acute liver insufficiency. Surgery 113(3):340–3.

50. Sussman NL, Kelly JH., 1993, Improved liver function following treatment with an extracorporal liver assist device. Artif–Organs 17(1):27–30.

51. Gerlach J, Stoll P, Schnoy N, Bücherl ESB., 1990, Membranes as substrate for hepatocyte adhesion in liver support bioreactors. Int. J. Artif. Org. 13/1:436–441.

52. Hynda KK, Mc Garvey ML, Liotta LA, Robbey PG, Tryggvason K, Martin GR., 1982, Isolation and characterisation of type IV procollagen, laminin and heparan sulfate proteoglycans from the EHS sarcoma. Biochemistry 21:6188–93.

53. Gerlach J, Schnoy N, Smith MD, Neuhaus P., 1994, Hepatocyte culture between woven capillary networks – a microscopy study. Int. Artif. Org. 18:226–230.

54. Gerlach J, Klöppel K, Stoll P, Vienken J, Müller Ch, Schauwecker HH., 1990, Gas supply across membranes in liver support bioreactors. Artif. Org. 14:328–333.

55. Gerlach J, Schauwecker HH, Klöppel K, Tauber R, Müller Ch, and Bücherl ES., 1989, Use of hepatocytes in adhesion and suspension cultures for liver support bioreactors. Int. J. Artif. Org. 12:788–793.

56. Gerlach J, Schauwecker HH, Hennig E, Bücherl ES., 1989, Endothelial cell seeding on different polyurethanes. Artif Org 13:144–147.

Hepatitis C Viral Infection after Orthotopic Liver Transplantation

Joaquín Berenguer, Martín Prieto, José Mir, Juan Cordoba, Miguel Rayón

Liver transplantation rapidly evolved throughout the 1980s into an effective treatment for end–stage liver disease. Most adult patients undergoing liver transplantation have cirrhosis and portal hypertension; however, the etiology of cirrhosis varies (1). Chronic hepatitis C virus (HCV) infection is a common cause of end–stage cirrhosis leading to the consideration of OLT (2). Many cirrhotic patients experience repeated bouts of encephalopathy despite therapy with lactulose/lactitol and/or neomycin. In fact, encephalopathy is the second most common quality–of–life indication of OLT in these patients (3). In our series, 29% of the cirrhotic patients undergoing OLT had had at least one episode of encephalopathy before transplantation.

Recurrent HCV infection is universal in patients with pretransplant HCV infection, but the consequences of post–transplantation HCV infection are yet to be defined. Our study reports data regarding evolution of HCV infection after transplantation from a series of patients undergoing OLT as treatment for end–stage cirrhosis related to chronic C virus infection.

1. Patients and Methods

From January 1991 through December 1993, 101 liver transplants were performed in 97 patients at our Hospital. One–year survival is currently 76%. Thirty–eight of these patients had chronic hepatitis C virus infection either as the only etiologic factor (n=28) or associated with other etiologies of liver disease (alcohol 6, hepatitis B virus 3, porphyria cutanea tarda 1) (figure 1). The mode of transmission of HCV infection on the basis of patient history was classified as sporadic in 47% of the cases, transfusion–associated in 50% and related to prior intravenous drug abuse in the remaining 3% of the cases. The diagnosis was reached by anti-HCV testing using a second–generation EIA test and/or presence of HCV–RNA in serum detected by PCR, using primers derived from the 5' non–coding region of the genome. Of these 97 patients, 39 were excluded because the follow–up was < 6 months or inadequate or, in the patients with HCV infection prior to OLT, because they were coinfected with hepatitis B virus. The remaining 58 patients were included in the study and divided into two groups, those with evidence of pretransplant HCV infection (n: 22, group 1), and those who were not infected with HCV before OLT (n: 36, group 2). The follow–up ranged from 9 to 36 months (mean ± s.d.: 19.6±6.9 months) after OLT. Patients received a standard triple immunosuppressive regimen including corticosteroids, cyclosporine and azathioprine. The first biopsy specimen was obtained during surgery after reperfusion of the graft. Protocol biopsies

Hospital Universitario La Fe. Valencia, SPAIN

Hepatic Encephalopathy, Hyperammonemia, and Ammonia Toxicity
Edited by V. Felipo and S. Grisolia, Plenum Press, New York, 1994

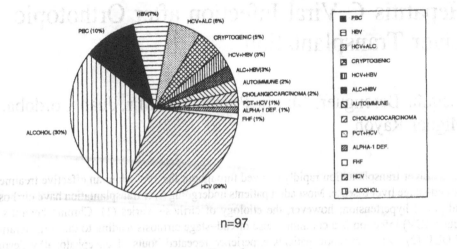

n=97

Figure 1.

were performed at day 10 after transplantation, then yearly, and at any time in case of abnormality of liver function tests.

Histological study.– Paraffin–embedded, code specimens, were stained with hematoxilin–eosin, Masson, and a periodic–acid Schiff reagent. The diagnosis of chronic hepatitis C was based on histological findings and abnormal aminotransferase levels, lasting at least 3 months, without evidence of rejection. For quantification of histological changes in biopsy samples with "hepatitis–like changes", the numerical scoring system, according to Knodell et al (4), was used. The criteria for acute rejection included lymphohistiocytic infiltration with endothelial inflammation in portal and central veins, occasional piece–meal necrosis, and lesions in bile duct epithelia (acute cholangitis).

2. Results

HCV infection recurred in 100% of the patients with HCV infection prior to OLT: 21 (95 %) were positive for both anti–HCV and serum HCV–RNA; one patient was positive only for serum HCV–RNA. By contrast, serum HCV–RNA was positive after OLT in only 2 (5 %) out of 36 patients without pretransplant HCV infection (p < 0,0001). At the time of their latest follow–up visit, serum ALT levels were within the normal range in 19% of group 1, compared with 55% of group 2 (p=0,04). Chronic hepatitis has developed in 12 out of 16 (75%) patients with HCV reinfection after OLT with a follow–up > 1 year. The histological distribution of chronic hepatitis cases is shown in figure 2. No single case of cirrhosis related to post–transplantation HCV infection has been observed so far. In three subjects with post–transplantation HCV infection, all of them with positive serum HCV–RNA, the liver histology was normal or showed minimal changes. Chronic hepatitis has not developed in any of the 2 patients with "de novo" HCV infection after OLT. No death in these series of patients could be related to HCV reinfection after OLT.

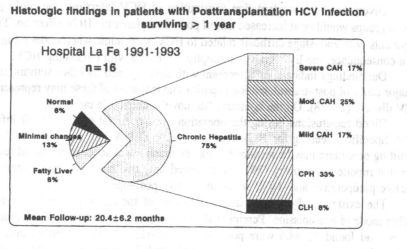

Histologic findings in patients with Posttransplantation HCV infection surviving > 1 year

Figure 2.

3. Discussion

Recent developments have provided serological diagnostic tests for infection by HCV (5). First–generation tests have documented antibody against HCV (anti–HCV) in 70% to 80% of patients with non–A, non–B hepatitis (6, 7). However, it soon became apparent that first generation anti–HCV tests may produce false–positive results (8, 9). Studies with second–generation tests have documented anti–HCV in about 90% of patients with chronic Non–A, Non–B hepatitis (10). Additionally, the polymerase chain reaction (PCR) assay, with specific primers for HCV, has allowed direct demonstration of the virus either in the serum or in the liver (11, 12). Studies with this technique have shown that HCV infection is present in more than 90% of patients with non–A, non–B hepatitis (13).

The high rate of chronic liver disease (~60%) after acute infection, regardless of how the disease was initially contracted: recipients of blood transfusions (14, 15), parenteral drug users (16), community acquired hepatitis C (sporadic infection) (17), accounts for the importance of HCV in patients with end–stage cirrhosis, the patient group most likely to be considered for liver transplantation.

Although no large study has addressed risk factors for HCV infection in OLT patients, some information is available. Ten out of 32 (31%) anti–HCV–positive liver transplantation recipients at the University of California, San Francisco, admitted prior parenteral drug use; 14 (38%) had a history of previous blood transfusions, and 4 (13%) had both risk factors. Only 4 (13%) recipients had no parenteral risk factors (18). Several reasons may explain the difference between risk factors in these patients compared to those in patients surveyed in broad epidemiologic studies (16). First, patients with end–stage cirrhosis undergoing liver transplantation may have been transfused following the onset of liver disease, thus the risk factor may be overestimated. Second, there may be a variation in the genotype, and, as a consequence, in the virulence of the infection among the different patient groups (19). HCV infection is frequently present in other groups of patients with chronic liver disease: 31% to 37% of patients with alcoholic cirrhosis, 12% to 55% of those with cirrhosis associated with HBV infection, 23% of those with autoimmune cirrhosis and 50% of those with cryptogenic cirrhosis (2, 20, 21). In contrast, HCV infection is rarely present in patients with primary biliary cirrhosis, hemochromatosis, primary sclerosing cholangitis, and fulminant hepatic failure unassociated with serologic markers of hepatitis A or B infection (2, 21, 22).

Given the pre–transplantation distribution of HCV infection, one could predict that certain groups would be at increased risk of post–transplantation HCV infection. The majority of patients with end–stage cirrhosis related to HCV are viremic when undergoing OLT (23). As a consequence, the liver graft is promptly reinfected with circulating HCV.

Our findings indicate, in agreement with data reported by other authors, that HCV is a major cause of post–transplantation hepatitis and that most of these may represent recurrent HCV disease (23–28). On the contrary, "de novo" infection is rare (23).

Blood transfusions during the operation are a potential cause of graft infection with HCV. Specific screening for HCV with anti–HCV ELISA test, and a careful blood donor recruiting procedure may be responsible for the much lower acquisition rate of recent studies than that reported previously (29). We observed only two patients who seroconverted from negative preoperative anti–HCV status to positive post–operative status.

The existence of chronic virus C infection of the donor has to be considered as a posible mode of transmission. Pereira et al (30) performed a retrospective study in 716 organ donors, and found 13 who were positive for anti–HCV (1,8%). Non A, non B hepatitis developed in 14 of 29 organ recipients (48%). HCV infection was the cause of post–transplantation liver disease in 12 of the 13 recipients (92%) for whom serum samples were available. No apparent relation existed between the type of transplantation procedure and the risk of hepatitis. In another study by the same group (31), they found that 7 of 26 organ recipients were HCV–RNA positive before transplantation and 23 of 24 (92%) after transplantation. HCV infection was detected in the 13 patients who received an organ from a HCV–RNA positive donor. In our series we found no evidence of preoperative HCV infection of the donor organ, except in one case.

Recent studies in CAH patients, treated with interferon, with complete response (definitive normalization of liver enzymes and loss of HCV–RNA in the serum, associated with histologic improvement) give some evidence that HCV may persist in the peripheral blood mononuclear cells and that it is able to replicate in these cells (32, 33). Therefore, these cells may constitute a reservoir for recurrent HCV infection. Extrahepatic sites of infection might gain significance if it were possible to eradicate the viremia successfully before transplantation. A possible way to approach this problem in the future might be to combine alfa–interferon with granulocyte colony–stimulating factor. This combination would enable increased doses of alfa interferon to be administered to patients with end–stage cirrhosis before OLT, and thus decisively reducing the risk of leukopenia and thrombocytopenia (34). Given the failure of OLT recipients to produce anti–HCV, now well documented (35), the prevalence of post–transplantation HCV infection is underestimated by anti–HCV testing (2, 30, 34). Comparison of three anti–HCV tests (first and second generation EIA, and second generation radio–immunoblot assay) with HCV–RNA in serum detected by PCR, demonstrated that antibody tests failed to diagnose HCV infection in 30% of patients (31). HCV–RNA may also be detected by b–DNA (36). Although both tests are reliable for detecting post–transplantation HCV infection, the later test is less cumbersome than PCR. The diagnosis has to be confirmed, in any case, by exclusion of HBV and other viral infections, such as cytomegaviral infection, and of acute rejection. Table 1 shows the major histological criteria for hepatitis C reinfection versus acute rejection. There is a considerable overlap between both causes of dysfunction of the liver graft, often making the histologic distinction between hepatitis and rejection difficult (37, 38).

HCV reinfection accounts for 60%, 90% and 96% of cases of post–transplantation hepatitis in three separate studies in which other viral infections were excluded (23, 30, 35). In a study from the University of California, San Francisco, that used both anti–HCV test and PCR to identify HCV–RNA, a clear association between pre–transplantation HCV and both post–transplantation viremia and hepatitis was shown (23). Recent evidence suggests that most patients with post–OLT HCV infection may have chronic infection without clinical and histological consequences. This means that in the inmuno–supressed transplant recipient, as in non–transplanted subjects (17, 40), a "healthy carrier state" of the virus may exist (18).

Table 1. Major histological criteria for hepatitis C reinfection versus acute rejection

Histological changes	Hepatitis reinfection	Acute rejection
Portal inflammation	+	+
Portal vein endothelitis	−	+
Acute cholangitis	−	+
Piecemeal necrosis	+	(+)[a]
Eosinophilic changes	+	−
Focal necrosis	+	(+)[a]
Central vein endothelitis	−	+

a mainly indicative of hepatitis reinfection but may also occur in acute rejection. From reference 27.

Acute hepatitis C after transplantation is frequently asymptomatic (24). Chronic hepatitis will develop within 12 to 24 months in a high proportion of the patients with pos–transplantation HCV infection (37), but progression to cirrhosis seems to be slow (24), although there is a discrepancy between different studies concerning this issue (37, 39).

Treatment of the non–transplanted patient with chronic HCV infection with alfa interferon unfortunately results in a complete response in only 15% of the patients (41, 42). There is only preliminary information about the efficacy of alfa interferon in the treatment of post–liver transplantation hepatitis (43, 44, 45). Of 11 patients with HCV and 6 with non–A, non–B hepatitis treated at the University of Pittsburgh with 3 million U three times per week for 6 months, only one patient (9%) of those with HCV and 18% with non–A, non–B hepatitis experienced complete normalization of liver enzymes (43). Samuel et al reported a complete response in only 2 (20%) of their 10 patients with chronic hepatitis C after transplantation (44). In contrast, an 80% response rate was recently observed by Villamil et al in a preliminary study (45).

The greatest concern about the use of interferon in post–liver transplantation patients has been the possibility of precipitating allograft rejection. Interferon increases expression of HLA class I and II antigens, which are involved in the cellular immune response in allograft rejection. Thus, there is a theoretical risk of increased rejection in patients treated with alfa interferon, even though no episode of rejection was attributable to interferon in the Pittsburgh series (43). On the contrary, rejection was observed in 3 (30%) out of the 10 patients treated by Samuel et al (44). However, given the histologic overlap between hepatitis and acute rejection, it is possible that allograft rejection is underestimated in patients with ongoing hepatitis. Controlled trials, comparing patients treated with interferon to a group of untreated patients, are required to demonstrate the safety and the efficacy of this drug.

References

1. Van Thiel DH, Schade RR, Gavaler JS, Shaw BW Jr, Iwatsuki S, Starzl TE. Medical aspects of liver transplatation. Hepatology 1984; **4** (suppl):79–83.
2. Read AE, Donegan E, Lake J et al. Hepatitis C in patients undergoing liver transplantation. Ann Intern Med 1991; **114**:282–284.
3. Lake JR. Changing indications for liver transplantation. Gastroenterol Clin North Am 1993; **22**: 213–229.

4. Knodell RG, Ishak KG, Black WC et al. Formulation and application of a numerical scoring system for assesing histological activity in chronic active hepatitis. Hepatology 1981; **1**:431–435.

5. Kuo G, Choo QL, Alter HJ et al. An assay for circulating antibodies to a major etiologic virus of human non–A, non–B hepatitis. Science 1989; **244**:362–364.

6. Alter HJ, Purcell RH, Shih JW et al. Detection of antibody to hepatitis C virus in prospectively followed transfusion recipients with acute and chronic non–A, non–B hepatitis. N Engl J Med 1989; **321**:1494–1500.

7. Tremolada F, Casarin C, Tagger A et al. Antibody to hepatitis C virus in post–transfusion hepatitis. Ann Intern Med 1991; **114**:277–289.

8. Theilmann L, Blazek M, Goeser T, Gmelin K, Kommerell B, Fiehn W. False positive anti–HCV tests in rheumatoid arthritis. Lancet 1990; **335**:1346.

9. Mc Farlane IG, Smith HM, Johnson PJ, Bray GP, Vergani D, Williams R. Hepatitis C virus antibodies in chronic active hepatitis: pathogenetic factor or false–positive results? Lancet 1990; **335**:754–757.

10. Mc Hutchinson JG, Person JL, Govindarajan S et al. Improved detection of hepatitis C virus antibodies in high–risk populations. Hepatology 1991; **13**:465–470.

11. Garson JA, Tedder RS, Briggs M et al. Detection of hepatitis C viral sequences in blood donations by "nested" polymerase chain reaction and prediction ofinfectivity. Lancet 1990; **335**:1419–1422.

12. Ulrich PP, Romeo JM, Lane PK, Kelly I, Daniel LJ, Vyas GN. Detection, semiquantitation, and genetic variation in hepatitis C virus sequences amplified from the plasma of blood donors with elevated alanine aminotransferase. J Clin Invest 1990; **86**:1609–1614.

13. Enomoto N, Takada N, Takase S, Takada A, Date T. Hepatitis C virus RNA genome in plasma of patients with non–A, non–B hepatitis. Gastroenterol J 1991; **26**:42–46.

14. Alberti A, Chemello L, Cavalleto D et al. Antibody to hepatitis C virus and liver disease in healthy blood donors. Ann Intern Med 1991; **114**:1010–1012.

15. Rakela J, Redeker AG. Chronic liver disease after acute non–A, non–B viral hepatitis. Gastroenterology 1979; **77**:1200–1202.

16. Alter MJ, Hadler SC, Judson FN et al. Risk factors for acute non–A, non–B hepatitis in the United States and association with hepatitis C infection. JAMA 1990; **264**:2231–2235.

17. Alter MJ, Margolis HS, Krawczynski K et al. The natural history of community–adquired hepatitis C in the United States. N Engl J Med 1992; **327**:1899–1905.

18. Wright TL. Liver transplantation for chronic C viral infection. Gastroenterol Clin North Am 1993; **22**:231–242.

19. Féray C, Gigou M, Samuel D et al. Direct evidence for a more pathogenic effect of HCV type II. The model of liver transplantation. J Hepatol 1993; **18** (suppl 1):S4.

20. Jeffers W, Hasan F, de Medina et al. Prevalence of antibodies to hepatitis C virus among patients with cryptogenetic chronic hepatitis and cirrhosis. Hepatology 1992; **15**:187–190.

21. Brown J, Dourakis S, Karayiannis P et al. Seroprevalence of hepatic C virus nucleocapsid antibodies in patients with cryptogenic chronic liver disease. Hepatology 1992; **15**:175–179.

22. Wright TL, Hsu H, Donegan E et al. Hepatitis C virus not found in fulminants non–A, non–B hepatitis. Ann Intern Med 1991; **115**:111–112.

23. Wright TL, Donegan E, Hsu HH et al. Recurrent and adquired hepatitis C viral infection in liver transplant recipients. Gastroenterology 1992; **103**:317–322.

24. Martin P, Muñoz SJ, Di Bisceglie AM et al. Recurrence of hepatitis C virus infection after orthotopic liver transplantation. Hepatology 1991; **13**:719–721.

25. Shah G, Demetris AJ, Gavaler JS et al. Incidence, prevalence, and clinical course of hepatitis C following liver transplantation. Gastroenterology 1992, **103**:323–329.

26. Féray C, Samuel D, Thiers V et al. Reinfection of liver graft by hepatitis C virus after liver transplantation. J Clin Invest 1992; **89**:1361–1365.

27. Konig V, Banditz J, Lobeck M et al. Hepatitis C virus reinfection in allografts after orthotopic liver transplantation. Hepatology 1992; **16**:1137–1143.

28. Gretch DR, De la Rosa C, Perkins J et al. HCV infection in liver transplant recipients: chronic reinfection is universal, de novo acquisition rare. Hepatology 1992; **16**:45A.

29. Donahue JG, Muñoz A, Ness, PM et al.The declining risk of post–transfusion hepatic C virus infection. N Engl J Med 1992; **327**:369–373.

30. Pereira BJG, Milford EL, Kirkman RL, Levi AS. Transmission of hepatic C virus by organ transplantation. N Engl J Med 1991; 325:454–460.

31. Pereira BJG, Milford EL, Kirkman et al. Prevalence of hepatitis virus RNA in organ donors positive for hepatitis C antibody and in the recipients of their organs. N Engl J Med 1992; 327: 910–915.

32. Berenguer M, Olaso V, Córdoba J, Benages R, Berenguer J. The presence of HCV–RNA in peripheral blood mononuclear cells in chronic hepatitis C patients with complete response to alfa–IFN treatment could explain the frequent recurrences. J Hepatol 1993; 18 (suppl l):S56.

33. Qian C, Camps J, Maluenda MD, Civeira MP, Prieto J. Replication of hepatitis C virus in peripheral blood mononuclear cells. Effect of alpha–interferon therapy. J Hepatol 1992, 16: 380–383.

34. Gurakar A, Gavaler JS, Wright HI et al. Granulocyte colony–stimulating factor (GCSF) treatment of cirrhotic patients with neuropenia due to hyperesplenism. Hepatology 1992, 16:A156.

35. Poterucha JJ, Rakela J, Lumeng L, Lee CH, Traswell HF, Wiesner RH. Diagnosis of chronic hepatitis C after liver transplantation by the detection of viral sequences with polymerase chain reaction. Hepatology 1992; 15:42–45.

36. Donegan E, Wright TL, Kim M et al. Diagnosis of hepatitis C viral (HCV) infection in liver transplant recipients. Hepatology 1992; 16:70A.

37. Ferrell LD, Wright TL, Roberts J et al. Pathology of hepatitis C viral infection in liver transplant recipients. Hepatology 1992, 16:865–876.

38. Mor E, Solomon H, Gibbs J et al. Acute cellular rejection following liver transplantation: clinical pathologic features and effect on outcome. Sem Liver Dis 1992; 12:28–40.

39 Belli LS, Alberti A, Rondinara GF et al. Recurrent HCV hepatitis after liver transplantation. Lancet 1993; 341:378–379.

40. Prieto M, Verdu RC, Gisbert C et al. Does the healthy hepatitis C virus carrier state really exist? An analysis through PCR. J Hepatol 1993; 18 (suppl l):S30.

41. Di Bisceglie AM, Martin P, Kassianides C et al. Recombinant interferon alfa therapy for chronic hepatitis C. A randomized, double–blind placebo controlled trial. N Engl J Med 1989; 321: 1506–1510.

42 Davis GL. Recombinant alpha–interferon treatment of non–A, non–B (type C) hepatitis:Review of studies and recommendations for treatment. J Hepatol 1990; 11 suppl 1:S72–74.

43. Wright HI, Gavaler JS, Van Thiel DH. Preliminary experience with alfa–2b–interferon therapy of viral hepatitis in liver allograft recipients. Transplantation 1992; 53:121–124.

44. Samuel D, Gigou M, Feray C et al. Recombinant alpha interferon for hepatitis C on the graft in liver transplant patients. Hepatology 1992; 16:48A.

45. Villamil F, Yu CH, Hu KQ, et al. Alfa 2b–interferon (2b–IFN) therapy of hepatitis C following liver transplantation (LT). Hepatology 1992; 16:48A.

Exercise–Induced Hyperammonemia: Skeletal Muscle Ammonia Metabolism and the Peripheral and Central Effects

Terry E. Graham

1. Introduction

The area of ammonia metabolism in skeletal muscle is a vast topic and one that involves both directly and indirectly carbohydrate, fat and protein. To gain an appreciation for hyperammonemia associated with exercise one must also understand the membrane-associated events as well as the clearance mechanisms for ammonia. These cannot be dealt with in detail in this paper and those who wish more information can refer to a variety of recent reviews by this author (1,2) and others (3,4,5,6). This manuscript will address the possible effects that exercise–induced ammonia hyperemia could have on the feelings of fatigue and also will address whether there are local effects within the active muscle. Attention will also be given to the clearance mechanisms that are active in association with exercise states both because they are critical to determining the circulating ammonia concentration and also since they represent aspects of how ammonia affects various tissues. However, before these issues can be addressed the basic aspects of ammonia metabolism in muscle will be reviewed.

There are many excellent studies using animal models and they form the bases for what we understand regarding ammonia metabolism in the human. However there are many qualitative and quantitative differences between humans and, for example, rodents in terms of both muscle and liver metabolism. Thus whenever possible I will base my statements on research with human subjects.

2. Overview of Skeletal Muscle Ammonia Metabolism

At rest skeletal muscle is consistently an ammonia consumer; in my experience the human quadriceps has an uptake of approximately 1 umol/min. This would mean that there is a clearance of approximately 0.3 umol/kg wet wt/min by resting muscle. Assuming that the body is 40% muscle then there would be 8 umol/min taken up by resting muscle. This is not insignificant since Eriksson (7) reported that splanchnic ammonia uptake at rest was 12 umol/min.

During exercise muscle rapidly shifts within 30 seconds to releasing ammonia. Originally it was believed that exercise intensity needed to be severe i.e. at least 80% VO_2 max before ammonia was produced. However we have found that at as little as 60% VO_2

Human Biology, University of Guelph, Guelph, Ontario, Canada, N1G 2W1. Phone: 519 824 4120 Ext. 3319, FAX: 519 767 1942

Hepatic Encephalopathy, Hyperammonemia, and Ammonia Toxicity
Edited by V. Felipo and S. Grisolia, Plenum Press, New York, 1994

Table 1. Cumulative Data for Single Leg Extensor Exercise.

Exercise Conditions		NH₃ "load"		Net Total flux (nmoles/kg)					
Intensity (% thigh max)	Duration (h)	Release (nmoles)	Δart NH₃[c] (uM)	NH₃	Gln	Ala	Glu	La	Pyr[a]
140	0.05	1.9	45	0.9	?	?	?	26.5	53[b]
80	1	4.4	38	1.5	1.2	0.9	0.6	33.6	166
70	1	5.0	15	1.4	1.4	1.2	0.3	58.0	181
65	1.5	8.4	25	3.0	2.2	1.7	0.6	64.0	132[b]
60	3	10.9	15	4.4	6.4	3.6	1.8	15.6	312

[a] (glucose uptake plus decrease in Glycogen) x 2 = pyruvate flux.
[b] Glucose uptake not considered.
[c] Δart NH₃ is the increase above rest in the arterial ammonia concentration.

max(an intensity that can be maintained for several hours) there is a continuous ammonia production. The arterial concentration is virtually constant (table 1) as clearance matches release and so if one does not measure release of ammonia directly the production would go undetected. It has not been determined what the minimum intensity of activity is in which there is no net ammonia release.

2.1. Ammonia from AMP Deamination

It is commonly believed that the source of ammonia is from AMP deamination and there is no question that it is the main source (perhaps the only source) when the exercise is brief (a few minutes or less) and intense (90% VO_2 max or greater). Under these conditions it has been shown that the rise in the product of AMP deamination, IMP is stoichiometrically matched very closely with the net ammonia production (7,8,9). However, even this well accepted statement must be accepted cautiously as most investigators have only measured the net increase in muscle ammonia as a reflection of production. As described below one needs to include the ammonia that is released during the exercise as well as that which is removed as glutamine and possibly as alanine in order to get an accurate measure of production.

Despite these reservations there is no question that AMP deaminase (reaction (c) figure 1) is the key enzyme in ammonia production during intense exercise. The fundamentals of the regulation of this process are well documented (1–6) and generally it appears that shifts in the energy status of the tissue resulting in an increase in AMP as well as rises in ADP and

Ammonia from AMP deamination

a) ATP -> ADP + Pi

b) 2ADP -> ATP + AMP

c) AMP -> IMP + NH₃

Figure 1. Ammonia from AMP deamination. A series of reactions take place during high metabolic stress to try to maintain a high ATP/ADP ratio. Myosin ATP'ase (and others) cause ATP to go to ADP (reaction (a)). As ADP accumulates adenylate kinase forms ATP and AMP (reaction (b)). To encourage ATP formation AMP is removed via AMP deaminase (reaction (c)) and ammonia is formed.

a) Asp + IMP + GTP -> GDP + Pi + S-AMP

b) S-AMP -> Fumarate + AMP

c) AMP -> IMP + NH_3

Net: Asp + GTP -> GDP + Pi + fumarate + NH_3

Figure 2. Ammonia from aspartate deamination. The purine nucleotide cycle is a series of 3 reactions IMP and aspartate form adenylosuccinate (S-AMP)and requires GTP in the adenylosuccinate synthase step (reaction (a)). This is converted to fumarate and AMP by adenylosuccinate lyase (reaction (b)). Finally, the AMP is deaminated to ammonia and IMP (reaction(c)). Thus the cycle results in the deamination of aspartate, the formation of fumarate and ammonia and requires GTP.

H+ and a decline in CP will increase the activity of the enzyme. Rundell and coworkers (10,11) have demonstrated that during intense exercise the AMP deaminase shifts to a bound form on myosin and this may be a critical factor in regulation. It is not clear what promotes the binding and recently we (12) have demonstrated that this may not be vital in human muscle. For example, while the percent of bound enzyme rose during moderate exercise (despite no change in the nucleotide pool) there was no further increase when the subjects increased their power output even though the ammonia production rapidly increased and fatigue occurred.

2.2. Ammonia from Aspartate Deamination

A second possible source of ammonia is the purine nucleotide cycle (PNC) (figure 2). AMP deaminase is one step of this process (reaction (c) figure 2) and is often referred to as the initial step. However, if the PNC is cycling it is difficult to identify a start and end. In the PNC AMP is deaminated to IMP and ammonia and the IMP is then processed by the "reaminating arm" of the cycle (reactions (a) and (b) of figure 2). The amino acid aspartate and IMP form adenylosuccinate and the step is energy (GTP) requiring (reaction (a) figure 2). The process is not fully understood, but it is inhibited by IMP, AMP, and Pi. Hence it is difficult to accept that this step would be active during exercise. The adenylosuccinate is then converted to fumarate, a TCA cycle intermediate and AMP (reaction (b) of figure 2). Thus when the PNC actually cycles the net effect would be aspartate being deaminated to fumarate with the production of ammonia and the consumption of GTP. The purpose of this cycle appears to be the anaplerotic effect for the TCA cycle (discussed below) and it is apparent that the process can not contribute to nucleotide management. In contrast when the deaminating step occurs with no further cycling then there should be a benefit to the nucleotide pool in that the removal of AMP would promote adenylate kinase activity in the ATP formation direction and so help to maintain a high ATP/ADP ratio (figure 1).

It is controversial whether cycling occurs during exercise; Terjung and coworkers argue that if it does then it is in fibers that have already fatigued and which are recovering even as the exercise continues (5,6). Broberg and coworkers (13) propose that cycling occurs in humans during moderate exercise. However, their evidence is very circumstantial and they

a) BCAA + α KG -> Glu + BCKA   (KIC, KIV, KMV)

b) BCKA + NAD$^+$ + CoA -> acyl CoA derivatives + NADH + CO_2

c) Acyl CoA derivatives -> acetoacetate, acetyl CoA, succinyl CoA

Figure 3. Ammonia from branched chain amino acid deamination. The three branched chain amino acids use alpha ketoglutarate to accept the amino group in a near equilibrium reaction (a) catalysed by branched chain amino transaminase. The keto acids are dehydrogenated by the key non-equilibrium enzyme branched chain keto acid dehydrogenase (reaction (b)), and depending on the original amino acid one of three acyl CoA derivatives is formed (alpha ketoisovalerate (KIV), alpha ketoisocaproate (KIC) and alpha keto 3–methylvalerate (KMV)). These are converted to TCA intermediates by a series of dehydrogenases and other reactions.

fail to consider factors such as branched chain amino acid deamination(see below). Recently Hood and Parent (14) have presented evidence that rat fast twitch red fibers do have cycling during prolonged activity. However, given that the metabolic characteristics of human muscle are not as distinctly differentiated between fiber types as that of the rat, one cannot generalize these findings to the human.

2.3. Ammonia from Branched Chain Amino acid Deamination

The third process by which skeletal muscle can produce ammonia is by the deamination of the branched chain amino acids (figure 3). Unlike the metabolism described above this takes place in the mitochondrial compartment. The three branched chain amino acids, leucine, isoleucine and valine can be deaminated to their respective keto acids with alpha ketoglutarate accepting the ammonia group and forming glutamate (reaction (a), figure 3). This is a near equilibrium reaction and the keto acids can either be released and transported to the liver for further oxidation or they can be catabolized to TCA intermediates in the muscle mitochondria and oxidized (reactions (b) and (c), figure 3). At rest the former appears to be dominant while during prolonged, steady state exercise the latter process is very active. In the latter case the key enzyme is branched chain keto acid dehydrogenase (BCKAD) (reaction (b) figure 3) and this exists in both an active and an inactive form. At rest the muscle form is very inactive but during prolonged exercise the activity increases considerably (4,12), presumably due to the increase in branched chain keto acids in the mitochondria. It has been suggested that a decline in mitochondrial ATP is also a factor (4), but we found that there is considerable BCKAD activation when there is no disturbance in the nucleotide pool (12).

2.4. Ammonia, Glutamine and Alanine

The glutamate produced by the branched chain amino acid deamination does not accumulate but in fact from the onset of exercise there is a marked drop in concentration to less than 50% of rest levels and it remains at this level throughout the exercise. Glutamate is the onlyamino acid to decline significantly in muscle during exercise and this occurs

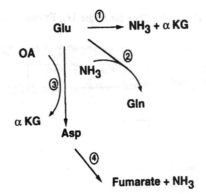

Figure 4. The fate of Glutamate. This illustrates some of the metabolic processes involving glutamate (Glu). It can be deaminated by glutamate dehydrogenase (reaction (1)). It can form glutamine (reaction 2)) via glutamine synthase. It can also be involved in transaminations. The one represented by reaction (3) is aspartate transaminase which uses oxaloacetate (OA) and forms aspartate (Asp). Asp can then be deaminated by the purine nucleotide cycle (4) to fumarate and ammonia. Note how frequently TCA cycle intermediates are involved.

despite the fact that the muscle is continuously taking up large quantities of glutamate. It is a very active amino acid involved in numerous reactions (figure 4). It can be deaminated by glutamate dehydrogenase to form ammonia and alpha ketoglutarate (reaction (1) of figure 4). It can also take on another ammonia group to form glutamine and it can take part in various transamination reactions. The two critical ones in muscle are alanine aminotransferase and aspartate aminotransferase. The former requires pyruvate and results in alanine leaving the muscle while the latter requires oxaloacetate and the aspartate can go to ammonia and fumarate via the PNC (reactions (3) and (4) of figure 4).

We do not know the importance of each of these processes but it appears that they are all active during exercise. This obviously complicates studies of ammonia metabolism. For example just to quantify the ammonia production one needs to evaluate the release and change in intramuscular concentration of not only ammonia but also glutamine and alanine. Very few scientists have done so and even when this is performed one cannot be certain whether the glutamine "counts" for one or two ammonia and whether alanine represents one or no ammonia. In order to establish this one has to know whether the glutamate that was used was synthesized from alpha ketoglutarate or whether it came from an existing glutamate pool. Nevertheless as reviewed below there is a large production and release of ammonia, glutamine and alanine in most forms of exercise.

There have been a number of measures of muscle ammonia during exercise. The values at the end of intense exercise are typically approximately 1 mmol/kg wet wt and at the end of prolonged exercise the concentration is usually about half of this value (2), while resting ammonia ranges from .15–.30 mmol/kg wet wt. The rise in plasma or blood concentration is also reasonably modest with typical values at exhaustion being 100–150 uM regardless of exercise intensity. There has been a report of values as high as 250 uM in one study of elite athletes (15) and as high as 3–400 uM in McArdle's patients (16). While changes in plasma concentration generally are a qualitative reflection of ammonia release and production there is no question that they cannot be used quantitatively (8,17). There have been very few measures of circulating ammonia concentrations in other species, but the horse appears to be able to generate greater levels of ammonia than that found in humans. During intense exercise

Table 2. Cumulative Data for Single Leg Extensor Exercise.

Exercise Conditions		Net total flux (umoles/kg-min)					
Intensity (% thigh max)	Duration (h)	NH_3	Gln	Ala	Glu	La	Pyr[a]
140	0.05	300	?	?	?	8,800	17,700[b]
80	1	25	20	15	10	560	2,800
70	1	23	23	20	5	970	3,000
65	1.5	33	24	19	7	710	1,470[b]
60	3	24	36	20	10	87	1,730

[a] (glucose uptake plus decrease in Glycogen) x 2 = pyruvate flux.
[b] Glucose uptake not considered.

lasting 1–4 minutes horses achieve values of 300–1000 uM (18,19). Furthermore based on the increase in muscle IMP (20) the intramuscular ammonia may be 3–4 mmol/kg wet wt. It is not clear whether this is due to the enzyme compliment of the animals or whether it is due to their tremendous sprinting power.

Rarely have studies reported the responses of ammonia, glutamine and alanine during exercise. We have been fortunate to be able to do so in a series of studies that have all used the same experimental model. We have studied humans exercising the quadriceps of one leg (the single leg knee extensor model) in brief, exhaustive exercise as well as during various intensities of prolonged exercise. Table 1 and 2 summarize these studies for both the rate of metabolite production as well as the total quantity of metabolite formed during the entire exercise. It can be seen that while intense exercise naturally has a higher rate of production the total quantity of formation is greater during prolonged exercise. Thus the latter state will place a greater demand on the supply and removal mechanisms even though the former may generate greater changes in plasma metabolites as reflected in the change in arterial ammonia. Unfortunately we did not measure alanine or glutamine release in the study in which the subjects worked at 140% VO_2 max (8) but Katz et al (9) found that humans released at least as much alanine and glutamine as ammonia during whole body exercise at 100% VO_2 max. It was not established whether this was due to production or a washout of intramuscular stores. It is clear that multiple measures are necessary to quantify ammonia production.

2.5. Plasma Clearance

Associated with the release of ammonia and alanine and glutamine there is a release of essential amino acids (17). This occurs even though there is no change in the intramuscular free pool of essential amino acids and so this must represent a net protein catabolism. It is impressive that the efflux of the various amino acids and ammonia are great enough to potentially produce huge changes in the circulating concentrations yet very little change is observed (17). This must mean that clearance mechanisms are very sensitive to plasma changes and they have a large capacity. It has been shown that the splanchnic clearance of amino acids is quite active during exercise and most are probably used for gluconeogenesis (21,22,23) and Carraro et al (24) have reported that the liver can also synthesize small, short-lived plasma proteins during exercise. This latter response would result in the conservation of amino acids and reduce the need to produce urea.

The clearance mechanisms for ammonia have not been clearly quantified or even identified (figure 5). As mentioned above resting muscle can clear ammonia but its role during exercise has not been quantified. The liver takes up ammonia but Eriksson and coworkers (7) could not show an increase in extraction during exercise. Sweat contains not only urea (25), but also ammonia (26). The magnitude of these processes have not been determined. In addition we demonstrated that the clearance of ammonia decreased very

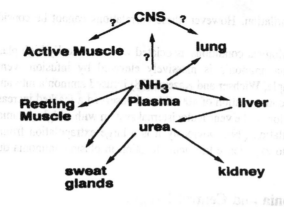

Actions of Plasma Ammonia

Figure 5. An illustration of how plasma ammonia may affect various tissues. It may be cleared by the lung, resting muscle, sweat glands and the liver. The latter forms urea which can be excreted in urine and sweat. In addition, plasma ammonia may affect the brain and in turn stimulate ventilation and/or cause fatigue. Because these are more speculative question marks are beside these arrows.

rapidly in the first few seconds of recovery and speculated that the lung could be an important clearance organ (8).

Thus it is evident that the ammonia production of exercise is associated with many metabolic processes and exits the muscle in several forms. As described below these events have been used to construct several theories of central (i.e. CNS) fatigue and peripheral fatigue. In addition the changes in plasma ammonia and assorted amino acids cause immediate changes in a variety of tissues that are involved in the clearance of these substances.

3. Central Effects of Ammonia and Associated Amino acids

In all considerations of ammonia and the central nervous system one must keep in mind that the exercise hyperammonemia rarely exceeds 150 uM and that these changes are very transient, lasting only minutes or perhaps even seconds. Furthermore Cooper and Plum (27) point out that while ammonia is metabolised in many compartments in the brain it is largely metabolized in the astrocytes, which act as a metabolic trap for ammonia. Ammonia can result in numerous changes in neural membranes, including depolarizing resting membrane potentials, inhibition of axonal action potentials, and depression of excitatory postsynaptic potentials (27). However, the ammonia concentrations and duration of exposure appear to be considerably greater than those that a person would encounter during exercise.

3.1. Ammonia and Ventilation

As discussed previously ventilation during exercise may serve as a means of reducing the ammonia load. In addition it has been suggested that the increase in plasma ammonia may act to stimulate the ventilatory response during exercise (figure 5). Certainly the temporal patterns in plasma ammonia during an exercise in which the power output rises rapidly (eg. a standard, progressive VO_2 max test) follow the curvilinear rise in ventilation. Similarly during prolonged, steady state exercise the plasma ammonia concentration tends to drift upwards as does ventilation. However, these correlations cannot be considered proof of a causal relationship.

In some pathological conditions associated with chronically high plasma ammonia as well as when plasma ammonia is massively elevated by infusion, ventilation may be stimulated. For example, Wichser and Kazemi (28) infused ammonia into anaesthetized dogs to a blood ammonia concentration of 400 uM and observed a marked increase in ventilation. Similarly direct infusion of the ventriculocisternal system with a high glutamate concentration also stimulated ventilation (29). Obviously it is a large extrapolation from such studies to conscious human who experience transient elevation in plasma ammonia during exercise.

3.2. Ammonia and Central Fatigue

Some investigators have demonstrated a correlation between plasma ammonia concentration and the perception of exertion (exertion is rated on a numerical scale) and from this observation have suggested that the ammonia is influencing the perception within the CNS (16,30) (figure 5). Similarly Banister and Cameron (31) speculate that plasma ammonia may cause ammonia toxicity which leads to a lack of coordinated movement, ataxia and stupor. There is no evidence to support any of these claims and given the transient nature of the moderate increases in plasma ammonia together with the protective role of the astrocytes these theories seem to be unlikely.

The second theory involving central fatigue that pertains to this discussion focuses not on ammonia but on the plasma amino acid profile (figure 6). This theory is included in this review since the branched chain amino acids are major factors in this theory. The hypothesis that has been put forward by Newsholme (32) is based on several well established facts. The neural transmitter serotonin or 5-hydroxytryptamine is known to cause impaired mental performance and to induce sleep. It is also clear that the synthesis of this monoamine is

BCAA and Central Fatigue

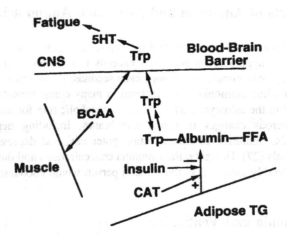

Figure 6. A scheme for how branched chain amino acids may cause fatigue (adapted from Newsholme (32). Tryptophan (Trp) is both free and bound to albumin in the plasma. During exercise catecholamines (CAT) rise and insulin falls causing a rise in free fatty acids (FFA). These displace the tryptophan from albumin. The rise in free amino acid allows it to enter the brain and stimulate the synthesis of serotonin (5HT).

dependent on the availability of its amino acid precursor, tryptophan. This amino acid is transported across the blood brain barrier by the same transport mechanism that carries the branched chain amino acids. Thus there is a competition for entry into the central nervous system and any stress that alters the ratio of these amino acids could also be reflected in a change in serotonin.

Tryptophan is not abundant in proteins so it is difficult to increase its plasma concentration with diet changes. However, one can increase the intake of branched chain amino acids and lower the tryptophan/branched chain amino acid ratio (TRP/BCAA). In addition tryptophan is unique among amino acids in that it is bound to plasma albumin, the same protein that carries free fatty acids. As a result there is a bound and free fraction of tryptophan in the plasma. Furthermore albumin prefers free fatty acids and the fraction of bound tryptophan varies inversely with the plasma fatty acid level and it is the free fraction that competes with the branched chain amino acids for entry into the brain. Newsholme (32) points out that when the plasma free fatty acid concentration exceeds approximately 1 mM there is a rise in free tryptophan. Importance is placed on factors that would either change the concentration of the branched chain amino acids or the free fatty acids. During intense exercise there would be little change in either factor but in prolonged exercise several aspects can change. It is well known that insulin levels decline and also that catecholamines increase. These can elevate free fatty acid levels and hence increase the free fraction of tryptophan. In addition the active muscle can extract plasma branched chain amino acids and so both actions could increase the TRP/BCAA ratio. Newsholme (32) proposes that the resulting shift increases the brain serotonin and promotes central perceptions of fatigue.

There is very limited experimental knowledge in this area. Blomstrand and coworkers (33) examined rats following sustained running to complete exhaustion. They found that the plasma TRP/BCAA ratio was elevated (due mainly to an increase in the free/bound tryptophan) and the serotonin concentration was increased 15% in the brain stem and hypothalamus. Of course it is speculative as to what is the functional significance of these changes. These workers subsequently studied humans running in a marathon. They administered branched chain amino acids to half of the runners prior to the race but they did not control the intake of fluids either as water or as carbohydrate/electrolyte solutions during the race. Thus the study is questionable. Furthermore performance was not improved unless only the slower runners(3:05–3:30 h) were examined separately. Even then there was only a 3% improvement. The administration of branched chain amino acids is probably not the best way in which to alter the TRP/BCAA ratio; while it certainly lowers the ratio it also results in a large increase in the plasma ammonia concentration (4,34) and we have recently observed that this is due to a large increase in the activation of BCKAD in the active muscle.

Davis et al (35) had cyclists ride to exhaustion and they ingested either a placebo or a 6 or a 12% carbohydrate solution both prior to and during the exercise. Carbohydrates resulted in an increase in endurance and in plasma insulin. There was also a lower concentration of plasma free fatty acids and together with this, less free tryptophan and a lower TRP/BCAA ratio. Of course it is unknown whether the endurance benefit came from the carbohydrate or from the TRP/BCAA shift. In contrast Madsen et al (unpublished observations) have recently completed a similar study. Their cyclists ingested either placebo or carbohydrate or carbohydrate plus branched chain amino acids. There was no difference in performance and the carbohydrate–branched chain amino acid trial had greater plasma ammonia levels.

This theory remains as a theory and since it involves the central nervous system it will be difficult to examine in any detail. Perhaps it will require the use of pharmacological treatments to influence the synthesis and degradation of serotonin to resolve the hypothesis in humans.

4. Peripheral Effects of Ammonia and Associated Amino acids

4.1. Possible Roles of Ammonia in Skeletal Muscle

There have traditionally been four possible roles attributed to ammonia formation in active skeletal muscle. In actual fact several of these should be proposed for the PNC or at least AMP deamination rather than to ammonia itself.

It has been suggested that ammonia will act as a buffer against metabolic acidosis. With a pKa of 9.3 it will be predominantly in the form of ammonium ion in physiological solutions. However, there is a large disparity in the capacity for ammonia and lactate production (table 1 and 2); for example in several minutes of strenuous exercise we estimated that the net ammonia formation was 2 mmoles while that of lactate was 127 mmoles (8) and corresponding values for an hour of moderately strenuous exercise were 4.4 and 92.6 mmoles (17). Thus the buffering capacity of ammonia must be very minor.

It has also been suggested that ammonia is a modulator of the key glycolytic enzyme, phosphofructokinase. However, it is not generally viewed as an important regulator and there are many examples where the rates of ammonia and lactate formation vary independent of each other. For example, we observed that ammonia formation continues to rise during prolonged exercise while lactate formation increases early in the activity and then decreases (17,36) and during the breathing of hyperoxic gas lactate formation is depressed while ammonia formation is not altered (36).

The third putative role is for the prevention of adenosine nucleotide degradation, i.e. by forming ammonia (and IMP) the accumulation of AMP is less. If AMP accumulates presumably some would be degraded to adenosine. However, this apparent advantage of conserving the adenosine nucleotide pool is more accurately attributed to the AMP deaminase process than to ammonia per se. Furthermore it would only be associated with ammonia if the ammonia is formed from AMP deamination (as opposed to amino acid degradation) and if there is no PNC cycling.

The fourth possible role is that of maintaining a high ATP/ADP ratio. As mentioned earlier the assumed purpose of AMP deamination is to attenuate the rise in AMP which in turn creates an environment in which ATP formation via adenylate kinase reaction would proceed. Again this is a property of the process of AMP deamination rather than something that can be directly attributed to ammonia. Furthermore it would not be associated with ammonia formed by amino acid deamination.

In addition to these commonly listed possible roles ammonia formation due to amino acid deamination is associated with anaplerotic actions for the TCA cycle both when aspartate goes to fumarate in the PNC (figure 2) or when branched chain amino acids are catabolized to succinyl CoA and/or acetyl CoA (figure 3). If these actions are important it is most likely to be during prolonged exercise as discussed below.

Besides these possible actions ammonia has been associated with fatigue processes within the muscle, i.e. local or peripheral fatigue. Brouns et al (15) examined endurance cyclists during extremely long rides and speculated that muscle cramps and fatigue were caused by ammonia influencing the muscle membrane potential. This is rather similar to the possibility that ammonia is influencing the central nervous system in that the muscle ammonia levels do not get very high compared to those of in vitro studies and the high levels only occur transiently. There is also the possibility that the muscle ammonia acts as a stimulant to the peripheral sensory nervous system. In addition to the Ia, Ib and II afferents which originate from muscle spindles, Golgi tendon organs and Pacinian corpuscles, skeletal muscle has group III and IV afferents. Their receptors are "free" nerve terminals or unencapsulated nerve endings. These receptors are responsible for reflex cardiovascular responses that occur with static contractions (37) and some of the receptors are termed nociceptors. These are activated by noxious chemical stimuli and are responsible for the sensation of muscle pain. Rotto and Kaufman (38) demonstrated that lactate, adenosine and inorganic phosphate were ineffective stimuli of these group III and IV afferents, while lactic acid and cyclo–oxygenase products (prostaglandins and thromboxanes) were potent stimuli. Lewis and Haller (39) speculated that ammonia would also be a stimulus since McArdle's patients have an exaggerated ammonia production and pressor responses to dynamic exercise. This is still open to speculation, but in a preliminary report they found that ammonia had little or no effect on these afferents (40).

In 1990 two investigators (4,41) proposed that a decrease in the TCA intermediates during prolonged exercise may be the main fatigue factor. This is a very interesting proposition and it is fascinating that while both scientists put forward the same theory and both link it to increased ammonia production and decreased carbohydrate supply, the fundamental nature of their proposed mechanisms is completely different!. Perhaps this is the best reflection of the controversy and complexity of this field when two excellent scientists propose similar explanations for fatigue but have very different mechanisms for the same factors. It is well documented that during prolonged exercise there is a continuous and progressive release of ammonia from active muscle (13,17). It has also been accepted for decades that carbohydrate supply, mainly as muscle glycogen is a major limiting factor in prolonged exercise, i.e. when the glycogen stores become low the person must stop or at least decrease the power output. Traditionally it has been stated that while there are abundant fat stores available the maximal rate of ATP supply from fats is limiting.

However, both of the present theories suggest that as fatigue approaches there is a progressive decline in TCA intermediates either because they are involved in other reactions or because there is a slowing of some of the anaplerotic reactions. This in turn might result in a decreased capacity to maintain a high rate of ATP production. Sahlin and coworkers (41) made a detailed study of the TCA intermediates during 75 minutes of exhaustive exercise. They found that there was an initial 10–fold rise in TCA intermediates and that this slowly decreased over the course of the exercise to only 68% of the initial rise. However, it was still 6–fold greater than the rest level. They propose that as the carbohydrate supply decreases, the rate of glycolysis declines. This results in less pyruvate and phosphoenolpyruvate being available for the synthesis of TCA cycle intermediates. The reduced flux through the TCA cycle and thus decreased aerobic ATP supply causes an increase in cytosolic ADP, AMP, Pi and creatine. These would both lead to a greater AMP deamination and ammonia production as well as stimulation of the regulatory enzymes of the TCA cycle by ADP and Pi. To a degree this argument seems circuitous and it hinges on the ammonia production being related to only AMP deamination. It is clear that the ammonia production during most of the duration of prolonged exercise is not associated with IMP accumulation and thus AMP deamination is not the source. Furthermore, it is clear that branched chain amino acids are oxidized in muscle during prolonged exercise (2,6) and this would provide TCA intermediates as would PNC cycling. Furthermore, one might expect to observe a decrease in VO_2 and an increase in NADH if mitochondrial function is impaired and these were not observed in the study by Sahlin. In addition we (42) found that at the point of exhaustion in prolonged exercise the muscle acetyl CoA concentration was 1.3–fold greater than rest. Thus it is difficult to accept that the TCA cycle is limiting.

Wagenmakers and coworkers (4,43) have made a proposal quite similar to that of Sahlin. They suggest that there is a depletion of TCA intermediates at exhaustion and that it is associated with ammonia metabolism. However, in their theory the ammonia is derived from the deamination of the branched chain amino acids. They have demonstrated that the activity of the BCKAD increases as the glycogen stores are depleted (43) and if carbohydrate is given during the exercise the enzyme's activity declines (4) as does plasma ammonia. We (44) have shown that giving a branched chain amino acid supplement results in increased plasma ammonia and recently (unpublished data) have found that there is an increase in ammonia production and a marked increase in BCKAD activity. This demonstrates that the rate of this pathway is sensitive to substrate supply. Since the branched chain aminotransferase requires alpha ketoglutarate Waganmakers suggests that this acts as a drain

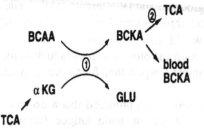

Figure 7. A scheme to illustrate how branched chain amino acid deamination could lower TCA intermediates (adapted from Wagenmakers (4,43)). When branched chain amino acids are transaminated they take alpha ketoglutarate from the TCA. The keto acids may leave the muscle or form TCA intermediates (reaction (2)). Depending on this and the fate of the glutamate (Glu) (see figure 4) there could be an impact on the TCA.

on the TCA cycle (figure 7). The fate of the products of the transamination are critical to this theory; if the branched chain keto acids leave the muscle and if the glutamate proceeds on to glutamine and is released (figure 4) then the theory would be supported. Our understanding of the fate of the keto acids is incomplete, but it appears that oxidation within the muscle is likely (45). This is supported by the increased activation of the BCKAD and the fact that it is greater when there is more branched chain amino acids available. If this is the case then the oxidation would provide succinyl CoA and acetyl CoA. The fate of the glutamate is more difficult to resolve. Certainly there is glutamine formation, but glutamate is also involved in alanine and aspartate synthesis. Both would regenerate the alpha ketoglutarate and the latter would also provide fumarate for the TCA cycle (figure 4). One could argue that the alanine formation would be a drain on pyruvate and thus indirectly a loss for the TCA cycle, but in prolonged exercise we estimated that at most 1% of the pyruvate goes to alanine (17) (table 1 and 2). In our experience active muscle releases similar amounts of glutamine, ammonia and alanine throughout prolonged exercise. Both of these theories are interesting and hopefully will stimulate more research. However, at this time it seems unlikely that either of them is correct. There have been two studies that have examined ammonia and fatigue in a more general manner. Miller–Graber and coworkers (46) administered ammonium acetate to horses and exercised them to exhaustion with an exercise intensity that lead to fatigue in 15–20 minutes. They observed no difference in exhaustion time even though the plasma ammonia was 200uM at exhaustion after the ammonium acetate rather than 110 uM as in the control; in fact there was a tendency for a longer endurance time with the ammonium load and the ventilation also tended to be lower not higher! Similarly Beaunoyer et al (47) infused monosodium glutamate into horses and ran them to exhaustion with intense exercise. The infusion resulted in almost 50% less increase in plasma ammonia and yet there was a nonsignificant decrease in exercise time (3:55 vs 3:30 minutes for control and treatment respectively). Neither of these studies suggest that ammonia has any relationship with any aspect of fatigue.

5. Concluding Remarks

The metabolism of ammonia in active skeletal muscle clearly elevates both the intramuscular and the plasma concentrations of ammonia. The roles of the various metabolic pathways in the production of ammonia are not clear. It is likely that AMP deamination is dominant in intense exercise lasting only a few minutes and that branched chain amino acid oxidation is a major factor in prolonged exercise. The rise in plasma ammonia is associated with rapid responses by tissues involved in clearance. However, even the relative importance of each of these tissues remains to be established. There have been suggestions about the possible roles of ammonia accumulation in muscle, but it is likely that it is a "necessary evil" and any functional roles are attributed to associated changes in metabolic modulators such as AMP and IMP and to increased production of TCA intermediates. Ammonia and some amino acids have been speculated to alter brain function, but there is little evidence for this. Similarly ammonia production has been suggested to result in fatigue in the active muscle during prolonged exercise, but again the evidence is lacking.

Acknowledgements: The work of the author has been supported by NSERC of Canada. The author gratefully acknowledges the outstanding support of Premila Sathasivam as research assistant as well as the excellent support of many collaborative scientists.

References

1. Graham, T. E., Rush, J. W. E., and MacLean, D. A. 1994, Skeletal muscle amino acid metabolism and ammonia production during exercise. Chapter 5 in Exercise Metabolism. Edited by M. Hargreaves. Human Kinetics, Champaign, Illinois, in press.
2. Graham, T.E., and MacLean, D.A. 1992, Ammonia and amino acid metabolism in human skeletal muscle during exercise. Can. J. Physiol. Pharmacol. **70**:132–141.
3. Lowenstein, J.M. 1990, The purine nucleotide cycle revised. Int. J. Sports Med. **11**:537–546.
4. Wagenmakers, A.J.M., Coakley, J.H., and Edwards, R.H.T. 1990, Metabolism of branched-chain amino acids and ammonia during exercise. Clues from McArdle's disease. Int. J. Sports Med. **11**:S101–S113.
5. Tullson, P.C., and Terjung, R.L. 1991, Adenine nucleotide metabolism in contracting skeletal muscle. Ex. Sports Sci. Rev. **19**:507–537.
6. Hood, D.A., and Terjung, R.L. 1990, Amino acid metabolism during exercise and following endurance training. Sports Med. **9**:23–35.
7. Eriksson, L.S., Broberg, S., Bjorkman, O., and Wahren, J. 1985, Ammonia metabolism during exercise in man. Clin. Physiol. (Oxf) **5**:325–336.
8. Graham, T.E., Bangsbo, J., Gollnick, P.D., Juel, C., and Saltin, B. 1990, Ammonia metabolism during intense dynamic exercise and recovery in humans. Am. J. Physiol. **259** (Endocrinol. Metab. 22):E170–E176.
9. Katz, A., Broberg, S., Sahlin, K., and Wahren, J. 1986, Muscle ammonia and amino acid metabolism during dynamic exercise in man. Clin. Physiol. (Oxf) **6**:365–379.
10. Rundell, K.W., Tullson, P.C., and Terjung, R.L. 1992, AMP deaminase binding in contracting rat skeletal muscle. Am. J. Physiol. **263**:C287–C293.
11. Rundell, K.W., Tullson, P.C., and Terjung, R.L. 1992, Altered kinetics of AMP deaminase by myosin binding. Am. J. Physiol. **263**:C294–C299.
12. Rush, J. W. E., MacLean, D. A., and Graham, T. E. 1993, Branched chain keto acid dehydrogenase and AMP deaminase activities in skeletal muscle. Can. J. Appl. Physiol. **18**:432P.
13. Broberg, S., and Sahlin, K. 1989, Adenine nucleotide degradation in human skeletal muscle during prolonged exercise. J. Appl. Physiol. **67**:116–122.
14. Hood, A. D., and Parent, G. 1991, Metabolic and contractile responses of rat fast-twitch muscle to 10-Hz stimulation. Am. J. Physiol. **260**:C832–C840.
15. Brouns, F., Beckers, E., Wagenmakers, A. J. M., and Saris, W. H. M. 1990, Ammonia accumulation during highly intensive long-lasting cycling: individual observations. Int. J. Sports Med. **11**(Suppl 2):S78–S84.

16. Coakley, J. H., Wagenmakers, A. J. M., and Edwards, R. H. T. 1992, Relationship between ammonia, heart rate, and exertion in McArdle's disease. Am. J. Physiol. **262**:E167–172.

17. Graham, T.E., Kiens, B., Hargreaves, M., and Richter, E.A. 1991, Influence of fatty acids on ammonia and amino acid flux from active human muscle. Am. J. Physiol. **261**:E168–E176.

18. Harris, R. C., Marlin, D. J., and Snow, D. H. 1991, Lactate kinetics, plasma ammonia and performance following repeated bouts of maximal exercise. Equine Exerc. Physiol. **3**:173–178.

19. Miller, P., Lawrence, L., Kline, K., Kane, R., Kurcz, E., Smith, J., Fisher, M., Siegel, A., and Bump, K. 1987, Plasma ammonia and other metabolites in the racing standardbred. Proceedings of the tenth equine nutrition and physiology symposium:397–402.

20. Sewell, D. A., and Harris, R. C. 1992, Adenine nucleotide degradation in the thoroughbred horse with increasing exercise duration. Eur. J. Appl. Physiol. **65**:271–277.

21. Ahlborg, G., Felig, P., Hagenfeldt, L., Hendler, R., and Wahren, J. 1974, Substrate turnover during prolonged exercise in man. J. Clin. Invest. **53**:1080–1090.

22. Felig, P., and Wahren, J. 1971, Amino acid metabolism in exercising man. J. Clin. Invest. **50**:2703–2714.

23. Wahren, J., Felig, P., and Hagenfeldt, L. 1976, Effect of protein ingestion on splanchnic and leg metabolism in normal man and in patients with diabetes mellitus. J. Clin. Invest. **57**:987–999.

24. Carraro, F., Stuart, C. A., Hartl, W. H., Rosenblatt, J., and Wolfe, R. R. 1990, Whole body and plasma protein synthesis in exercise and recovery in human subjects. Am. J. Physiol. **259**:E821–E831.

25. Lemon, P.W.R. 1987, Protein and exercise: update. 1987, Med. Sci. Sports **19**:S179–S190.

26. Czarnowski, D., and Gorski, J. 1991, Sweat ammonia excretion during submaximal cycling exercise. J. Appl. Physiol. **70**:371–374, 1991.

27. Cooper, A.J.L., and Plum, F. 1987, Biochemistry and physiology of brain ammonia. Physiol. Rev. **67**:440–519.

28. Wichser, J., and Kazemi, H. 1974, Ammonia and ventilation: site and mechanism of action. Resp. Physiol. **20**:393–406.

29. Chiang, C–H., Pappagianopoulos, P., Hoop, B., and Kazemi, H. 1986, Central cardiorespiratory effects of glutamate in dogs. J. Appl. Physiol. **60**:2056–2062.

30. Spodaryk, K., Szmatlan, U., and Berger, L. 1990, The relationship of ammonia and lactate concentrations to perceived exertion in trained and untrained women. Eur. J. Appl. Physiol. **61**:309–312.

31. Banister, E.W., and Cameron, B.J.C. 1990, Exercise–induced hyperammonemia: peripheral and central effects. Int. J. Sports Med. **11**(Suppl 2):S129–S142.

32. Newsholme, E. A., Calder, P., and Yaqoob, P. 1993, The regulatory, infomational, and immunomodulatory roles of fat fuels. Am. J. Clin. Nutr. **57**(suppl):738S–&51S.

33. Blomstrand, E., Perrett, D., Parry–Billings, M., and Newsholme, E. A. 1989, Effect of sustained exercise on plasma amino acid concentrations and on 5–hydroxytryptamine metabolism in six different brain regeons in the rat. Acta Physiol. Scand. **136**:473–481.

34. MacLean, D.A., and Graham, 1993, T.E. Branched chain amino acid supplementation augments plasma ammonia responses during exercise in humans. J. Appl. Physiol. **74**:2711–2717.

35. Davis, J. M., Bailey, S. P., Woods, J. A., Galiano, F. J., Hamilton, M. T., and Bartoli, W. P. 1992, Effects of carbohydrate feedings on plasma free tryptophan and branched–chain amino acids during prolonged cycling. Eur. J. Appl. Physiol. **65**:513–519.

36. Graham, T.E., Pedersen, P.K., and Saltin, B. 1987, Muscle and blood ammonia and lactate responses to prolonged exercise with hyperoxia. J. Appl. Physiol. **63**:1457–1462.

37. Mitchell, J.H. 1990, Neural control of the circulation during exercise. Med. Sci. Sports Exerc. **22**:141–154.

38. Rotto, D.M., and Kaufman, M.P. 1988, Effect of metabolic products of muscular contraction on discharge of group III and IV afferents. J. Appl. Physiol. **64**:2306–2313.

39. Lewis, S.F., and Haller, R.G. 1986, The pathopohysiology of McArcle's disease: clues to regulation in exercise and fatigue. J. Appl. Physiol. **61**:391–401.

40. Lewis, S.F., and Kaufman, M.P. 1985, Lack of pressor response to ammonium chloride injections in cat hindlimb. Physiologist **28**:292.

41. Sahlin, K., Katz, A., and Broberg, S. 1990, Tricarboxylic acid cycle intermediates in human muscle during prolonged exercise. Am. J. Physiol. **259:**C834–C841.

42. Spriet, L.L., MacLean, D.A., Dyck, D.J., Hultman, E., Cederblad, G., and Graham, T.E. 1992, Caffeine ingestion and muscle metabolism during prolonged exercise in humans. Am. J. Physiol. **262:**E891–898.

43. Wagenmakers, A. J. M., Beckers, E. J., Brouns, F., Kuipers, H., Soeters, P. B., Van Der Vusse, G., and Saris, W. H. M. 1991, Carbohydrate supplementation, glycogen depletion, and amino acid metabolism during exercise. Am. J. Physiol. **260:**E883–890.

44. MacLean, D.A., Spriet, L.L., Hultman, E., and Graham, T.E. 1991, Plasma and muscle amino acid and ammonia responses during prolonged exercise in humans J. Appl. Physiol. **70:**2095–2103.

45. Rennie, M.J., Edwards, R.H.T., Krywawych, S., Davies, C.T.M., Halliday, D., Waterlow, J.C., and Millward, D.J. 1981, Effect of exercise on protein turnover in man. Clin. Sci. **61:**627–639.

46. Miller–Graber, P., Lawrence, L., Fisher, M., Bump, K., Foreman, J., and Kurcz, E. 1991, Metabolic responses to ammonium acetate infusion in exercising horses. Cornell Vet. **81:**397–410.

47. Beaunoyer, D. E., Jackson, S. G., Gillespie, J. R., and Baker, J. P. 1991, The effect of monosodium glutamate infusion on time to fatigue. Equine Exerc. Physiol. **3:**209–214.

Possible Role of Ammonia in the Brain in Dementia of Alzheimer Type

Siegfried Hoyer

1. Introduction

Dementia of Alzheimer type (DAT) is not a single homogenous disorder. A distinction should necessarily be made between the genetically induced (1,2,3) and the sporadically induced forms. However, a common pathobiochemical feature was found in the drastically reduced cerebral metabolic rate (CMR) of glucose. The diminution in cerebral glucose utilization was more prominent in cerebral association cortex in early–onset genetically induced DAT, whereas in late–onset sporadic DAT, CMR glucose was rather globally reduced (4,5).

In the mature, healthy, nonstarved mammalian brain, glucose is the only substrate for oxydation (6,7), and thus for the formation of energy in the form of ATP (8) to maintain normal cellular work. Also, glucose carbon is rapidly transferred into amino acids via the tricarboxylic acid cycle. Glutamate, glutamine, aspartate and GABA are formed in largest quantities (9). At least two compartments of these acidic amino acids, one of which is a storage compartment, are postulated in the brain. The glucoplastic amino acids may serve in part as a fuel reserve for emergency conditions when glucose is lacking. Moreover, glutamate and aspartate function as excitatory, and GABA and glycine as inhibitory amino acid neurotransmitters.

Thus, it may be supposed that any change in glucose supply to the brain, and any perturbation in neuronal glucose metabolism is able to vary considerably the formation of ATP, and the metabolism of amino acids mentioned.

In this short overview, perturbations in cerebral oxidative energy metabolism, and in related amino acid metabolism in incipient DAT states are demonstrated. The abnormalities in cerebral ammonia metabolism are discussed with respect to its impacts on brain morphology and pathobiochemistry.

2. Subjects and Methods

2.1. Subjects

The groups of subjects studied were as follows:
1. Physically and mentally healthy young adult volunteers (HYAV): n=15; age 24 ± 2 yr; mostly medical students (7).

Professor for Experimental Neurology & Psychiatry. Brain Metabolism Group, Department of Pathochemistry & General Neurochemistry, University of Heidelberg, 69120 Heidelberg, FRG

Hepatic Encephalopathy, Hyperammonemia, and Ammonia Toxicity
Edited by V. Felipo and S. Grisolia, Plenum Press, New York, 1994

197

2. Healthy middle–aged controls (HMAC): n=11; age 44 ± 11 yr; subjects with a complete check–up (10).

3. Early–onset dementia of Alzheimer type (EODAT): n=20; age 46 ± 9 yr; incipient cases with histories of about 4 mo; four patients with suspected "familial" DAT (10).

4. Late–onset dementia of Alzheimer type (LODAT), subdivided into incipient (inc.) and stable advanced (adv.) LODAT: inc. LODAT: n=11; age 66 ± 5 yr; history going back less than 2 yr; adv. LODAT: n=7; age 75 ± 5 yr (I), during the second study 75.5 ± 5 yr (II); history of 8–12 yr (4).

All DAT patients suffered from severe rather than moderate dementia symptoms, which had been verified by a battery of psychometric tests. Patients with EODAT and inc. LODAT underwent EEG, CT of the brain, and intensive physical examinations. The latter revealed no risk factors, no endocrine abnormalities, no vitamin deficits, and so forth. In particular, normoglycemia and normoketonemia were present in incipient EODAT and LODAT (medical records endorsed: physically healthy except for brain function). In advanced LODAT normoglycemia existed. During the measurement of cerebral blood flow and the respective cerebral metabolic rates, all subjects studied were in a steady state of individual arterial normotension, of arterial normoglycemia, normocapnia, and normoxemia and in normothermia. For further detailed diagnostic criteria, ascertainment of diagnosis, inclusion criteria, exclusion criteria, and consent procedure, see (4,10).

Since we did not have a group of healthy elderly controls above the age of 60 yr in our sample of normal subjects, the data reported for normal elderly men (NEM; n=26; age 71 ± 1 yr) were taken from the literature (1,12) and were also used in calculation of the ATP production rate.

2.2. Methods

The CMRs of oxygen, CO_2, glucose and lactate and also cerebral blood flow were studied in the subjects detailed earlier by means of a modified Kety–Schmidt technique (13). The cerebral arteriovenous differences for amino acids and ammonia were obtained by the same procedure. Their concentrations were determined by the method of Moore and Stein (14,15). For further methodological details see (10).

Statistical significances were tested by means of Student's two–tailed t–test. Statistical significance was assumed at $p < 0.05$.

3. Results

In Table 1, the CMRs of oxygen, CO_2, oxidized glucose, the formation rate of ATP and the glucose oxidation ratio of the different subject groups studied are listed.

The above data demonstrate that the cerebral oxidative energy metabolism is maintained over a long period of life. In contrast, glucose metabolism and ATP formation are severely perturbed in all states of DAT studied. It also became obvious that in incipient DAT, glucose utilization was more marked damaged than oxygen utilization. Otherwise, in advanced disease states, the fall in oxygen utilization was more drastic than in glucose utilization. The findings on the CMR of oxygen as related to the CMR of glucose, also show that both parameters are balanced in the control groups but that not all oxygen utilized for glucose oxidation, utilized by the brain, is used for this purpose in DAT. It is assumed that the oxygen "surplus" is used to oxidize substrates other than glucose to improve the ATP formation (Table 2). The changes found in cerebral amino acid metabolism are listed in Table 3.

Table 1. CMR of oxygen (O_2), CMR of CO_2, CMR of oxidized glucose ($Gluc_{ox}$), ATP formation rate from glucose and glucose oxidation ratio (GOR) in mentally healthy and demented subjects

	O_2	CO_2	$GLUC_{ox}$	ATP	GOR
HYAV	1.58	1.68	0.26	9.36	0.99
HMAC	1.54	1.67	0.26	9.36	1.01
NEM	1.49		0.24	8.64	
inc.EODAT	1.45	1.50	0.12*	4.32*	0.50*
inc.LODAT	1.27*	1.24*	0.14*	5.04*	0.66*
adv.LODAT I	1.03*	1.13*	0.11*	3.96*	0.64*
adv.LODAT II	0.73*	0.78*	0.09*	3.24*	0.74*

Mean values and statistically significant differences have been taken from (16). For calculation procedures, see also (16). Data except GOR in mol/gxmin.
*$p < 0.05$ from HMAC

4. Discussion

With respect to the cerebral glucose/energy metabolism, there are striking similarities in the pathobiochemical features of both EODAT and LODAT in incipient states although there is clear evidence that the energy deficit due to the lacking glucose can be compensated nearly completely by the oxidation of substrates other than glucose in EODAT. The proportion of the latter was found to be 50% in incipient EODAT, more than 30% in incipient LODAT, and between 30% and 25% in advanced LODAT (Table 2). Evidence was provided that fatty acids derived from phospholipid breakdown were among the substitution substrates (17,18). With respect to amino acids, the glutamate concentration was diminished predominantly in temporal cerebral cortex but the concentrations of aspartate, alanine and serine were enhanced in the same area (19,20,21,22,23). These data may coincide with the results presented in Table 3. Glutamate can be assumed to be utilized in the aspartate aminotransferase reaction to form alpha–ketoglutarate and aspartate, the latter being enhanced in tissue (22) and cerebral venous blood (24). Otherwise, amino acids such as alanine, serine, and glycine, which are related to the alanine aminotransferase reaction, were found to be augmented in tissue and released from the brain. Since this reaction needs pyruvate as a substrate which is less available in DAT brain, it can be assumed that these amino acids are not utilized under these abnormal conditions. The massive release of ammonia from DAT brain (25), its possible sources and impacts on cellular metabolism will be discussed below in more detail.

The data presented in Table 3 clearly show that ammonia was taken up by the brain in a smaller amount under normal conditions (group HYAV), but was released from the brain in a high amount under the condition of incipient DAT in normoammonemia (7,25). It was concluded that ammonia was formed in the brain in the latter condition, which is different

Table 2. ATP formation in DAT brain from substrates other than glucose, and total amount of ATP formation. DATA from (16); *$p < 0.05$ from HMAC

	O_2 surplus	Substrates other than glucose. μ mol/g x min	ATP formation	Total glucose/other substrates
inc.EODAT	0.73	4.38	8.70	1:1
inc.LODAT	0.43	2.58	7.62*	2:1
inc.LODAT I	0.37	2.22	6.18*	2:1
inc.LODAT II	0.19	1.14	4.38*	3:1

Table 3. CMRs of amino acids in HYAV and incipient EODAT. Values are expressed as amino-N.

	HYAV	inc. EODAT	Ratio HYAV/DAT
glutamate	−0.030	−0.124	1:4 n.s.
serine	−0.111	−0.572	1:5 n.s.
aspartate	−0.008	−0.139	1:17*
alanine	+0.000	−0.394	*
glycine	−0.022	−0.455	1:21*
ammonia	+0.059	−0.121	*
total	−0.009	−0.293	1:33*

+: cerebral uptake
−: cerebral release
ns: not significant
*p < 0.05 between the groups studied

from chronic dementia states in which an only very small amount of ammonia was found to be released from the brain (26). When arterial ammonia was enhanced due to liver cirrhosis, cerebral glucose utilization increased markedly. In a subgroup of the patients studied, a release of glutamate (less pronounced) and of glutamine (more pronounced) was found. Patients with an additional reduced CMR of oxygen and EEG abnormalities had a poor prognosis in respect to life expectancy (27,28). The data indicate that, in principle, the brain is able to detoxify ammonia by binding to alpha-ketoglutarate and glutamate to form glutamine which is released from the brain (29). Different sources of ammonia formation are conceivable in incipient DAT brain. The most probable one is glutamine which is deaminated to form glutamate and ammonia. The activity of glutaminase was found not to be varied in DAT brain (22) whereas the activity of glutamine synthetase was diminished subsequent to excess protein oxidation (30). With respect to the consequence of the perturbed glucose metabolism, different experimental designs provided clear evidence that lacking glucose is substituted by glutamate which is metabolized in the aspartate aminotransferase reaction first. When CMR of glucose had dropped to 54% of control, the energy metabolism was fully maintained by way of glutamate substitution. However, when neuroglucopenia sustained for four hours, glutamate is also metabolized in the alanine aminotransferase reaction (31,32). In either case, ammonia formation increased steadily and was 15-fold, and glutamate concentration fell in the same manner, and was only 22% of control after four hours of absence of glucose (31).

Another important source of ammonia formation is assumed to be the purine nucleotide cycle (33). The catabolism of both AMP and adenosine yields ammonia. When CMR of glucose was around 40% of control, cerebral energy formation could not be maintained in spite of intense catabolism of amino acids. Energy turnover and AMP formation increased markedly (32). The latter may be assumed not to be recharged which also held true after ischemic stress during the postischemic recirculation period (34). The metabolic feature discussed above may be assumed to be also present in incipient DAT brain as can be deduced from the data presented in Table 3, and from the increased concentrations of xanthine and uric acid in the cerebrospinal fluid (35). In contrast, dopamine may not play a decisive role as a source of ammonia in DAT brain because this monoaminergic catecholamine is less involved in the pathobiochemistry of this disorder (36).

Morphological consequences related to increased ammonia concentration in cerebral tissue occur mostly in astrocytes in general. Alzheimer type II astrocytes have been found in gray matter showing an enlarged clear appearance with a large vesicular nucleus. With respect to DAT, Alzheimer himself described glial cells with enlarged nuclei and an enhanced formation of fibrillary glial cells, particularly in deeper cortical layers (37). More recently, laminar gliosis of the layers II, III, and V in cerebral association cortex has been reported in DAT (38). Interestingly, these layers were found to be particularly involved in DAT (39,40). In the very early phase preceding neuronal drop–out, paired astrocytic nuclei and reactive fibrillary astrocytes have been frequently found (41). Reactive gliosis is a common feature after damage to the brain (42), and reactive astrocytes characterized by enormous glial fibrillary acidic protein positive cell bodies and thick, long, intensely stained processes expressed the amyloid precursor protein (APP) (43). Although reactive gliosis is present due to enhanced ammonia concentration, no increase in glial fibrillary acidic protein was found (44,45). As yet, no studies have been performed to investigate APP expression at enhanced ammonia concentration although the latter has been demonstrated to influence the cleavage of APP (46,47).

In numerous studies, the divers effects of ammonia on brain metabolism have been described (for review 48,49). Here, it is focused on abnormalities occurring in oxidative glucose/energy metabolism in the CNS. However, it has to be determined that the results diverge in part considerably because of the different experimental designs used: acute or chronic enhancement of ammonia, in vivo and in vitro studies. This has to be taken into consideration for the discussion of the following data. Cerebral glucose consumption was found not to be impaired in the absence of net glutamine synthesis (50). Although the activities of pyruvate dehydrogenase, isocitrate dehydrogenase, alpha–ketoglutarate dehydrogenase and succinate dehydrogenase were shown to be enhanced (51), the formation of energy–rich phosphates is diminished (52,53). In contrast to the above discussed possibility that the activities of aspartate aminotransferase and alanine aminotransferase increase when glucose is lacking, ammonia augmentation led to a reduction in the activity of aspartate aminotransferase (51,54). From the neurotransmitter systems involved (55), the variations found in the acetylcholinergic system are of particular significance. The increase in brain ammonia content raised the activity of acetylcholinesterase in isolated synaptosomes (56). More generally, the changes which became obvious in neurotransmitter systems were assumed to be due to alterations in the biophysical properties of membranes (57,58).

From the data discussed above, it may be deduced that the enhanced ammonia concentration in the brain irrespective of its extracerebral or intracerebral source may contribute to divers pathobiochemical abnormalities also present in DAT brain. In contrast to other investigations (59,60), we did not find an increased level of arterial ammonia in well–nursed DAT patients included in our studies. Therefore, the augmentation in brain ammonia concentration is based on inherent cerebral sources. As was demonstrated in Tables 1 and 2, ATP production is drastically reduced in incipient DAT states obviously due to reduced activities in enzyme complexes with dehydrogenating capacity (for review see 16,61). As mentioned above, such enzyme activities are not decreased and are rather increased subsequent to enhanced ammonia concentration so that the possible effect of ammonia on energy production will have to be clarified. The assumed alterations in the biophysical properties of membranes are suspicious to be due to variations in the phospholipid composition of membranes. In DAT brain, evidence has been provided that a membrane defect exists due to a loss in phosphatidylcholine and phosphatidylethanolamine (18). It is as yet unresolved whether or not ammonia induces alterations in the phospholipid composition of membrane of same kind. In DAT brain, acetylcholine synthesis is diminished to 47% of control (62) which contributes considerably to the predominance of the clinical symptoms memory loss and cognition disturbances. Therefore, one of the goals in DAT therapy is to lower acetylcholine catabolism by means of blocking the activity of the enzyme acetylcholine esterase. Enhanced brain ammonia concentration increased the activity of acetylcholine esterase (see above) and thus catabolism of acetylcholine what may result in a deterioration of the reduced memory and cognition capacities.

4.2. Conclusion

Ammonia exerts a variety of detrimental effects on neuronal function. With respect to incipient DAT, ammonia is formed in the brain and may be supposed to deteriorate the disease-originated disturbances in membrane stability and neurotransmission mediated by acetylcholine. Thus, ammonia is an important pathobiochemical factor in the cascade of cell damaging events occurring in DAT (63,64). However, further studies are necessary to evaluate the exact contribution of ammonia to this damage.

References

1. St.George-Hyslop, P.H., Haines, J.L., Farrer, L.A., Polinsky, R., van Broeckhoven, C., Goate, A., Crapper McLachlan, D.R., Orr, H., Bruni, A.C., Sorbi, S., et al., 1990, Genetic linkage studies suggest that Alzheimer's disease is not a single homogenous disorder, Nature 347:194–197.

2. Pericak-Vance, M.A., Bebout, J.L., Gaskell jr., P.C., Yamaoka, L.H., Hung, W.Y., Alberts, M.J., Walker, A.P., Bartlett, R.J., Haynes, C.A., Welsh, K.A., Earl, N.L., Heyman, A., Clark, C.M. and Roses, A.D., 1991, Linkage studies in familial Alzheimer disease: evidence for chromosome 19 linkage, Am.J.Hum.Genet.48:1034–1050.

3. Schellenberg, G.D., Bird, T.D., Wijsman, E.M., Orr, H.T., Anderson, L., Nemens, E., White, J.A., Bonnycastle, L., Weber, J.L., Alonso, M.E., Potter, H., Heston, L.L., and Martin, G.M., 1992, Genetic linkage evidence for a familial Alzheimer's disease locus on chromosome 14, Science 258:668–671.

4. Hoyer, S., Nitsch, R., and Oesterreich, K., 1991, Predominant abnormality in cerebral glucose utilization in late-onset dementia of the Alzheimer type: a cross-sectional comparison against advanced late-onset and incipient early-onset cases, J.Neural Transm. (P-D Sect) 3:1–14.

5. Mielke, R., Herholz, K., Grond, M., Kessler, J., and Heiss, W.D., 1992, Differences of regional cerebral glucose metabolism between presenile and senile dementia of Alzheimer type, Neurobiol. Aging 13:93–98

6. Cohen, J.P., Alexander, S.C., Smith, T.C., Reivich, M., and Wollman, H., 1967, Effects of hypoxia and normocarbia on cerebral blood flow and metabolism in conscious man, J.Appl.Physiol.23:183–189.

7. Hoyer, S., 1970, Der Aminosäurenstoffwechsel des normalen menschlichen Gehirns, Klin.Wochenschr. 48:1239–1243.

8. Erecinska, M., and Silver, I.A., 1989, ATP and brain function, J.Cereb. Blood Flow Metab. 9:2–19.

9. Wong, K.L., and Tyce, G.M., 1983, Glucose and amino acid metabolism in rat brain during sustained hypoglycemia, Neurochem.Res.8:401–415.

10. Hoyer, S., Oesterreich, K., and Wagner, O., 1988, Glucose metabolism as the site of the primary abnormality in early-onset dementia of Alzheimer type ?, J.Neurol. 235:143–148.

11. Dastur, D.K., Lane, M.H., Hansen, D.B., Kety, S.S., Butler, R.N., Perlin, S., and Sokoloff, L., 1963, Effect of aging on cerebral circulation and metabolism in man, in Birren, J.E., Butler, R.N., Greenhouse, S.W., Sokoloff, L., and Yarrow, M.R. (eds.), US Department of Health, Education, and Welfare (DHEW publication no. 986), Washington DC, pp. 59–76.

12. Dastur, D.K., 1985, Cerebral blood flow and metabolism in normal human aging, pathological aging, and senile dementia, J.Cereb.Blood Flow Metab.5:1–9.

13. Kety, S.S., and Schmidt, C.F., 1948, The nitrous oxide method for the quantitative determination of cerebral blood flow in man: theory, procedure and normal values, J.Clin.Invest.27:476–483.

14. Moore, S., and Stein, W.H., 1954, Procedures for the chromatographic determination of amino acids on four per cent cross-linked sulfonated polystyrene resins, J.Biol.Chem.211:893–906.

15. Moore, S., and Stein, W.H., 1954, A modified ninhydrin reagent for the photometric determination of amino acids and related compounds, J.Biol.Chem. 211:907–913.

16. Hoyer, S., 1992, Oxidative energy metabolism in Alzheimer brain. Studies in early-onset and late-onset cases, Mol.Chem.Neuropathol.16:207–224.

17. Farooqui, A.A., Liss, L., and Horrocks, L.A., 1988, Neurochemical aspects of Alzheimer's disease: Involvement of membrane phospholipids, Metabol.Brain Dis. 3:19–35.

18. Nitsch, R.M., Blusztajn, J.K., Pittas, A.G., Slack, B.E., Growdon, J.H., and Wurtman, R.J., 1992, Evidence for a membrane defect in Alzheimer disease brain, Proc.Natl.Acad.Sci. USA **89**:1671–1675.

19. Arai, H., Kobayashi, K., Ichimiya, Y., Kosaka, K., and Iizuka, R., 1984, A preliminary study of free amino acids in the postmortem temporal cortex from Alzheimer–type dementia patients, Neurobiol. Aging **5**:319–321.

20. Ellison, D.W., Beal, M.F., Mazurek, M.F., Bird, E.D., and Martin, J.B., 1986, A postmortem study of amino acid neurotransmitters in Alzheimer's disease, Ann. Neurol. **20**:616–621.

21. Sasaki, H., Muramoto, O., Kanazawa, I., Arai, H., Kosaka, K., and Iizuka, R., 1986, Regional distribution of amino acid transmitters in postmortem brains and senile dementia of Alzheimer type, Ann.Neurol.**19**:263–269.

22. Procter, A.W., Palmer, A.M., Francis, P.T., Lowe, S.L., Neary, D., Murphy, E., Doshi, R., and Bowen, D.M., 1988, Evidence of glutamatergic denervation and possible abnormal metabolism in Alzheimer's disease, J.Neurochem. **50**:790–802.

23. Lowe, S.L., Bowen, D.M., Francis, P.T., and Neary, D., 1990, Ante mortem cerebral amino acid concentrations indicate selective degeneration of glutamate–enriched neurons in Alzheimer's disease, Neuroscience **38**:571–577.

24. Hoyer, S., and Nitsch, R., 1989, Cerebral excess release of neurotransmitter amino acids subsequent to reduced cerebral glucose metabolism in early–onset dementia of Alzheimer type, J.Neural Transm. **75**:227–232.

25. Hoyer, S., Nitsch, R., and Oesterreich, K., 1990, Ammonia is endogenously generated in the brain in the presence of presumed and verified dementia of Alzheimer type, Neuroscie. Lett.**117**:358–362.

26. Hoyer, S., 1969, Cerebral blood flow and metabolism in senile dementia, in Brock, M., Fieschi, C., Ingvar, D.H., Lassen, N.A., and Schürmann, K. (eds.), Cerebral blood flow. Clinical and experimental results, Springer, Berlin Heidelberg New York, pp. 235–236.

27. Hoyer, S., Papenberg, J., Berendes, K., and Peddinghaus, W.D., 1975, Störungen des Hirnstoffwechsels bei Leberkrankheiten, in Holm, E. (ed.), Ammoniak und hepatische Enzephalopathie, Fischer, Stuttgart, pp. 27–32.

28. Papenberg, J., Lanzinger, G., Kommerell, B., and Hoyer, S., 1975, Comparative studies of the electroencephalogram and the cerebral oxidative metabolism in patients with liver cirrhosis, Klin.Wochenschr. **53**:1107–1113.

29. Berl, S., Takagaki, G., Clarke, D., and Waelsch, H., 1962, Metabolic compartments in vivo. Ammonia and glutamic acid metabolism in brain and liver, J.Biol.Chem. **237**:2562–2569.

30. Smith, C.D., Carney, J.M., Starke–Reed, P.E., Oliver, C.N., Stadtman, E.R., Floyd, R.A. and Markesbery, W.R., 1991, Excess brain protein oxidation and enzyme dysfunction in normal aging and in Alzheimer disease, Proc.Natl.Acad.Sci. USA **88**:10540–10543.

31. Benjamin, A.M., and Quastel, J.H., 1975, Metabolism of amino acids and ammonia in rat brain cortex slices in vitro: a possible role of ammonia in brain function, J.Neurochem.**25**:197–206.

32. Norberg, K., and Siesjö, B.K., 1976, Oxidative metabolism of the cerebral cortex of the rat in severe insulin–induced hypoglycaemia, J.Neurochem. **26**:345–352.

33. Lowenstein, J.M., 1972, Ammonia production in muscle and other tissues: the purine nucleotide cycle, Physiol.Rev.**52**:382–414.

34. Hoyer, S., and Betz, K., 1988, Abnormalities in glucose and energy metabolism are more severe in the hippocampus than in cerebral cortex in postischemic recovery in aged rats, Neurosci. Lett. **94**:167–172.

35. Degrell, I., and Niklasson, F., 1988, Purine metabolites in the CSF in presenile and senile dementia of Alzheimer type, and in multi infarct dementia, Arch.Gerontol.Geriatr.**7**:173–178.

36. Riederer, P., Sofic, E., Moll, G., Freyberger, A., Wichart, I., Gsell, W., Jellinger, K., Hebenstreit, G., and Youdim, M.B.H., 1990, Senile dementia of Alzheimer's type and Parkinson's disease: neurochemical overlaps and specific differences, in Dostert, P., Riederer, P., Strolin Benedetti, M., and Ronucci, R., (eds.), Early markers in Parkinson's and Alzheimer's disease, Springer, Wien New York, pp. 221–232.

37. Alzheimer, A., 1911, Über eigenartige Krankheitsfalle des späteren Alters, Ztschr.Ges.Neurol.Psychiat. **4**:356–385.

38. Beach, T.G:, Walker, R., and McGeer, E.G., 1989, Patterns of gliosis in Alzheimer's disease and aging cerebrum, Glia **2**:420–436.

39. Davies, C.A., Mann, D.M.A., Sumpter, P.Q., and Yates, P.O., 1987, A quantitative morphometric analysis of the neuronal and synaptic content of the frontal and temporal cortex in patients with Alzheimer's disease, J.Neurol.Sci.**78**:151-164.

40. Masliah, E., Terry, R.D., DeTeresa, R.M., and Hansen, L.A., 1989, Immunohistochemical quantification of the synapse-related protein synaptophysin in Alzheimer disease, Neurosci.Lett. **103**:234-239.

41. Brun, A., and Englund, E., 1981, Regional pattern of degeneration in Alzheimer's disease: neuronal loss and histopathological grading, Histopathology **5**:549-564.

42. Duffy, P.E., 1983, Astrocytes: Normal, reactive, and neoplastic, Raven, New York.

43. Siman, R., Card, J.P., Nelson, R.B., and Davis, L.G., 1989, Expression of beta-amyloid precursor protein in reactive astrocytes following neuronal damage, Neuron **3**:275-285.

44. Norenberg, M.D., Neary, J.T., Norenberg, L.O., and McCarthy, M., 1990, Ammonia induced decrease in glial fibrillary acidic protein in cultured astrocytes, J.Neuropathol.Exp.Neurol.**33**:422-435.

45. Bodega, G., Suarez, I., Boyano, M.C., Rubio, M., Villalba, R.M., Arilla, E., Gonzales-Guijarro, L., and Fernandez, B., 1993, High ammonia diet: Its effect on the glial fibrillary acidic protein (GFAP), Neurochem.Res. **18**:971-975.

46. Caporaso, G.L., Gandy, S.E., Buxbaum, J.D., and Greengard, P., 1992, Chloroquine inhibits intracellular degradation but not secretion of Alzheimer beta-A4 amyloid precursor protein, Proc.Natl.Acad.Sci.USA **89**:2252-2256.

47. Golde, T.E., Estus, S., Younkin, L.H., Selkoe, D.J., and Younkin, S.G., 1992, Processing of the amyloid protein precursor to potentially amyloidogenic derivatives, Science **255**:728-730.

48. Cooper, A.J.L., and Plum, F., 1987, Biochemistry and physiology of brain ammonia, Physiol.Rev. **67**:440-519.

49. Seiler, N., 1993, Is ammonia a pathogenetic factor in Alzheimer's disease?, Neurochem.Res.**18**:235-245.

50. Hawkins, R.A., and Jessy, J., 1991, Hyperammonaemia does not impair brain function in the absence of net glutamine synthesis, Biochem.J. **277**:697-703.

51. Ratnakumari, L., and Murthy, C.R.K., 1989, Activities of pyruvate dehydrogenase, enzymes of citric acic cycle, and aminotransferases in the subcellular fractions of cerebral cortex in normal and hyperammonemic rats, Neurochem.Res.**14**:221-228.

52. Hindfelt, B., 1983, Ammonia intoxication and brain energy metabolism, in Kleinberge, G., and Deutsch, E. (eds.), New aspects of clinical nutrition, Karger, Basel, pp. 474-484.

53. Kauppinen, R.A., Williams, S.R., Brooks, K.J., and Bachelard, H.S., 1991, Effects of ammonium on energy metabolism and intracellular pH in guinea pig cerebral cortex studied by 31P and 1H nuclear magnetic resonance spectroscopy, Neurochem.Int. **19**:495-504.

54. Faff-Michalak, L., and Albrecht, J., 1991, Aspartate aminotransferase, malate dehydrogenase, and pyruvate carboxylase activities in rat cerebral synaptic and non synaptic mitochondria: Effects of in vitro treatment with ammonia, hyperammonemia and hepatic encephalopathy, Metabol.Brain Dis.**6**:187-197.

55. Rao, V.L.R., Murthy, C.R.K., and Butterworth, R.F., 1992, Glutamatergic synaptic dysfunction in hyperammonemic syndromes, Metabol.Brain Dis.**7**:1-20.

56. Devi, R.P.R., and Murthy, C.R.K., 1993, Ammonia-induced alterations in the activities of synaptosomal cholinesterases of rat brain under in vitro and in vivo conditions, Neurosci.Lett. **159**:131-134.

57. O'Connor, J.E., Guerri, C., and Grisolia, S., 1984, Effects of ammonia on synaptosomal membranes, Biochem.Biophys.Res.Commun. **119**:516-523.

58. Rao, V.L.R., Agrawal, A.K., and Murthy, C.R.K., 1991, Ammonia-induced alterations in glutamate and muscimol binding to cerebellar synaptic membranes, Neurosci.Lett.**130**:251-254.

59. Fisman, M., Gordon, B., Felcki, V., Helmes, E., Appell, J., and Rabhern, K., 1985, Hyperammonemia in Alzheimer's disease, Am.J.Psychiatry **142**:71-73.

60. Branconnier, R.J., Dessain, E.C., McNiff, M.E., and Cole, J.O., 1986, Blood ammonia and Alzheimer's disease, Am.J.Psychiatry **143**:1313.

61. Hoyer, S., 1993, Intermediary metabolism disturbance in AD/SDAT and its relation to molecular events, Prog.Neuro-Psychopharmacol.Biol.Psychiat.**17**:199-228.

62. Sims, N.R., Bowen, D.M., and Davison, A.N., 1981, (14C) acetylcholine synthesis and (14C) carbon dioxide production from (U-14C) glucose by tissue prims from human neocortex, Biochem.J. **196:**867–876.

63. Hoyer, S., 1988, Glucose and related brain metabolism in dementia of Alzheimer type and its morphological significance, Age **11:**158–166.

64. Hoyer, S., 1991, Abnormalities of glucose metabolism in Alzheimer's disease, Ann.N.Y. Acad.Sci. **640:**53–58.

CONTRIBUTORS

ALVAREZ, L.
Instituto de Investigaciones Biomédicas
CSIC
Arturo Duperier, 4
28029 Madrid
Spain

ALBRECHT, J.
Medical Research Centre
Polish Academy of Sciences
00-784 Warsaw
Poland

ANDREOLETTI, M.
ICGM, INSERM U380
22 rue Mechain
75014 Paris
France

BASILE, A. S.
Laboratory of Neuroscience
NIDDK
National Institutes of Health
Bethesda, Maryland
U.S.A.

BENNOUN, M.
ICGM, INSERM U380
22 rue Mechain
75014 Paris
France

BERENGUER, J.
Servicio de Medicina Digestiva
Hospital La Fe
Valencia
Spain

BIRGISSON, S.
Division of Gastroenterology
MetroHealth Medical Center
Case Western Reserve University
Cleveland, Ohio
U.S.A.

BOSMAN, D. K.
Dept. Experimental Internal Medicine
Academic Medical Centre
University of Amsterdam
1105 AZ Amsterdam
The Netherlands

BOVÉE, W. M. M. J.
Dept. Applied Physics
Delft University
Delft
The Netherlands

BRIAND, P.
ICGM, INSERM U380
22 rue Mechain
75014 Paris
France

BUTTERWORTH, R. F.
Neuroscience Research Unit
Hôpital Saint-Luc
University of Montreal
Montreal, Quebec
H2X 3J4 Canada

CASKEY, C. T.
Howard Hughes Medical Institute
Baylor College of Medicine
Houston, Texas 77030
U.S.A.

CHAMULEAU, R. A. F. M.
Lab. Experimental Internal Medicine
Academic Medical Centre
University of Amsterdam
1105 AZ Amsterdam
The Netherlands

CHEDID, A.
Dept. of Pathology
Finch University of Health Sciences
The Chicago Medical School
North Chicago
Illinois, 60064
U.S.A.

COLOMBO, J. P.
Dept. of Clinical Chemistry
Inselspital
University of Berne
3010 Berne
Switzerland

CONJEEVARAM, H.
Division of Gastroenterology
MetroHealth Medical Center
Case Western Reserve University
Cleveland, Ohio
U.S.A.

CORDOBA, J.
Servicio de Medicina Digestiva
Hospital La Fe
Valencia
Spain

DEJOSEPH, M. R.
Dept. Physiology and Biophysics
Finch University of Health Sciences
The Chicago Medical School
North Chicago
Illinois, 60064
U.S.A.

DURAN, C.
Instituto de investigaciones Biomédicas
CSIC
Arturo Duperier, 4
28029 Madrid
Spain

FAFF, L.
Medical Research Centre
Polish Academy of Sciences
00-784 Warsaw
Poland

FELIPO, V.
Instituto de Investigaciones Citológicas
Fundación Valenciana de
Investigaciones Biomédicas
Amadeo de Saboya, 4
46010 Valencia
Spain

FERENCI, P.
Dept. Internal Medicine IV
Gastroenterology and Hepatology
University of Vienna
A-1090 Wien
Austria

FRANCO, D.
Service de Chirurgie
Hôpital A. Beclère
92141 Clamart
France

GACAD, R. C.
Division of Gastroenterology
MetroHealth Medical Center
Case Western Reserve University
Cleveland, Ohio
U.S.A.

GERLACH, J. C.
Chirurgische Klinik
Universitätsklinikum Rudolf Virchow
Freie Universität Berlin
D-14050 Berlin 19
Germany

GEROK, W.
Medizinische Universitätsklinik
Hugstetterstrasse 55
D-79106 Freiburg
Germany

GRAHAM, T. E.
Human Biology
University of Guelph
Guelph, Ontario
N1G 2W1 Canada

GRISOLIA, S.
Instituto de Investigaciones Citologicas
Fundación Valenciana de
Investigaciones Biomédicas
Amadeo de Saboya, 4
46010 Valencia
Spain

HÄUSSINGER, D.
Medizinische Universitätsklinik
Hugstetterstrasse 55
D-79106 Freiburg
Germany

HAWKINS, R. A.
Dept. Physiology and Biophysics
Finch University of Health Sciences
The Chicago Medical School
North Chicago
Illinois, 60064
U.S.A.

HERNETH, A.
Dept. Internal Medicine IV
Gastroenterology and Hepatology
University of Vienna
A-1090 Wien
Austria

HOYER, S.
Dept. Pathochemistry and
General Neurochemistry
University of Heidelberg
Heidelberg 69120
Germany

JESSY, J.
Dept. Physiology and Biophysics
Finch University of Health Sciences
The Chicago Medical School
North Chicago
Illinois, 60064
U.S.A.

JONES, E. A.
Department of Health
London
United Kingdom

KOSENKO, E.
Institute of Theoretical and
Experimental Biophysics
Pushchino 142 292
Russia

MANS, A. M.
Dept. Physiology and Biophysics
Finch University of Health sciences
The Chicago Medical School
North Chicago
Illinois 60064
U.S.A.

MARCAIDA, G.
Instituto de Investigaciones Citologicas
Fundación Valenciana de
Investigaciones Biomédicas
Amadeo de Saboya, 4
46010 Valencia
Spain

MAS, A.
Liver Unit
Hospital Clinic i Provincial
Universitat de Barcelona
Barcelona
Spain

MATO, J. M.
Instituto de Investigaciones Biomédicas
CSIC
Arturo Duperier, 4
28029 Madrid
Spain

MINGORANCE, J.
Instituto de Investigaciones Biomédicas
CSIC
Arturo Duperier, 4
28029 Madrid
Spain

MIÑANA, M. D.
Instituto de Investigaciones Citológicas
Fundación Valenciana de
Investigaciones Biomédicas
Amadeo de saboya, 4
46010 Valencia
Spain

MIR, J.
Servicio de Medicina Digestiva
Hospital La Fe
Valencia
Spain

MORSY, M. A.
Department of Molecular
and Human Genetics
Baylor College of Medicine
Houston, Texas 77030
U.S.A.

MULLEN, K. D.
Division of Gastroenterology
MetroHealth Medical center
Case Western University
Cleveland, Ohio
U.S.A.

ORTIZ, P.
Instituto de Investigaciones Biomédicas
CSIC
Arturo Duperier, 4
28029 Madrid
Spain

PAGES, J. C.
ICGM, INSERM U380
22 rue Mechain
75014 Paris
France

PAJARES, M.
Instituto de Investigaciones Biomédicas
CSIC
Arturo Duperier, 4
28029 Madrid
Spain

PRIETO, M.
Servicio de Medicina Digestiva
Hospital La Fe
Valencia
Spain

PÜSPÖK, A.
Dept. Internal Medicine IV
Gastroenterology and Hepatology
University of Vienna
A-1090 Wien
Austria

RAABE, W.
Neurology
VA Medical Center
Deps. Neurology and Physiology
University of Minnesota
Minneapolis 55417
U.S.A.

RAYON, M.
Servicio de Medicina Digestiva
Hospital La Fe
Valencia
Spain

RODES, J.
Liver Unit
Hospital Clinic i Provincial
Universitatde Barcelona
Barcelona
Spain

SALMERON, J. M.
Liver Unit
Hospital Clinic i Provincial
Universitat de Barcelona
Barcelona
Spain

SILIPRANDI, N.
Dept. Chimica Biologica
Università di Padova
Padova
Italia

STEINDL, P.
Dept. Internal Medicine IV
Gastroenterology and Hepatology
University of Vienna
A-1090 Wien
Austria

TASSANI, V.
Dept. Research and Development
Sigma Tau Ind. Farm. Riun.
Pomezia
Roma
Italia

VENERANDO, R.
Dept. Chimica Biologica
Università di Padova
Padova
Italia

WEBER, A.
ICGM, INSERM U380
22 rue Mechain
75014 Paris
France

YURDAYDIN, C.
Department of Gastroenterology
University of Ankara
Ankara
Turkey

WÜNER, A.
ICGM INSERM U380
22, rue Méchain
75014 Paris
France

YURDAYDIN, C.
Department of Gastroenterology
University of Ankara
Cebeci
Ankara
Turkey

INDEX